The Use of Motion Analysis for Diagnostics

The Use of Motion Analysis for Diagnostics

Editors

**Carlo Ricciardi
Francesco Amato
Mario Cesarelli**

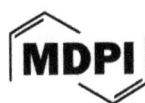

Basel • Beijing • Wuhan • Barcelona • Belgrade • Novi Sad • Cluj • Manchester

Editors

Carlo Ricciardi
University of Naples Federico II
Naples
Italy

Francesco Amato
University of Naples Federico II
Naples
Italy

Mario Cesarelli
University of Sannio
Benevento
Italy

Editorial Office
MDPI AG
Grosspeteranlage 5
4052 Basel, Switzerland

This is a reprint of articles from the Special Issue published online in the open access journal *Diagnostics* (ISSN 2075-4418) (available at: https://www.mdpi.com/journal/diagnostics/special_issues/Motion_Analysis_Diagnostics).

For citation purposes, cite each article independently as indicated on the article page online and as indicated below:

Lastname, A.A.; Lastname, B.B. Article Title. *Journal Name* **Year**, *Volume Number*, Page Range.

ISBN 978-3-7258-1509-8 (Hbk)
ISBN 978-3-7258-1510-4 (PDF)
doi.org/10.3390/books978-3-7258-1510-4

© 2024 by the authors. Articles in this book are Open Access and distributed under the Creative Commons Attribution (CC BY) license. The book as a whole is distributed by MDPI under the terms and conditions of the Creative Commons Attribution-NonCommercial-NoDerivs (CC BY-NC-ND) license.

Contents

About the Editors vii

Preface ix

Jaehwang Seol, Kicheol Yoon and Kwang Gi Kim
Mathematical Analysis and Motion Capture System Utilization Method for Standardization Evaluation of Tracking Objectivity of 6-DOF Arm Structure for Rehabilitation Training Exercise Therapy Robot
Reprinted from: *Diagnostics* **2022**, *12*, 3179, doi:10.3390/diagnostics12123179 1

Anna Hadamus, Michalina Błażkiewicz, Aleksandra J. Kowalska, Kamil T. Wydra, Marta Grabowicz, Małgorzata Łukowicz, et al.
Nonlinear and Linear Measures in the Differentiation of Postural Control in Patients after Total Hip or Knee Replacement and Healthy Controls
Reprinted from: *Diagnostics* **2022**, *12*, 1595, doi:10.3390/diagnostics12071595 24

Cathy M. Craig, James Stafford, Anastasiia Egorova, Carla McCabe and Mark Matthews
Can We Use the Oculus Quest VR Headset and Controllers to Reliably Assess Balance Stability?
Reprinted from: *Diagnostics* **2022**, *12*, 1409, doi:10.3390/diagnostics12061409 35

Wojciech Kukwa, Tomasz Lis, Jonasz Łaba, Ron B. Mitchell and Marcel Młyńczak
Sleep Position Detection with a Wireless Audio-Motion Sensor—A Validation Study
Reprinted from: *Diagnostics* **2022**, *12*, 1195, doi:10.3390/diagnostics12051195 47

Anna Boryczka-Trefler, Małgorzata Kalinowska, Ewa Szczerbik, Jolanta Stępowska, Anna Łukaszewska and Małgorzata Syczewska
Effect of Plano-Valgus Foot on Lower-Extremity Kinematics and Spatiotemporal Gait Parameters in Children of Age 5–9
Reprinted from: *Diagnostics* **2022**, *12*, 2, doi:10.3390/diagnostics12010002 56

Sang-Keun Woo, Byung-Chul Kim, Eun Kyoung Ryu, In Ok Ko and Yong Jin Lee
Low-Dose PET Imaging of Tumors in Lung and Liver Regions Using Internal Motion Estimation
Reprinted from: *Diagnostics* **2021**, *11*, 2138, doi:10.3390/diagnostics11112138 67

Benyameen Keelson, Luca Buzzatti, Jakub Ceranka, Adrián Gutiérrez, Simone Battista, Thierry Scheerlinck, et al.
Automated Motion Analysis of Bony Joint Structures from Dynamic Computer Tomography Images: A Multi-Atlas Approach
Reprinted from: *Diagnostics* **2021**, *11*, 2062, doi:10.3390/diagnostics11112062 80

Pedro Albuquerque, João Pedro Machado, Tanmay Tulsidas Verlekar, Paulo Lobato Correia and Luís Ducla Soares
Remote Gait Type Classification System Using Markerless 2D Video
Reprinted from: *Diagnostics* **2021**, *11*, 1824, doi:10.3390/diagnostics11101824 97

Mirjam Bonanno and Rocco Salvatore Calabrò
Robot-Aided Motion Analysis in Neurorehabilitation: Benefits and Challenges
Reprinted from: *Diagnostics* **2023**, *13*, 3561, doi:10.3390/diagnostics13233561 110

Sani Salisu, Nur Intan Raihana Ruhaiyem, Taiseer Abdalla Elfadil Eisa, Maged Nasser, Faisal Saeed and Hussain A. Younis
Motion Capture Technologies for Ergonomics: A Systematic Literature Review
Reprinted from: *Diagnostics* **2023**, *13*, 2593, doi:10.3390/diagnostics13152593 124

Jennifer Bosserman, Sonia Kelkar, Kristen D. LeBlond, Jessica Cassidy and Dana B. McCarty
Postural Control Measurements to Predict Future Motor Impairment in Preterm Infants: A Systematic Review
Reprinted from: *Diagnostics* **2023**, *13*, 3473, doi:10.3390/diagnostics13223473 . . . . **140**

Giuseppe Cesarelli, Leandro Donisi, Armando Coccia, Federica Amitrano, Giovanni D'Addio and Carlo Ricciardi
The E-Textile for Biomedical Applications: A Systematic Review of Literature
Reprinted from: *Diagnostics* **2021**, *11*, 2263, doi:10.3390/diagnostics11122263 . . . . **152**

About the Editors

Carlo Ricciardi

Carlo Ricciardi was born in Salerno (Italy) in 1993. He received his master's degree in biomedical engineering from the University of Naples in 2017 and his PhD degree in 2021 from the University Hospital of Naples. He was a Research Fellow at the University of Naples Federico II during 2021, and at the end of the same year, he became Assistant Professor at the Department of Electrical Engineering and Information Technology. He is currently a Tenure Track Assistant Professor in Biomedical Engineering. His main fields of research are gait analysis, with a particular focus on the study of neurological diseases (i.e., Parkinson's disease, Progressive Supranuclear Palsy, etc.); biosignal and bioimage processing, including applications of machine learning; and healthcare management, with focus on Health Technology Assessment and Lean Six Sigma. The scientific activity of Carlo in the above-mentioned fields allowed him to publish 92 papers in international journals and conference proceedings, and one book chapter in "Handbook of Surgical Planning and 3D Printing: Applications, Integration, and New Directions". He serves as reviewer for several journals in the field of Bioengineering, and is an Editorial Board Member of the Journal "Sensors" (MDPI).

Francesco Amato

Francesco Amato was born in Naples on February 2, 1965. He received his laurea and PhD degrees in electronic engineering from the University of Naples in 1990 and 1994, respectively. From 2001 to 2003, he was a Full Professor of Automatic Control at the University of Reggio Calabria. In 2003, he moved to the University of Catanzaro as Full Professor of Automatic Control and, from 2010 to 2018, as Full Professor of Bioengineering. At the University of Catanzaro, he has been the Dean of the School of Computer and Biomedical Engineering, the Coordinator of the Doctorate School in Biomedical and Computer Engineering, and Director of the Biomechatronics Laboratory. In 2018, he moved to the University of Naples Federico II as a Full Professor of Bioengineering, where he currently is the dean of the School of Biomedical Engineering. The research activity of Francesco Amato has developed in the fields of systems and control theory, computational biology, and the modeling and control of biomedical systems. He has published approximately 370 papers in international journals and conference proceedings, and three monographies, two with Springer Verlag and one with Wiley. He has participated in several financed projects in the context of Biomedical Engineering. He serves as a reviewer for many important journals in the field of Bioengineering and Automatic Control, and has overseen many research projects both at the national and international level.

Mario Cesarelli

Mario Cesarelli was born in Naples, Italy, in 1955. He received his Italian degree in Electronic Engineering from the University of Naples in 1979 and his post-graduate specialization in Biomedical Technologies from the University of Naples. From 1981 to 1989, he was a Scientific Technician at the Faculty of Medicine and Surgery of University of Naples. From 1989 to 1992, he was a researcher in Biomedical Engineering at the Department of Electronic Engineering of the University of Naples. From 1992 to 2018, he was an Associate Professor of Biomedical Engineering. At this university, he served as the coordinator of both the bachelor's and master's degrees in biomedical engineering. Since 2018, he has been full professor at the University of Naples Federico and, in 2022, he moved to the University of Sannio (Benevento, Italy). His main fields of research are biomedical instrumentation, bio-signal and image analysis, and health care information systems; this has allowed him to publish 293 contributions to international journals and conference proceedings, including some book chapters.

Preface

The aim of this Special Issue was to explore the latest research and innovations in motion analysis, offering unique insights and perspectives that advance knowledge within the field. Both clinical and engineering researchers have investigated the gait, balance, and joint kinematics in individuals affected by movement disorders, which can stem from musculoskeletal, neurological, or other bodily system dysfunctions. Artificial intelligence (AI) approaches can be utilized to facilitate scientists in the efficient management of complex datasets.

We would like to thank Eng. Noemi Pisani and Eng. Michela Russo for their collaborative efforts.

Carlo Ricciardi, Francesco Amato, and Mario Cesarelli
Editors

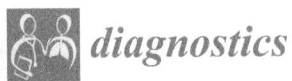

Article

Mathematical Analysis and Motion Capture System Utilization Method for Standardization Evaluation of Tracking Objectivity of 6-DOF Arm Structure for Rehabilitation Training Exercise Therapy Robot

Jaehwang Seol [1,2,†], Kicheol Yoon [2,3,†] and Kwang Gi Kim [1,2,3,4,*]

1. Department of Biomedical Engineering, College of Health Science, Gachon University, 191 Hambak-Moero, Yeonsu-gu, Incheon 21936, Republic of Korea
2. Medical Devices R&D Center, Gachon University Gil Medical Center, 21, 774 Beon-gil, Namdong-daero, Namdong-gu, Incheon 21565, Republic of Korea
3. Department of Biomedical Engineering, College of Medicine, Gachon University, 38-13, 3 Beon-gil, Dokjom-ro 3, Namdong-gu, Incheon 21565, Republic of Korea
4. Department of Health Sciences and Technology, Gachon Advanced Institute for Health Sciences and Technology (GAIHST), Gachon University, 38-13, 3 Beon-gil, Dokjom-ro, Namdong-gu, Incheon 21565, Republic of Korea
* Correspondence: kimkg@gachon.ac.kr; Tel.: +82-32-458-2880
† These authors contributed equally to this work.

Abstract: A treatment method for suppressing shoulder pain by reducing the secretion of neurotransmitters in the brain is being studied in compliance with domestic and international standards. A robot is being developed to assist physical therapists in shoulder rehabilitation exercise treatment. The robot used for rehabilitation therapy enables the training of patients to perform rehabilitation exercises repeatedly. However, the biomechanical movement (or motion) of the shoulder joint should be accurately designed to enhance efficiency using a shoulder rehabilitation robot. Furthermore, safely treating patients by accurately evaluating biomechanical movements in compliance with domestic and international standards is a major task. Therefore, an in-depth analysis of shoulder movement is essential for understanding the mechanism of shoulder rehabilitation using robots. This paper proposes a method for analyzing shoulder movements. The rotation angle and range of motion (ROM) of the shoulder joint are measured by attaching a marker to the body and analyzing the inverse kinematics. The first motion is abduction and adduction, and the second is external and internal rotation. The location information of the marker is transmitted to an application software through an infrared camera. For the analysis using an inverse kinematics solution, five males and five females participated in the motion capture experiment. The subjects did not have any disability, and abduction and adduction were repeated 10 times. As a result, ROM of the abduction and adduction were 148° with males and 138.7° in females. Moreover, ROM of the external and internal rotation were 111.2° with males and 106° in females. Because this study enables tracking of the center coordinates of the joint suitably through a motion capture system, inverse kinematics can be accurately calculated. Additionally, a mathematical inverse kinematics equation will utilize follow-up study for designing an upper rehabilitations robot. The proposed method is assessed to be able to contribute to the definition of domestic and international standardization of rehabilitation robots and motion capture for objective evaluation.

Keywords: shoulder pain; rehabilitation robot; motion capture system; inverse kinematics; range of motion; standardization evaluation

1. Introduction

Motor nerves transmit signals from the brain to muscles to induce movement of the shoulder and arm. In particular, when shoulder pain is induced, the muscle can be relaxed by physically stimulating it to relieve pain. Therefore, research is being conducted in compliance with domestic and international standards (IEC 80601-2-78:2019 and SC43) to suppress shoulder pain by reducing the neurotransmitter secretion in the brain. Shoulder pain is a common complication that can be caused by adhesive capsulitis and hemiplegia induced by a stroke [1]. In particular, the adhesive capsulitis causes shoulder pain due to the thickening of the joint capsule and the adhesion of tendons or ligaments [1]. Adhesive capsulitis also causes additional complications due to rotator cuff tears. Therefore, shoulder pain can be reduced through stretching and passive and active joint exercise treatment [1].

Shoulder pain in hemiplegia and adhesive capsulitis requires nonsurgical treatment and shoulder rehabilitation (SR). Rehabilitation exercises have been enabled through conventional manual therapy by physical therapists. However, owing to the development of biomedical engineering technology, the research and development of medical robots for rehabilitation treatment continues through the convergence of physical therapy and engineering [2–7]. The advantage of a rehabilitation robot is that therapists are able to train the patient, such that a male or female can repeatedly perform rehabilitation exercises [8,9]. The safety requirements of robots for rehabilitation exercise therapy are extremely important, as specified in the international standards (IEC 80601-2-78:2019). A representative requirement of international standardization of the safety of robots for rehabilitation exercise therapy is that when a hemiplegic or speech-impaired person is trained in a robot system to receive SR, communication between the therapist and the patient must be established [8]. However, it is difficult for a patient with a disability to convey meaning to the therapist, and if an emergency occurs, the paralyzed person must deliver a message to the therapist. However, it is difficult for these patients to convey a clear message. Therefore, these problems lead to medical accidents, making it necessary to establish domestic and international standardization of computer interfaces through which patients and therapists can communicate. Consequently, it is necessary to introduce an intelligent rehabilitation treatment robot to be able to deliver a message in an emergency and monitor the patient's condition.

In addition, the characteristics of the SR robot enable repetitive exercise training through the automation system, reducing the fatigue of the therapist who needs to perform extensive work, and can guide SR exercise training more accurately [9,10]. However, it is important to accurately implement the biomechanical movement (or motion) of the shoulder joint to enhance the efficiency of using a shoulder rehabilitation robot. The accurate movement of the SR robot can ensure patient safety and prevent accidents [9,10]. Therefore, an in-depth analysis of shoulder movement is essential for understanding the mechanism of SR robots. Various studies on the mechanism of shoulder movement have been conducted [11–16].

Wu et al., from the International Society of Biomechanics, proposed a shoulder model based on the definition of the shoulder joint coordinate system (JCS). In particular, the proposed method presented the standardization of the JCS for the shoulder, elbow, wrist, and hand [14], thereby contributing to smooth communication between researchers and clinicians regarding kinematics. However, during the repetitive experiment, the standard position of the joint is not constant and has limitations [14]. Jackson et al. analyzed shoulder kinematics by attaching a marker to the skin to fix the standard joint position. In particular, the method using the chain model and Kalman filter reconstructs the shoulder kinematics by tracking the trajectory of the marker. Therefore, the burden is reduced to an extent that it is unnecessary for the reconstruction of the mathematical model for the determination of the range of motion (ROM) [15]. Zhang et al. proposed a kinematic model using a Vicon motion capture system and markers. In particular, the shoulder elevation and depression phases, and the movement coupling relationship between the displacement of the glenohumeral (GH) joint center with respect to the thoracic coordinate system and elevation of the humerus was investigated. As a result, a new design model for an upper extremity rehabilitation robot consistent with the actual situation of the human body structure was developed [16].

Similar to previous studies, this study proposes a method for analyzing shoulder movements. The rotation angle and ROM of the shoulder joint were measured by attaching a marker to the body and analyzing the inverse kinematics. In particular, a rigid body was designated through a marker to accurately determine the internal center point of the joint. For the experiment, subjects of this study (five males and five females) without any functional disability in the body participated in the motion capture test. Based on the information, which was obtained by tracking the position of the marker, the ROM of each joint was analyzed using inverse kinematics. Consequently, motion analysis using inverse kinematics will be applied to the mechanism of rehabilitation robots. In addition, ROM information of a normal subject can be used as a database for utilizing an SR robot for rehabilitation exercises.

2. Analysis of Motion Capture

In the process of using the robot system for rehabilitation-based training treatment, patients receiving treatment for shoulder pain disease with hemiplegia or speech impairment can communicate with the therapist using a computer, as shown in Figure 1a [8].

Quadriplegic, deaf, blind, and speech-impaired patients cannot express themselves accurately to therapists during exercise training programs for rehabilitation treatment [17]. Therefore, if emergencies occur during the course of training and treatment using treatment instruments, the therapist may not recognize the patient's condition and a medical accident can occur. Brain computer interface (BCI) defines a technology for interaction between the brain and a computer [18]. This technology refers to a control technology that provides a service so that a computer can grasp the thoughts intended by humans and move objects [19]. In other words, BCI detects brain waves so that computers can grasp cognition, learning, and reasoning similarly to the human brain [20]. Therefore, it is predicted that the use of BCI technology will be high for quadriplegic, hearing-impaired, visually-impaired, and speech-impaired patients who need rehabilitation exercise. BCI technology uses a camera to capture the movement of the patient, and accurately reads an EEG from the patient. It then analyzes the data obtained from the camera and EEG diagnosis to identify the patient's movement pattern. Therefore, it is possible to predict the treatment outcome by understanding the patient's requirements and condition.

It is desirable to use a robotic system in which such brain-computer interface (BCI) standardization (SC43) has been established. The most important aspect when moving the arm of the robot in the process of robot motion is matching the movement of the patient's shoulder. Therefore, an objective evaluation is important to match the patient's shoulder movement when the robot's arm moves, and domestic or international standardization work for this evaluation method is highly important [8]. In considering the movement of the robot arm and patient shoulder to establish standardization, it is important to study the construction of a motion capture-based monitoring system for objective evaluation and a mathematical algorithm analysis method for verifying the objective evaluation. In this way, it is possible to provide a safe rehabilitation robot therapy (IEC 80601-2-78:2019) to patients.

Figure 1b shows the setup environment for the motion capture experiment. The overall movement, such as position data of the arm, was tracked through motion capture, and the value of the end effector was obtained. In this study, the wrist was designated as an end effector and utilized as input data to interpret the inverse kinematics. Accordingly, the position and direction vectors of the wrist were tracked in real time through the motion capture system.

The subjects wore stretchy suits to demonstrate that the markers could be attached to the skin. The markers were coated with a material that reflects infrared light, which transmits the position data of the markers to the application software (Motive) using an infrared camera (Flex13, OptiTrack). Consequently, the position vector and direction vector of the markers were extracted in real time based on the absolute coordinate system in the software. In this study, the position data of the markers were analyzed by tracking the two rehabilitation motions. The first motion is abduction and adduction, and the second is external and internal rotation.

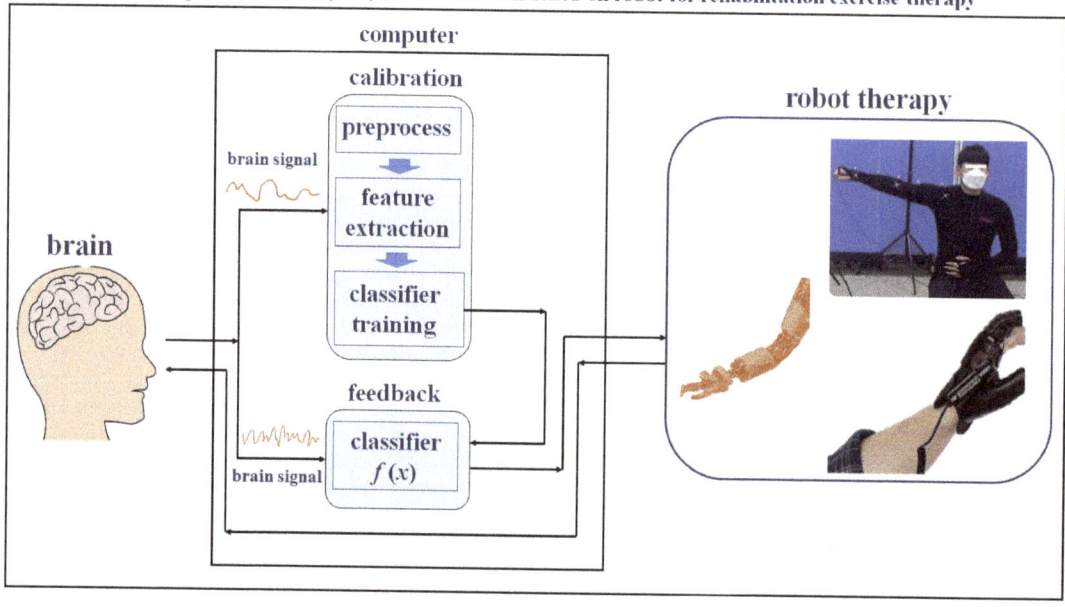

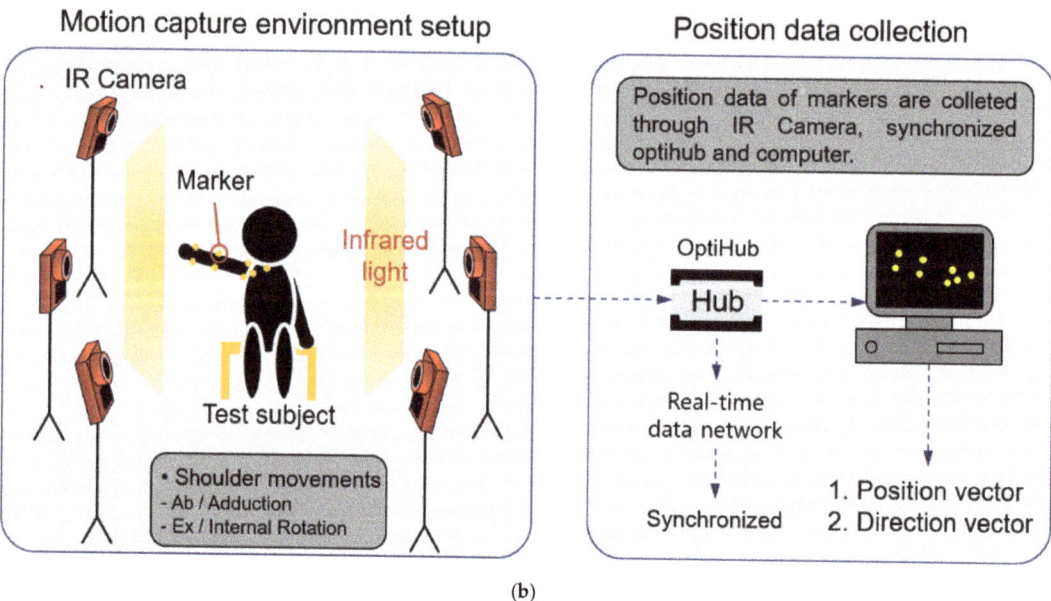

Figure 1. Configuration of a motion capture system for standardized rehabilitation exercise therapy. (**a**) Definition of the brain–computer interface (BCI). (**b**) Experimental environment setup for the motion capture and tracking markers.

Figure 2 shows the location of the markers that were attached to the elastic suit. As shown in Figure 2a, the markers were attached to the clavicle, shoulder, elbow, and wrist. The joints of the arms are located internally and contribute to the rotation of the bones. Therefore, the markers were attached with the center position coinciding with the internal center of the joint. While attaching the markers to designate the subjects' joint center points, the accuracy was increased by attaching the markers with help of an on-site physical therapist.

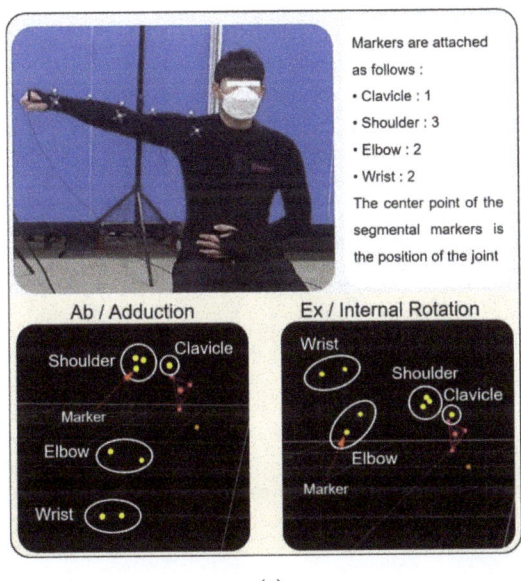
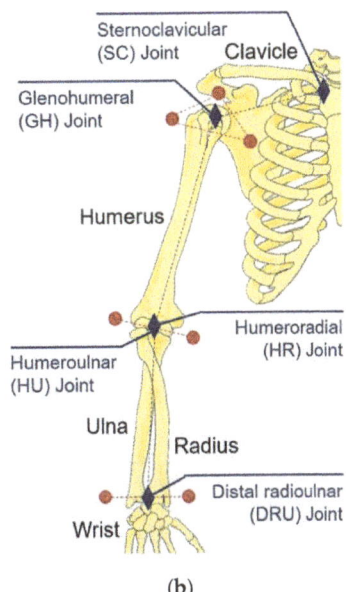

Figure 2. Photograph of the motion capture. (**a**) Abduction/adduction and external/internal rotation was performed to obtain the position and direction data of the markers. (**b**) The markers were attached to the skin to coincide with the central coordinate of the joint.

Figure 2b shows the locations of the marker attachments and central coordinates of the bone structure of the right arm. The sternoclavicular (SC) protrudes because the muscular membrane and skin covering the joint are thinner than other areas of the body. Therefore, one marker was attached without calculating the central coordinate. Three markers were attached to the shoulder to designate the glenohumeral (GH) joint as the central coordinate system. Two markers were attached to the elbow and wrist, and the humeroulnar (HU) joint and distal radioulnar (DRU) joint were designated as the center coordinates.

3. Mechanism and Mathematical Analysis

3.1. Forward Kinematics

Before interpreting an inverse kinematics solution, forward kinematics was analyzed and defined as a homogeneous transformation matrix [21]. Figure 3 shows the forward kinematics modeling of the right arm that is expressed based on the rotation joint.

Figure 3a shows the rotation joints contributing to the movement of the arm at each central joint position. In particular, points O, S, E, and EE (indicated by the blue dashed circle) are the center points of the joint coordinate system and represent the center coordinates of the joint rotation designated through motion capture. Point O (SC joint) comprises a two-axis rotation joint that involved the vertical and horizontal rotation of the clavicle. Point O is designated as the base point in the kinematics model. Point S (GH joint) is composed of three-axis rotation joints that involved the roll, pitch, and yaw rotation. Point

E (HU and HR joint) is composed of a uniaxial rotation joint that involved the flexion and extension of the arm. Finally, point EE (DRU joint) is designated as the end effector of the forward kinematics. In the following kinematics analysis process, the central coordinates of the clavicle, shoulder, elbow, and wrist are expressed as points O, S, E, and EE, respectively.

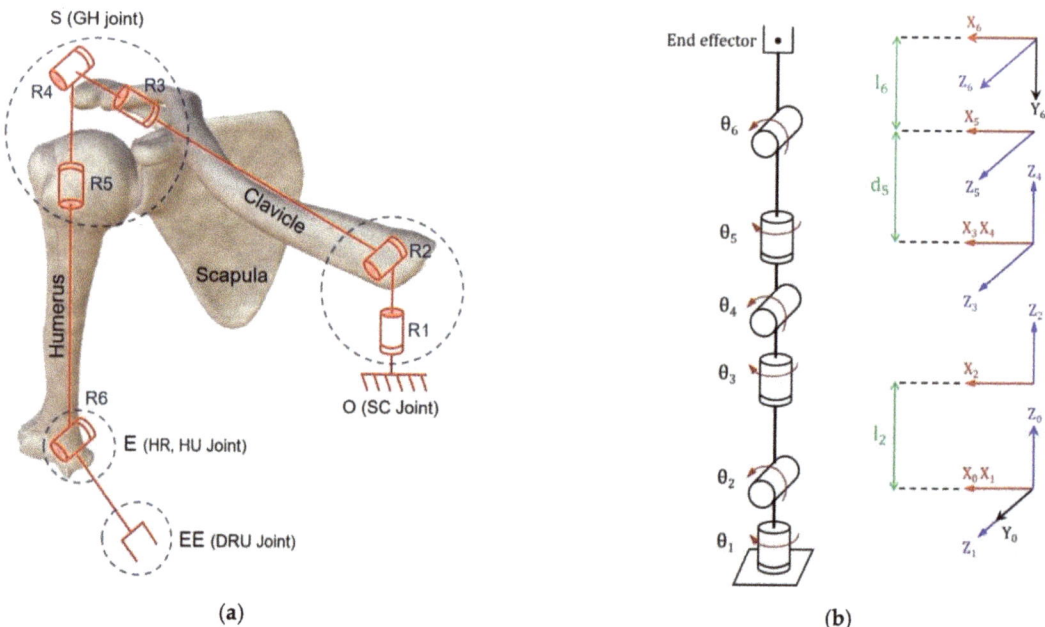

Figure 3. Shoulder complex modeling. (**a**) Mechanism of the shoulder complex model with rotation joints. (**b**) Forward kinematics modeling of the shoulder complex with a relative position coordinate system.

Figure 3b shows the forward kinematics model of the shoulder with the moving coordinate system. In each joint, the X_i, Y_i, and Z_i $(i=0\ to\ 6)$ axes that are the movement coordinate systems were mapped to the joint θ_i. The links and rotation parameters based on the forward kinematics are shown in Table 1 and were determined from the Denavit–Hartenberg proof [22,23]. In particular, θ_i is the rotation joint and directly concerns the rehabilitation exercise. Therefore, it is an important to measure θ_i and ROM in this study.

Table 1. Denavit–Hartenberg Table.

Joint	Link Angle θ_i (rad)	Link Offset d_i (mm)	Link Length l_i (mm)	Link Twist a_i (rad)
1	θ_1	0	0	$-\frac{\pi}{2}$
2	θ_2	0	l_2	$\frac{\pi}{2}$
3	θ_3	0	0	$-\frac{\pi}{2}$
4	θ_4	0	0	$\frac{\pi}{2}$
5	θ_5	d_5	0	$-\frac{\pi}{2}$
6	θ_6	0	l_6	0

The link offset and length (e.g., humerus or radius) are from different subjects. Therefore, the links can be calculated through the distance formula between two points in 3-dimensional space to substitute inverse kinematics as a constant value. Equation (1) represents the distance formula of links (d_i or l_i) based on the arbitrary 3-dimensional position from the X_n, Y_n and Z_n (n=natural number) position. To reflect the links that change in real time in the forward and inverse kinematics, a MATLAB tool was used.

$$l_i = d_i = \sqrt{(X_i - X_{i-1})^2 + (Y_i - Y_{i-1})^2 + (Z_i - Z_{i-1})^2} \tag{1}$$

$$^0T_1 = \begin{bmatrix} C_1 & 0 & -S_1 & 0 \\ S_1 & 0 & C_1 & 0 \\ 0 & -1 & 0 & 0 \\ 0 & 0 & 0 & 1 \end{bmatrix}, \quad {}^1T_2 = \begin{bmatrix} C_2 & 0 & S_2 & l_2C_2 \\ S_2 & 0 & -C_2 & l_2S_2 \\ 0 & 1 & 0 & 0 \\ 0 & 0 & 0 & 1 \end{bmatrix}, \quad {}^2T_3 = \begin{bmatrix} C_3 & 0 & -S_3 & 0 \\ S_3 & 0 & C_3 & 0 \\ 0 & -1 & 0 & 0 \\ 0 & 0 & 0 & 1 \end{bmatrix},$$

$$^3T_4 = \begin{bmatrix} C_4 & 0 & S_4 & 0 \\ S_4 & 0 & -C_4 & 0 \\ 0 & 1 & 0 & 0 \\ 0 & 0 & 0 & 1 \end{bmatrix}, \quad {}^4T_5 = \begin{bmatrix} C_5 & 0 & -S_5 & 0 \\ S_5 & 0 & C_5 & 0 \\ 0 & -1 & 0 & d_5 \\ 0 & 0 & 0 & 1 \end{bmatrix}, \quad {}^5T_6 = \begin{bmatrix} C_6 & -S_6 & 0 & l_6C_6 \\ S_6 & C_6 & 0 & l_6S_6 \\ 0 & 0 & 1 & 0 \\ 0 & 0 & 0 & 1 \end{bmatrix} \tag{2}$$

Based on the information in Table 1, a homogeneous transformation matrix of each rotation joint is shown in Equation (2). Among the components of the matrix, the 3 × 3 matrix (row: 1 to 3, column: 1 to 3) represents the rotation matrix, and the 3 × 1 matrix (row: 1 to 3, column: 4) represents the position vector.

$$^0T_6 = {}^0T_1 {}^1T_2 {}^2T_3 {}^3T_4 {}^4T_5 {}^5T_6 = \begin{bmatrix} R_{11} & R_{12} & R_{13} & P_x \\ R_{21} & R_{22} & R_{23} & P_y \\ R_{31} & R_{32} & R_{33} & P_z \\ 0 & 0 & 0 & 1 \end{bmatrix} \tag{3}$$

$$^0T_5 = {}^0T_1 {}^1T_2 {}^2T_3 {}^3T_4 {}^4T_5 = \begin{bmatrix} r_{11} & r_{12} & r_{13} & X_e \\ r_{21} & r_{22} & r_{23} & Y_e \\ r_{31} & r_{32} & r_{33} & Z_e \\ 0 & 0 & 0 & 1 \end{bmatrix} \tag{4}$$

Equation (3) represents the multiplication of the matrix from points O to EE. The direction vectors are expressed as R_{ij} (i,j=1 to 3) and the position vectors are expressed as P_i (i=x, y, z). Equation (4) represents the multiplication of the matrix from point O to point E. Similarly, the direction vectors are included as r_{ij} (i,j=1 to 3) and the position vectors are included as I_e (I=X, Y, Z).

3.2. Inverse Kinematics

3.2.1. Position Vector Analysis

The end effector is defined as a homogeneous transformation matrix through motion capture. Subsequently, the position vector of the elbow is calculated utilizing the end effector data. Figure 4 shows the position and direction vector of each point. As shown in Equation (5), the position vector of point E (X_e, Y_e, Z_e) is calculated through the x-axis direction vector of the end effector and link l_6.

$$EE = \begin{bmatrix} P_x \\ P_y \\ P_z \end{bmatrix}, \quad E = EE - l_6 R \begin{bmatrix} 1 \\ 0 \\ 0 \end{bmatrix} = \begin{bmatrix} P_x - l_6 R_{11} \\ P_y - l_6 R_{21} \\ P_z - l_6 R_{31} \end{bmatrix} \tag{5}$$

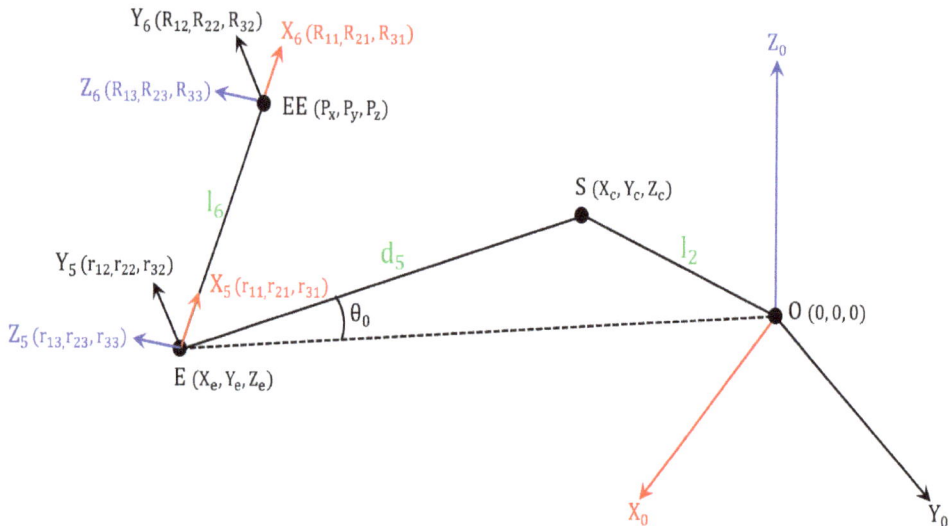

Figure 4. Position vector and direction vector of points E and EE.

In particular, $R_{ij\ (i,j=1\ to\ 3)}$ represents the rotation matrix of the end effector. Therefore, the direction vector of the x-axis is analyzed by multiplying the transposition matrix $[1\ 0\ 0]^T$ with the R matrix, and the links (l_6) are multiplied to calculate the magnitude of the x-axis direction. Consequently, the position vector of point E (X_e, Y_e, Z_e) is calculated by subtracting, as shown in Equation (5).

$$\vec{ES} = \vec{OS} - \vec{OE} = \langle X_c - X_e, Y_c - Y_e, Z_c - Z_e \rangle \quad (6)$$

$$\vec{R_z} = \langle R_{13}, R_{23}, R_{33} \rangle \quad (7)$$

$$\vec{ES} \cdot \vec{R_z} = \left| \vec{ES} \cdot \vec{R_z} \right| \cdot \cos \frac{\pi}{2} = 0 \quad (8)$$

$$\vec{ES} \cdot \vec{EO} = \left| \vec{ES} \cdot \vec{EO} \right| \cdot \cos \theta_0 = \langle X_c - X_e, Y_c - Y_e, Z_c - Z_e \rangle \cdot \langle -X_e, -Y_e, -Z_e \rangle \quad (9)$$

$$R_{13}X_c + R_{23}Y_c + R_{33}Z_c = \alpha, \quad (\alpha = R_{13}X_e + R_{23}Y_e + R_{33}Z_e) \quad (10)$$

$$X_e X_c + Y_e Y_c + Z_e Z_c = \beta, \quad (\beta = X_e^2 + Y_e^2 + Z_e^2 - |\vec{ES}| \cdot |\vec{EO}| \cdot \cos \theta_0) \quad (11)$$

$$\cos \theta_0 = \frac{d_5^2 + (X_e^2 + Y_e^2 + Z_e^2) - l_2^2}{2 \cdot d_5 \cdot \sqrt{X_e^2 + Y_e^2 + Z_e^2}} \quad (12)$$

In Equation (6), the $\vec{ES}$ vector is calculated by subtracting the vectors $\vec{OS}$ and $\vec{OE}$. In Equation (7), the vector $\vec{R_z}$ is defined as the z-axis direction vector of the end effector. Equations (8) and (9) show the dot product formula between vectors $\vec{ES}$ and $\vec{EO}$. As shown in Equation (8), vectors $\vec{ES}$ and $\vec{R_z}$ are always perpendicular, and the magnitude of the dot product always converges to zero. Equation (9) shows the left and right mathematical expression that represent the identities. Equations (8) and (9) can be induced and arranged into Equations (10) and (11). In particular, α and β are substituted variable values for constant value through the position and direction vector of EE and E. Consequently, $\cos \theta_0$ is obtained by calculating the internal angle through $\overrightarrow{ES}$ and $\overrightarrow{EO}$ in $\triangle OSE$.

$$(R_{23} - \frac{Y_e}{X_e}R_{13})Y_C + (R_{33} - \frac{Z_e}{X_e}R_{13})Z_C = \alpha - \frac{R_{13}}{X_e}\beta \rightarrow p_1 Y_c + q_1 Z_c = r_1 \quad (13)$$

$$(R_{13} - \frac{X_e}{Y_e}R_{23})X_C + (R_{33} - \frac{Z_e}{Y_e}R_{23})Z_C = \alpha - \frac{R_{23}}{Y_e}\beta \rightarrow p_2 X_c + q_2 Z_c = r_2 \quad (14)$$

Equations (10) and (11) are combined and expressed as a simultaneous equation and induced to Equations (13) and (14). In particular, the argument of X_C, Y_C, Z_C, and right mathematical expression are defined as constant values in Equations (5)–(12). Therefore, p_1, q_1, and r_1 are respectively defined as variable values of X_C, Y_C, and Z_C in Equation (13). Similarly, Equation (14) defines the variable value as p_2, q_2, and r_2.

$$X_c^2 + Y_c^2 + Z_c^2 = l_2^2 \quad (15)$$

$$(\frac{q_1^2}{p_1^2} + \frac{q_2^2}{p_2^2} + 1)Z_C^2 - 2(\frac{q_1 r_1}{p_1^2} + \frac{q_2 r_2}{p_2^2})Z_C + (\frac{r_1^2}{p_1^2} + \frac{r_2^2}{p_2^2}) = l_2^2, \ (Z_C > 0) \quad (16)$$

Equation (15) is the equation of a sphere that has center point from point O. The distance between points S and O represents the radius of the sphere and is equal to link l_2. Therefore, by substituting Equations (13)–(15), Equation (16) can be expressed as a quadratic equation for Z_C.

Figure 5 shows the mathematical relationship between Equations (10), (11), (15), and (16) in 3D coordinate space. It is possible to geometrically interpret a quadratic equation that Z_C is a variable. In particular, Equations (10) and (11) are presented by a three-dimensional plane. Therefore, the two planes are crossed and make an intersection line, and the intersection line passes through the sphere to obtain the two intersection points. Consequently, the two intersection points have a potential to be solutions of Equation (16), being the z-axis position vector of point S.

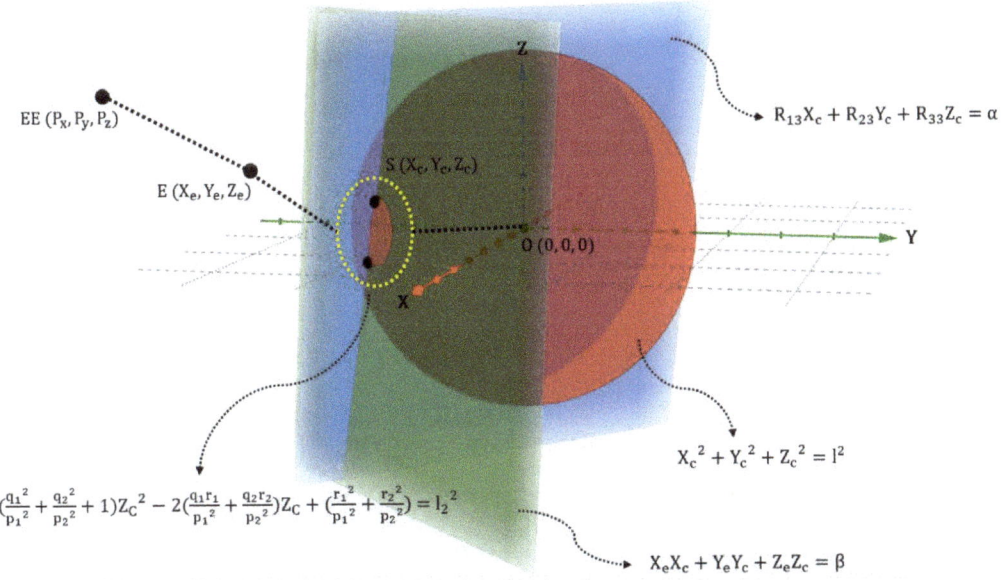

Figure 5. Two shoulder position vectors that are expressed through three-dimensional space.

Two solutions are obtained in Equation (16). According to the joint structure of the upper limb, one solution is selected by considering the normal biomechanical movement. Figure 6 shows the biomechanical relationship between the shoulder and the acromioclavicular joint. In Figure 6a, the head of the humerus is covered by the glenohumeral joint and the subacromial bursa. The head of the humerus relaxes or contracts through the supraspinatus and becomes the axis of shoulder rotation. Simultaneously, with the rotation of the shoulder, the clavicle rotates through the sternal end that becomes the axis of rotation. Therefore, the rotary direction of the shoulder and clavicle are the same, as shown in the normal state in Figure 6b. In contrast, the rotation of the shoulder and clavicle are in opposite directions in the abnormal state shown in Figure 6b. Therefore, the movement of the shoulder has the potential to create friction between the humeral head and the acromion.

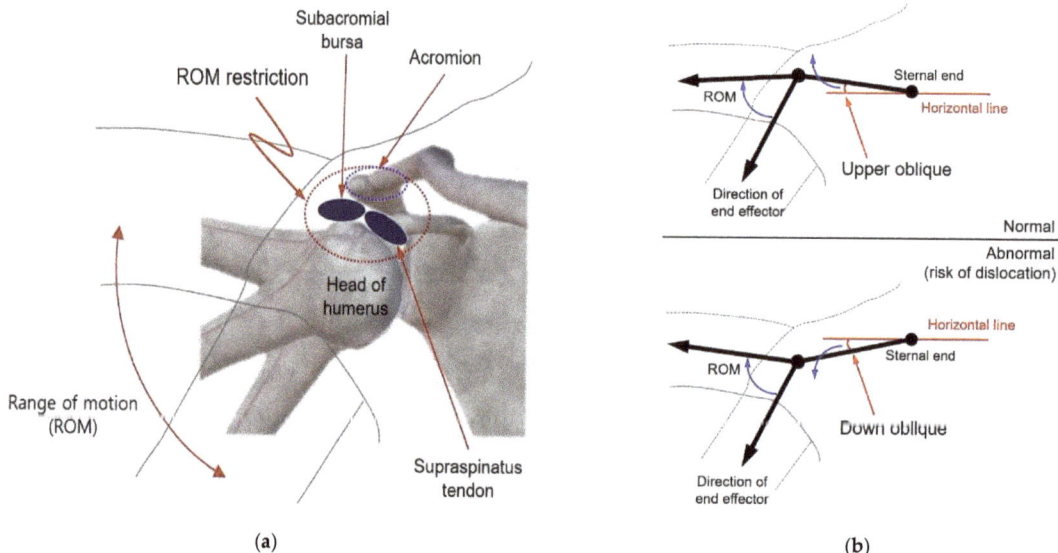

Figure 6. The biomechanical relationship between the shoulder and the acromioclavicular joint. (**a**) Anatomical structure of the shoulder joint and the acromioclavicular joint. (**b**) Normal or abnormal correlation of the inclination of the clavicle and shoulder rotation.

Two solutions of Equation (16) determine Z_C as the position vectors of point S. According to biomechanical analysis, the calculation of Equation (16) can add two conditions. A comparison is possible when it is assumed that two Z_C values are expressed as Z_{C1} and Z_{C2}. If $Z_{C2} > Z_{C1}$ and Z_{C1} is selected as the solution, the center coordinate of the shoulder is always located below the horizontal line. Therefore, the clavicle has a downward oblique angle and an abnormal state, as shown in Figure 6b. In contrast, if Z_{C2} is selected as the solution, point S is located above the horizontal line. Therefore, the clavicle maintains the upper oblique angle and a normal state, as shown in Figure 6a. As a result, a condition is ensured to select Z_{C2} when the condition is added, such as $Z_{C2} > 0 > Z_C$.

Based on Equations (13) and (14), the position values of X_C and Y_C were calculated using the selected Z_C. The head of the humerus is attached to the acromion and fixed by the pectoralis major, supraspinatus, and infraspinatus. Therefore, when determining X_C, the condition $X_C > 0$ is ensured, based on point O (sternoclavicular). As a result, when determining Z_C, the conditions that $Z_{C2} > 0 > Z_C$ and $X_C > 0$ can be added.

Figure 7 shows the results when the conditions ($Z_C > 0$ and $X_C > 0$) are violated by the simulation (Robo analyzer). The position and direction vector of the end effector are inputted, and the angle of the rotation joint is calculated. In abduction, the Z_C and X_C

values are negative, causing shoulder dislocation, as shown in Figure 7A. Similarly, if Z_C is negative during external rotation, shoulder dislocation occurs, as shown in Figure 7B. In summary, the position vector of points EE, E, and S are calculated by adding appropriate conditions. Based on the proper position vector, the angle of the rotation joint will be obtained.

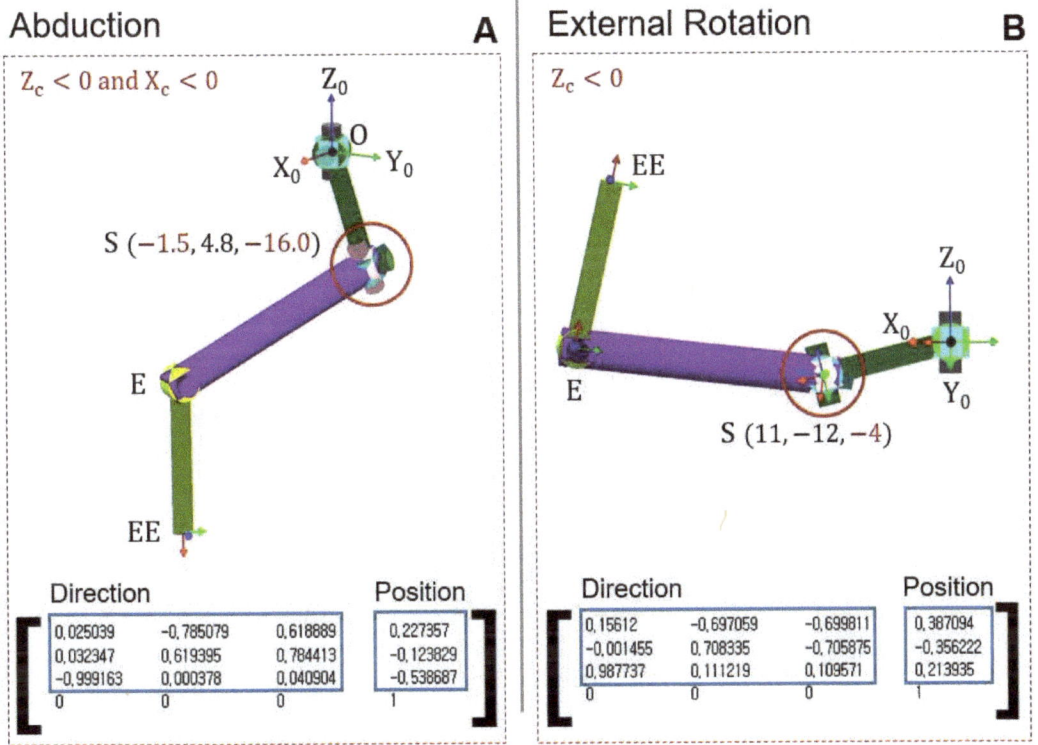

Figure 7. Simulation of shoulder movement based on the position vector of the end effector. (**A**) Math condition violation in abduction ($Z_C < 0$ and $X_C < 0$). (**B**) Math condition violation in external rotation ($Z_C < 0$).

3.2.2. Joint Angle Analysis

The joint rotation angles are analyzed to calculate the ROM of each rehabilitation motion. In particular, the inverse kinematics solution of the 6-degree of freedom (DOF) is obtained by solving the position vectors of points E and S in advance [19]. This study used the Mathematica tool (Wolfram Alpha) to solve complex trigonometric functions. In this section, $\cos\theta_n$ and $\sin\theta_n$ are replaced by the C_n and S_n (n = positive number).

Equations (17) and (18) show the calculation process for the joint angle θ_1. In Equation (17), X_C and Y_C are the position vectors of point S. In particular, because the coordinate of one point is included in the spherical coordinate system, X_C and Y_C are expressed as l_2, C_1, C_2, and S_1. Therefore, θ_1 is calculated by dividing the two position vectors. Arctan2 is used to consider the sign of the angle.

$$X_C = l_2 C_2 C_1, \quad Y_C = l_2 C_2 S_1 \tag{17}$$

$$\theta_1 = \operatorname{atan2}(Y_C, \quad X_C) \tag{18}$$

Equations (19)–(21) show the calculation process for the joint angle θ_2. Because the left and right mathematical expressions of Equation (19) constitute the same homogeneous transformation matrix, both sides of the matrix have equal element values. Therefore, Equations (20) and (21) are derived through the comparison of the element (row: 1 column: 4) and (row: 2 column: 4) by the homogeneous transformation matrix. As a result, θ_2 is calculated through dividing $l_2 S_2$ and $l_2 C_2$. Similar to the calculation process for θ_2, the remaining joint angle is solved by comparing the element from both sides of the homogeneous transformation matrix.

$$\left(^0 T_1\right)^{-1} \cdot {^0T_2} = {^1T_2} \tag{19}$$

$$C_1 X_C + S_1 Y_C = l_2 C_2 \tag{20}$$

$$-Z_C = l_2 S_2 \tag{21}$$

$$\theta_2 = \operatorname{atan2}(-Z_C,\ C_1 X_C + S_1 Y_C) \tag{22}$$

In Equation (23), both sides of the element values of (row: 1 column: 4) and (row: 2 column: 4) are compared. Equations (24) and (25) are the left element equation and are substituted with characteristics such as a and b. Subsequently, characteristics a and b are multiplied by C_3 and S_3 to derive Equation (26), which is expressed in a simultaneous equation with Equations (27) and (28). Similarly, both sides of the element values of (row: 1 column: 1) and (row: 2 column: 1) are compared. Equations (27) and (28) are the left element equation and are substituted with c and d. After respectively multiplying c and d by C_3 and S_3, Equation (29) can be expressed through a simultaneous equation. As a result, Equations (26) and (29) are pressed by comparing both sides of the element and divided to derive θ_3.

$$\left(^0 T_2\right)^{-1} \cdot {^0T_6} = {^2T_6} \tag{23}$$

$$a = C_1 C_2 P_x + C_2 S_1 P_y - S_2 P_z - l_2 \tag{24}$$

$$b = -S_1 P_x + C_1 P_y \tag{25}$$

$$l_6 C_6 S_5 = -a S_3 + b C_3 \tag{26}$$

$$c = C_1 C_2 R_{11} + C_2 S_1 R_{21} - S_2 R_{31} \tag{27}$$

$$d = -S_1 R_{11} + C_1 R_{21} \tag{28}$$

$$C_6 S_5 = -c S_3 + d C_3 \tag{29}$$

$$\theta_3 = \operatorname{atan2}(b - l_6 d,\ a - l_6 c) \tag{30}$$

In Equation (31), the element values of (row: 1, column: 3) and (row: 2 and column: 3) are compared. The left and right mathematical expression of the matrix element are replaced by P and Q, as shown in Equations (32) and (33). As a result, θ_4 is calculated by dividing Q and P.

$$\left(^0 T_3\right)^{-1} \cdot {^0T_6} = {^3T_6} \tag{31}$$

$$P = (C_1 C_2 C_3 - S_1 C_3) R_{13} + (C_2 C_3 S_1 + C_1 S_3) R_{23} - C_3 S_2 R_{33} = -C_4 S_5 \tag{32}$$

$$Q = -C_2 S_2 R_{13} - S_1 S_2 R_{23} - C_2 R_{33} = -S_4 S_5 \tag{33}$$

$$\theta_4 = \operatorname{atan2}(Q,\ P) \tag{34}$$

In the left mathematical expression of Equation (35), the element values of (row: 1, column: 1), (row 1, column 2), and (row 1, column 3) are substituted with α, β, and γ, respectively. On the right side, (row 2, column 1), (row 2, column 2), and (row 2, column 3) are substituted with a, b, and c, respectively. As a result, Equations (36) and (37) are divided to calculate θ_5.

$$\left(^0T_4\right)^{-1} \cdot {}^0T_6 = {}^4T_6 \tag{35}$$

$$\alpha R_{11} + \beta R_{21} + \gamma R_{31} = S_5 C_6 \tag{36}$$

$$a R_{11} + b R_{21} + c R_{31} = C_5 C_6 \tag{37}$$

$$\theta_5 = \text{atan2}(\alpha R_{11} + \beta R_{21} + \gamma R_{31}, \quad a R_{11} + b R_{21} + c R_{31}) \tag{38}$$

Finally, θ_6 compares the element values of (row 1, column 1) and (row 2, column 1) in the left and right terms of Equation (39). In matrix $\left(^0T_5\right)^{-1}$, (row 1, column 1), (row 1, column 2), and (row 1, column 3) are replaced by U_1, U_2, U_3, respectively. Additionally, (row 2, column 1), (row 2, column 2), and (row 2, column 3) are replaced by V_1, V_2, and V_3, respectively. Consequently, Equations (40) and (41) are divided to calculate θ_6.

$$\left(^0T_5\right)^{-1} \cdot {}^0T_6 = {}^5T_6 \tag{39}$$

$$U_1 R_{11} + U_2 R_{21} + U_3 R_{31} = C_6 \tag{40}$$

$$V_1 R_{11} + V_2 R_{21} + V_3 R_{31} = S_6 \tag{41}$$

$$\theta_6 = \text{atan2}(V_1 R_{11} + V_2 R_{21} + V_3 R_{31}, \quad U_1 R_{11} + U_2 R_{21} + U_3 R_{31}) \tag{42}$$

4. Experiment Results and Discussion

4.1. Abduction and Adduction

Prior to the analysis, five randomized males and five randomized females participated in the motion capture experiment. The subjects did not show any disability. Abduction and adduction motions were repeated 10 times. Figure 8 shows the joint rotation angle, ROM, and simulation results from abduction and adduction.

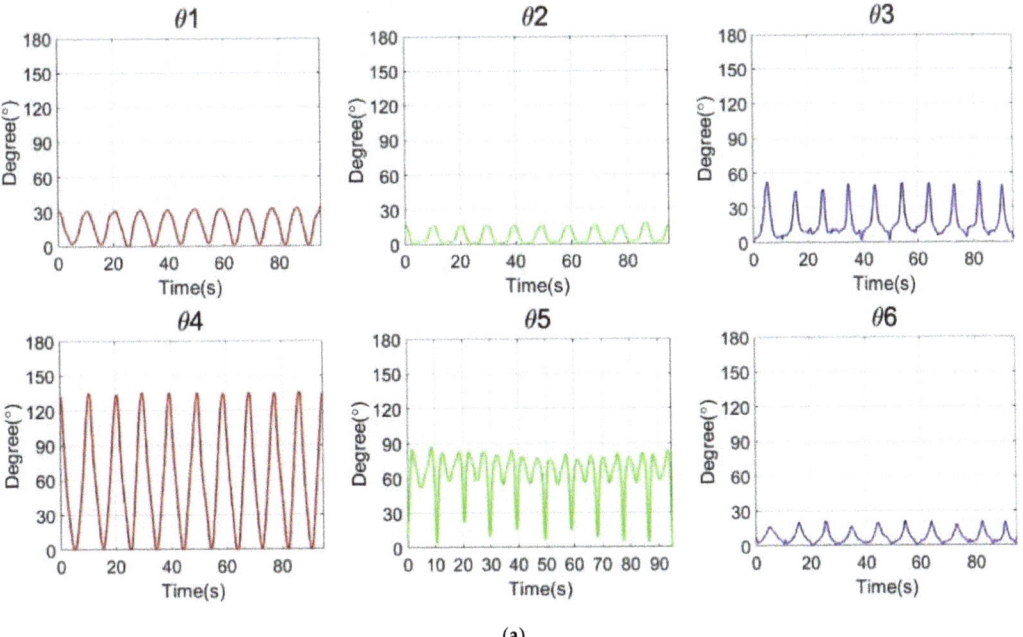

(a)

Figure 8. *Cont.*

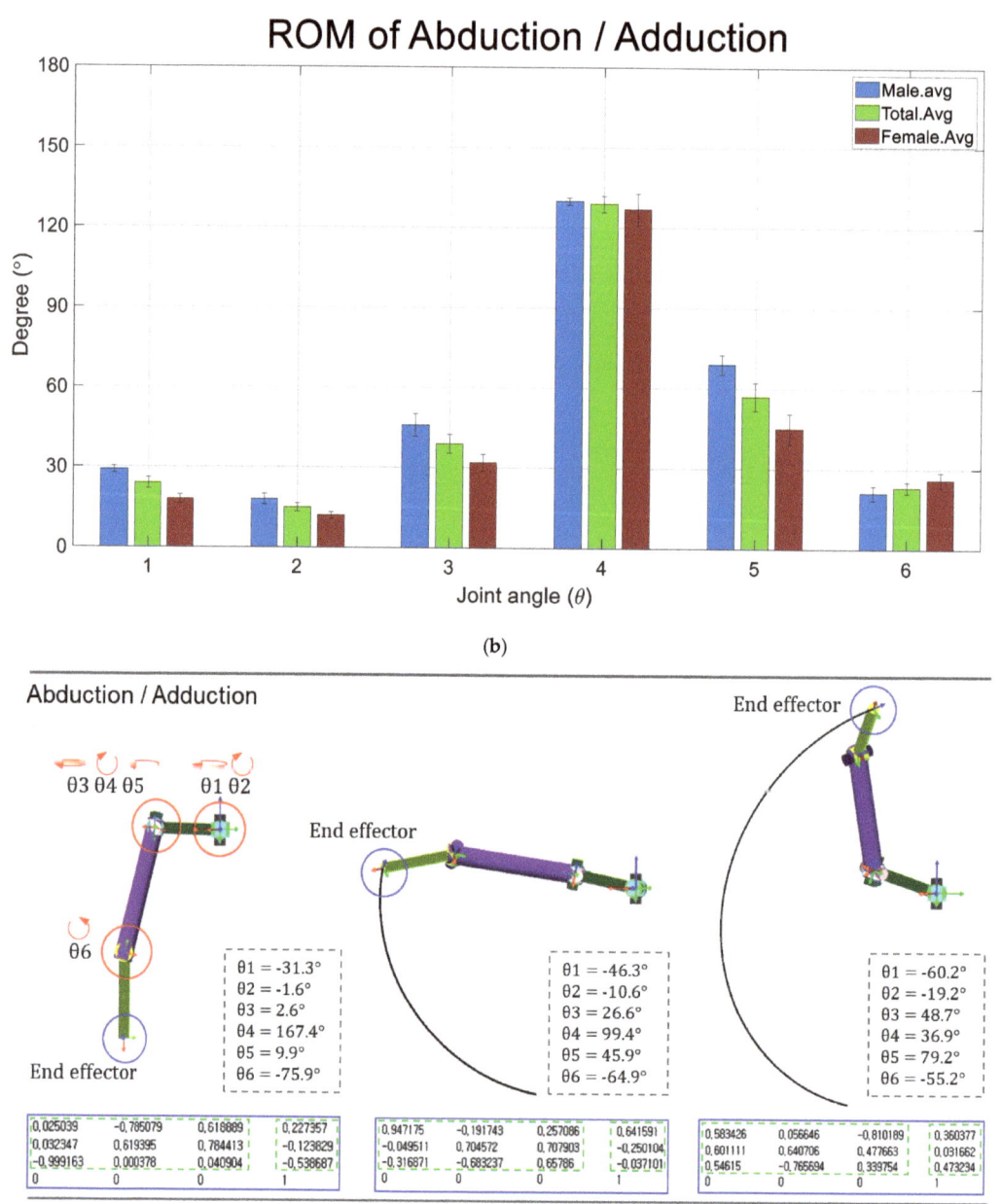

Figure 8. Cont.

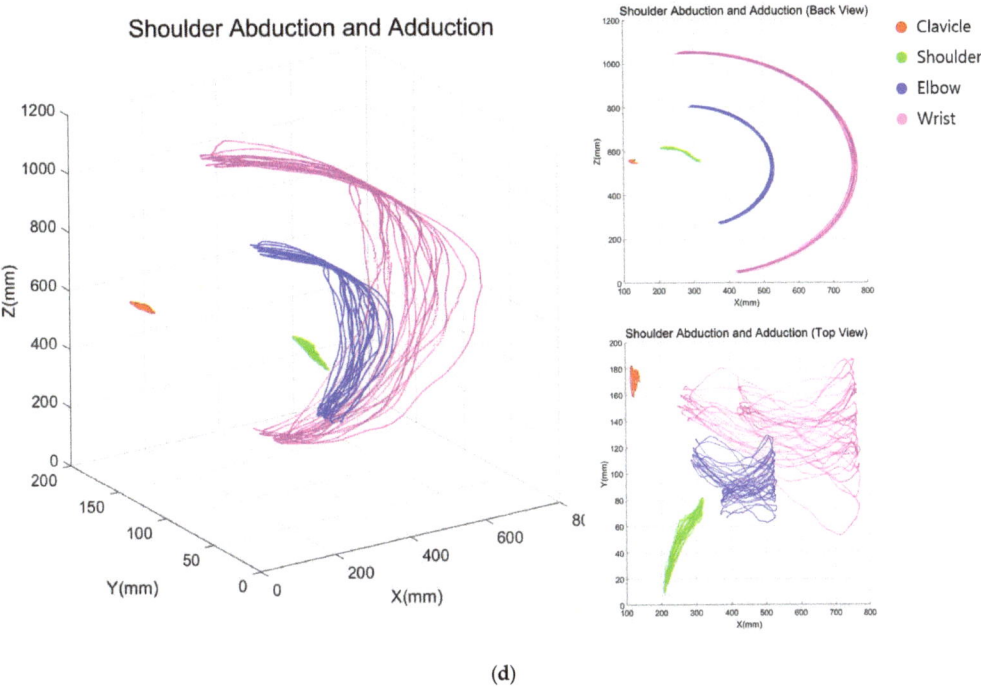

(d)

Figure 8. Joint rotation angle with ROM and simulation by analysis of the inverse kinematics. (**a**) Realized rotation degree variation. (**b**) Average ROM of males and females in abduction and adduction. (**c**) Simulation results of abduction and adduction. (**d**) Joint-centered trajectory graph in a 6-axis arm structure.

Figure 8a shows the joint rotation pattern of a subject who performed the abduction and adduction. While each subject performed the exercise 10 times, the similar pattern of the joint angle appeared from θ_1 to θ_6. In particular, the shoulder joint (θ_4) has the largest variation degree. Simultaneously, the clavicle joint (θ_2) rotates in the same direction with θ_4. All subjects have different ROM, and the quantitative ROM information is listed in Table 2.

Table 2 shows the ROM of males (M) and females (F) in abduction and adduction. The average ROM for the horizontal angle of the clavicle (θ_1) was 28.9° and 18.3° for males and females, respectively, and the ROM for the vertical angle of the clavicle (θ_2) was 17.6° and 11.5°, respectively. Therefore, both θ_1 and θ_2 average ROM for males was higher than that of females. Roll (θ_3), pitch (θ_4), and yaw (θ_5) of the shoulder joint contribute to the shoulder rotation. The average ROM of roll (θ_3) was 46.1° and 31.9° for males and females, respectively, and yaw (θ_5) was 69.3° and 44.8° for males and females, respectively, indicating that the ROM of males was higher than that of females. In particular, the ROM of pitch (θ_4) was 130.4° and 127.2°. Therefore, θ_3, θ_4, and θ_5 values for the males were higher than the females. Elbow joint (θ_6) was 20.7° and 26.2° for males and females, respectively. As a result, males have higher average ROM in the clavicle and shoulder than females, whereas females have higher average ROM in the elbow. For the average ROM by rotation angle of 10 subjects, the standard deviation (σ) was calculated. The standard deviation of θ_2 and θ_4 that significantly contributes the abduction and adduction is 4.8 and 10.0.

Table 2. Data collection for ROM (°) for males and females (abduction and adduction).

	Height (mm)	θ_1	θ_2	θ_3	θ_4	θ_5	θ_6
M.avg	177	28.9	17.6	46.1	130.4	69.3	20.7
M_1	170	33.1	18.1	44.5	127.3	79.9	26.4
M_2	174	30.8	15.9	45.3	133.7	72.0	18.3
M_3	177	24.8	25.9	43.9	130.4	69.8	24.0
M_4	190	29.1	14.9	33.8	134.3	54.8	10.5
M_5	172	26.8	13.4	63.1	126.4	70.1	24.5
SD	7.1	2.9	4.4	9.5	3.2	8.1	5.8
SEM	3.2	1.3	2.0	4.2	1.4	3.6	2.6
F.avg	160	18.3	11.5	31.9	127.2	44.8	26.2
F_1	161	21.5	11.3	26.0	132.9	48.2	24.9
F_2	159	14.4	12.4	25.8	116.1	23.5	33.7
F_3	165	13.5	6.6	33.1	108.2	63.6	28.0
F_4	160	21.7	14.8	45.2	146.4	42.5	14.5
F_5	154	20.3	12.5	29.2	132.5	46.3	29.9
SD	3.5	3.6	2.7	7.2	13.5	12.9	6.5
SEM	1.6	1.6	1.2	3.2	6.0	5.7	2.9
T.avg		23.6	14.6	39.0	128.8	57.1	23.5
SEM		2.0	1.5	3.5	3.1	5.2	2.1

SD (σ): Standard deviation. SEM: Standard error of the mean. T.avg: Total average.

Figure 8b graphically shows the average ROM for 10 subjects through an analysis of Table 2. Rounding was performed to the first decimal place. The angles of θ_1 and θ_2 that contributed to the movement of the clavicle were 24° and 15°, respectively. Moreover, angles of θ_3, θ_4, and θ_5 that are involved in shoulder movement were 39°, 129°, and 57°, respectively. The elbow movement (θ_6) has 23° in abduction and adduction. Figure 8c shows the simulation of the abduction and adduction based on the average ROM. The standing motion was set to the initial position that reflects initial angle value in the parameter of Figure 8c. Consequently, robot simulation shows the accurate trajectory that starts from the initial point and end point of the rotation angle with six-axis joints.

Figure 8d shows the joint-centered trajectory graph in a 6-axis arm structure based on the authors' motion capture experiment. In the figure, the clavicle maintains a relatively constant position. On the other hand, the shoulder, elbow, and wrist have repetitive movements. Based on the figure, we can analyze the one difference between the simulation and movement of humans in Figure 8c,d. The robot simulation gives a certain angle to form repetitive ROM in one caption line. However, in the human movement based on the motion capture data, the ROM was obtained through repetitive motion in various caption lines, as shown in Figure 8d. The caption line of abduction and adduction changes within 45 degrees and moves to maintain a constant ROM.

4.2. External and Internal Rotation

Figure 9 shows the joint rotation angle, ROM, and simulation results from external rotation and internal rotation.

Figure 9a shows the joint rotation pattern of a subject who performed the external and internal rotation. As with abduction and adduction, each subject performed the exercise 10 times, and the similar pattern of the joint angle appeared from θ_1 to θ_6. In particular, the shoulder joint (θ_5) has the largest degree of variation. Furthermore, all the joints, except the elbow joint (θ_6), showed relatively small movement. As for abduction and adduction, Table 3 summarizes the ROM for the ten subjects in an external and internal rotation experiment.

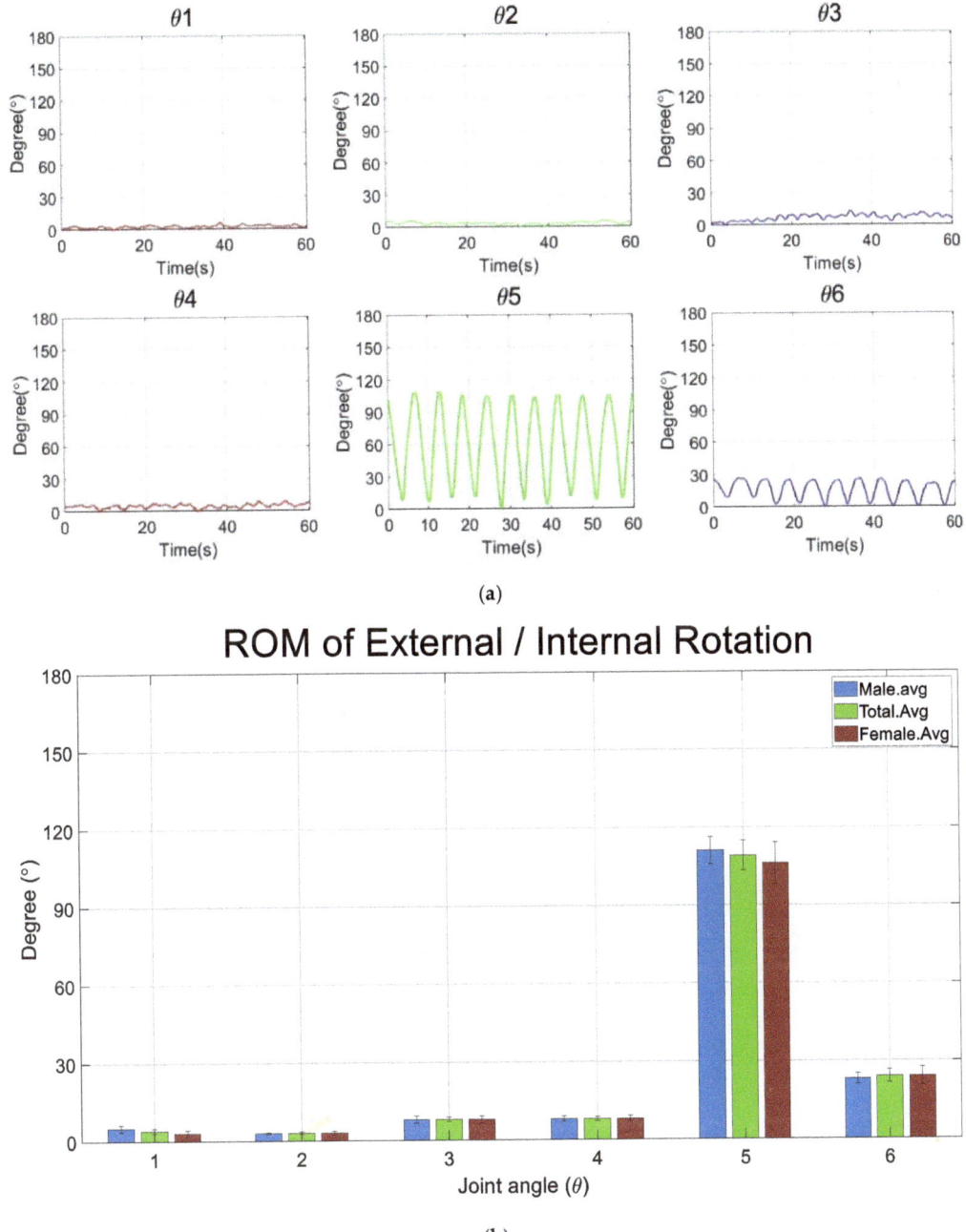

Figure 9. *Cont.*

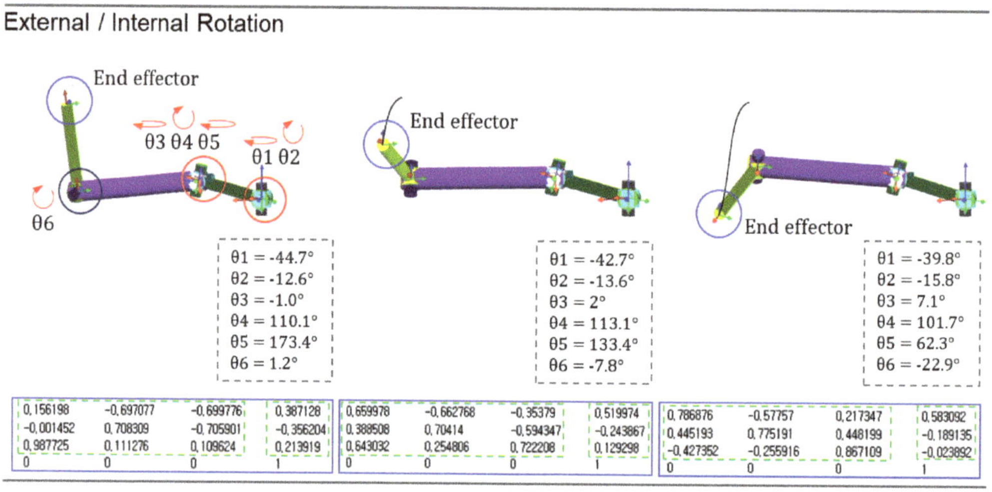

Figure 9. Joint rotation angle with ROM and simulation. (**a**) Realized rotation degree variation in external and internal rotation. (**b**) Average ROM for males and females. (**c**) Simulation results of external and internal rotation. (**c,d**) Simulation results of abduction and adduction. (**d**) Joint-centered trajectory graph in a 6-axis arm structure.

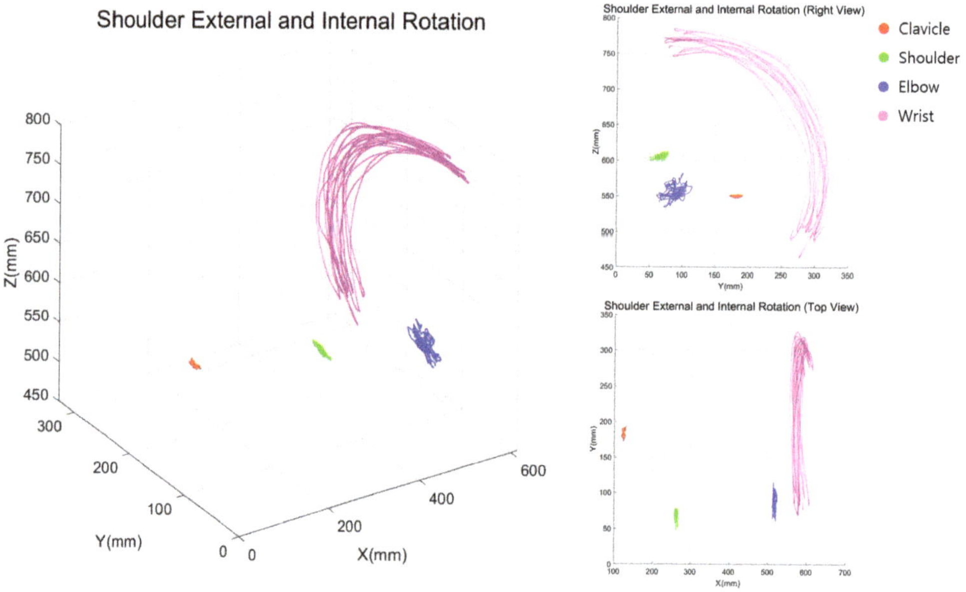

The average ROM for the horizontal angle of the clavicle (θ_1) was 4.9° and 2.9° for males and females, respectively, and the ROM for the vertical rotation (θ_2) was 3.2° and 3.4°, respectively. Therefore, the θ_1 degree for males is significantly higher than females. However, degree θ_2 for females is significantly higher than males. The average ROM of roll (θ_3) was 8.0° and 7.9° for males and females, respectively, and pitch (θ_4) was 8.5° and

7.5° for males and females, respectively, indicating that both ROM for males was slightly higher than females. In particular, the average ROM of yaw (θ_5) was 111.1° and 106.0°. Therefore, degree θ_5 for the males is significantly higher than females. The ROM of the elbow (θ_6) was almost same in males and females at 23.4° and 23.6°, respectively. The standard deviation of the average ROM (σ) was calculated, and the standard deviation of θ_5, which significantly contributes the external and internal rotation, is 18.2.

Table 3. Data collection for the ROM (°) for males and females (external and internal rotation).

	Height	θ_1	θ_2	θ_3	θ_4	θ_5	θ_6
M.avg	177	4.9	3.2	8.0	8.5	111.1	23.4
M_1	170	2.6	3.4	8.5	9.4	109.9	18.8
M_2	174	2.8	2.9	3.5	3.9	97.5	22.1
M_3	177	2.0	2.2	5.4	9.3	99.5	20.6
M_4	190	9.0	4.4	11.5	10.2	125.9	32.1
M_5	172	8.0	3.3	11.2	9.5	122.7	23.6
SD	7.1	3.0	0.7	3.2	2.3	11.6	4.6
SEM	3.2	1.3	0.3	1.4	1.0	5.2	2.1
F.avg	160	2.9	3.4	7.9	7.5	106.0	23.6
F_1	161	6.6	6.9	12.3	8.8	138.5	42.9
F_2	159	1.3	1.0	5.6	5.1	79.7	22.3
F_3	165	1.2	1.8	5.7	4.4	89.9	19.2
F_4	160	3.4	4.5	7.5	8.4	122.4	19.5
F_5	154	2.0	3.0	8.4	10.9	90.3	13.9
SD	7.1	2.0	2.1	2.4	2.4	22.4	10.0
SEM	3.2	0.9	0.9	1.1	1.1	10.0	4.5
T.avg		3.9	3.3	8.0	8.0	107.6	23.5
SEM		0.9	0.5	0.9	0.8	5.7	2.5

SD (σ): Standard deviation. SEM: Standard error of the mean. T.avg: Total average.

Figure 9b graphically shows the average ROM for 10 subjects through an analysis of Table 3. Rounding was performed to the first decimal place. Angle of θ_1 and θ_2 that contributed to movement of clavicle were 4° and 3°, respectively. Moreover, angle of θ_3, θ_4 and θ_5 that involved in shoulder movement were 8°, 8° and 109°. The elbow movement (θ_6) has 24° in external and internal rotation. Figure 9c shows the simulation of the external and internal based on the average ROM. The standing motion was set to the initial position that reflects initial angle value in the parameter of the Figure 8c. Consequently, robot simulation shows the accurate trajectory that starts from initial point and end point of the rotation angle with six-axis joints. Figure 8d shows the joint-centered trajectory graph in 6-axis arm structure. In the figure, clavicle and shoulder maintain a relatively constant position. On the other hand, wrist have repetitive movements with axis of radius. As a result, we analyzed that both the simulation and the subject maintain a constant scription line, repeating the movement.

4.3. Discussion

This study measured the joint angle degree and ROM of the 6-DOF for two SR motions of the subjects. The joint angles (θ_4) that are most significantly involved in abduction and adduction were 130.4° and 127.2° for males and females, respectively. Therefore, the ROM of abduction and adduction is calculated by adding θ_2 with θ_4, and obtained 148° and 138.7° for males and females, respectively. The joint angles (θ_5), which are most significantly involved in external and internal rotation movements, were 111.10° and 105.96° for males and females, respectively. Therefore, the ROM of external and internal rotation is calculated by θ_5, and obtained 111.1° and 106° for males and females, respectively. In conclusion, the average ROM of ten subjects for abduction/adduction and external/internal rotation was, respectively, 143.4° and 108.6°. In abduction and adduction, males showed significantly higher ROM than females. Moreover, the elbow angle (θ_6) of females was higher than males. Therefore, it is judged that females use the elbow more when moving in abduction and adduction than males to tracking motion trajectory.

Unlike external and internal rotation, there are θ_2 and θ_4 that are centrally involved in the ROM of the shoulder in abduction and adduction. Besides θ_2 and θ_4, the rotation angles of θ_3, θ_5, and θ_5 stand out. θ_3 represents the left and right rotation of the shoulder. We think that this is likely due to the shoulder rotation working together with the help of the scapula during the rotation process of the shoulder. θ_5 represents the rotation of the radius or ulna. In the posture of performing the initial movement, the direction vector of the palm faces the center of the body, but as ROM increases, it rotates outward and moves away from the center of the body. θ_6 represents extension and flexion of the elbow. In the course of abduction and adduction exercise through motion capture, the exercise standard is 10 circular movements in a 180-degree range of motion. Therefore, in the process of exercising with the wrist in a half-moon-shaped orbit, if the ROM of the shoulder is limited, it is determined that the rotation follows the half-moon-shaped trajectory by flexion of the elbow.

Ropars classified shoulder hypersensitivity using a motion capture system and physical therapy goniometer. As a result, in the process of measuring standard data for the general public, the average ROM of the shoulder abduction and adduction was 129.9° ± 7.4°. Furthermore, the average external and internal rotational ROM of the shoulder was 94.3° ± 14.1 [24]. To analyze the scapular–humerus rhythm, Bagg, S. measured the movement of the scapula and humerus in abduction and adduction. As a result, the average ROM was 104.3° and a maximum movable range was 111.8° [25]. Barnes analyzed the ROM of shoulder movement using linear regression analysis and studied the age, gender, and dominance as comparative subjects. As a result, abduction and adduction was 180.1° ± 18.2 in males and 187.6° ± 16.1 in females, and the external and internal rotation was 101.2° ± 11.6 in males and 104.9° ± 12.0 in females. [26]. Rigoni validated an IMU for measuring shoulder range of motion in healthy adults. Each movement was assessed with a goniometer, and the IMU by two testers independently. Therefore, the compared agreements were assessed with intra-class correlation coefficients (ICC) and Bland–Altman 95% limits of agreement (LOA). As a result, the ROM of abduction and adduction were measured as 151.4 and 152.2, respectively; and internal and external rotation were measured as 141.1 and 142.3 with intra-class correlation (≥ 0.90) [27].

The last thing to consider is the accuracy of the function of the motion capture (OptiTrack) system. Motion capture (OptiTrack) is very important for the accuracy of the sensor's response when an object moves. Therefore, we can present the excellence of the accuracy of the proposed method by analyzing [28–33]. The method of this study and the methods of studies from [28–33] have different objects of observation and different quantities of sensors. However, since all of them used the same motion capture, it is possible to present an average value of accuracy for the function of motion capture. The average value for accuracy is recorded in Table 4, and it can be seen that the accuracy of this study improved by more than 10% compared to [28–33].

Table 4. Comparison for accuracy of proposed system and others.

Reference	Average Accuracy [%]	Performance of a Motion Capture
this work	97.6	OptiTrack
[28]	94.8	optical motion capture method (DeepMoCap)
[29]	93.6	multi-person pose estimation
[30]	95.9	OptiTrack
[31]	95.0	IMU Sensor (mobilityILab system)
[32]	85.3	multiple Kinect sensors
[33]	70.0	kinect V2 and captiv sensor

5. Conclusions

Based on the results of this study, the kinematics solution for 6-DOF of ROM could be determined through the standardized motion of the SR exercise, starting with the clavicle as the base point. In particular, based on the end effector information, we tried to solve the homogeneous transformation matrix of Equations (2) and (3) at first. However, because the constant values for the parameters (shoulder position) could not be solved, we changed the direction of the study to obtain the shoulder position first, then calculate the inverse kinematics formula. As a result, our approach differs compared to the commonly known 6-DOF inverse kinematics solution that combines 3-DOF of the wrist and the other joint angle of the 3-DOF. Through solving the 6-DOF inverse kinematics, future research and development of the 6-axis rehabilitation robot will be conducted. In the follow-up study, we will consider collecting the end effector data through force and torque sensors instead of using a motion capture system. If the end effector data is collected, the rehabilitation robot follows the trajectory of the patient's motion through a kinematics solution. At the same time, the robot measures the maximum ROM of the patients, and it is envisaged that the patient will be able to perform stretching or passive or active-assisted exercises through the designated ROM.

Upper limb joints are structurally deeper than skin tissue, muscle tissue, and cartilage tissue. The existing research methods have limitations in objective evaluation because they do not select and analyze the central coordinates of the joint. However, because inverse kinematics can be automatically calculated by determining the center of the joint through motion capture, we think that it is extremely advantageous to suitably interpret the center coordinates of the joint, and the study results are more accurate and superior. Additionally, in order to reduce the standard deviation of the ROM and increase the accuracy of the experimental data, additional experiments should be conducted with increased subjects sample size.

If the cause of the difference in ROM is identified in the same rehabilitation motion, it is expected to make a great contribution to the analysis of rehabilitation exercise and human body mechanics. We think of two reasons why errors occur, even after repeating the same motion 10 times and obtaining an average ROM. The first is the degree of flexibility according to the ROM and muscle mass according to the patient's own body shape. The second is judged to be a relative error of the center position according to the attachment position of the marker, even if it is purely the same operation.

The movement of the SR robot must be the same as the human rehabilitation motion. Therefore, the proposed mathematical analysis method is sufficiently applicable because it is an analysis method for the objective evaluation of the movement of the rehabilitation robot. In conclusion, this study shows that a person will be able to exercise efficiently by wearing the rehabilitation robot with suggested kinematics model. Additionally, this study facilitated the determination of the ROM in the rehabilitation robot considering the ROM of normal subjects. Using the proposed model, it is possible to increase the accuracy of the trajectory of the rehabilitation robot and contribute to the improvement in safety. Comprehensively, utilizing the mathematical inverse kinematics equation that were debuted in this study, we will fabricate an upper rehabilitation robot through designing the mechanism instructor and motor in a follow-up study. In addition, because the rehabilitation exercise training-guided robot is linked to brain-related diseases, it contributes to the definition of domestic and international standardization of rehabilitation robots, affording universal training methods, accurate results, and objective evaluation for the safe treatment of patients.

Author Contributions: Design and experiment: J.S., analysis and fabrication: K.Y., and guidance and supervisor: K.G.K. All authors have read and agreed to the published version of the manuscript.

Funding: This research was supported by the GRRC program of the Gyeonggi province (No. GRRC-Gachon2020 (B01)) and suported by Gachon University (GCU-202205980001).

Institutional Review Board Statement: Not applicable.

Informed Consent Statement: Not applicable.

Data Availability Statement: The data presented in this study are available upon request from the corresponding author. The data are not publicly available because of privacy and ethical re-strictions.

Acknowledgments: Jaehwang Seol and Kicheol Yoon equally contributed to this work. Jaehwang Seol and Kicheol Yoon are the co-first (lead) authors.

Conflicts of Interest: The authors declare no conflict of interest.

References

1. Cho, C.H.; Bae, K.C.; Kim, D.H. Treatment strategy for frozen shoulder. *Clin. Orthop. Surg.* **2019**, *11*, 249–257. [CrossRef] [PubMed]
2. Cho, K.H.; Song, W.K. Robot-assisted reach training for improving upper extremity function of chronic stroke. *Tohoku J. Exp. Med.* **2015**, *237*, 149–155. [CrossRef] [PubMed]
3. Kang, B.; Lee, H.; In, H.; Jeong, U.; Chung, J.; Cho, K.J. Development of a polymer-based tendon-driven wearable robotic hand. In Proceedings of the IEEE International Conference on Robotics and Automation (ICRA) 2016, Stockholm, Sweden, 16–21 May 2016.
4. Woo, H.; Lee, J.; Kong, K. Gait assist method by wearable robot for incomplete paraplegic patients. *J. Korea Robot. Soc.* **2017**, *12*, 144–151. [CrossRef]
5. Lee, K.S.; Park, J.H.; Beom, J.; Park, H.S. Design and evaluation of passive shoulder joint tracking module for upperlimb rehabilitation robots. *Front. Neurorobot.* **2018**, *12*, 1–14. [CrossRef]
6. Cho, K.H.; Song, W.K. Robot-assisted reach training with an active assistant protocol for long term upper extremity impairment poststroke: A randomized controlled trial. *Arch. Phys. Med. Rehabil.* **2019**, *100*, 213–219. [CrossRef] [PubMed]
7. Yang, Q.; Pan, X.; Guo, Y.; Qu, H. Design of rehabilitation medical product system for elderly apartment based on intelligent endowment. *ASP Trans. Internet Things* **2022**, *2*, 1–9.
8. Wolpaw, J.R. Brain-computer interface technology: A review of the first international meeting. *IEEE Trans. Rehabil. Eng.* **2000**, *8*, 164–173. [CrossRef]
9. Yang, H.E.; Kyeong, S.; Lee, S.H.; Lee, W.J.; Ha, S.W.; Kim, S.M. Structural and functional improvements due to robot-assisted gait training in the stroke-injured brain. *Neurosci. Lett.* **2017**, *637*, 114–119. [CrossRef]
10. Mehrholz, J.; Thomas, S.; Kugler, J.; Pohl, M.; Elsner, B. Electromechanical-assisted training for walking after stroke. *Cochrane Database Syst. Rev.* **2020**, *10*, CD006185.
11. Carpinella, I.; Lencioni, T.; Bowman, T. Effects of robot therapy on upper body kinematics and arm function in persons post stroke: A pilot randomized controlled trial. *J. Neuroeng. Rehabil.* **2020**, *17*, 1–19. [CrossRef]
12. Pereira, S.; Silva, C.C.; Ferreira, S. Anticipatory postural adjustments during sitting reach movement in post-stroke subjects. *J. Electromyogr. Kinesiol.* **2014**, *24*, 165–171. [CrossRef] [PubMed]
13. Kim, J. A Study on the Therapeutic Effect of the Upper Limb Rehabilitation Robot "Camillo" and Improvement of Clinical Basis in Stroke Patients with Hemiplegia. Master's Thesis, Dongguk University, Seoul, Republic of Korea, 2021.
14. Wu, G.; Helm, V.D.; Veeger, F.C.; Makhsous, H.E.; Van Roy, M.; Anglin, P.; Nagels, C.; Karduna, J.; McQuade, A.R.; Wang, K.; et al. ISB Recommendation on definitions of joint coordinate systems of various joints for the reporting of human joint motion–Part II: Shoulder, elbow, wrist and hand. *J. Biomech. Int. Soc. Biomech.* **2005**, *38*, 981–992. [CrossRef] [PubMed]
15. Jackson, M.; Michaud, B.; Tétreault, P.; Begon, M. Improvements in measuring shoulder joint kinematics. *J. Biomech.* **2012**, *45*, 2180–2183. [CrossRef] [PubMed]
16. Zhang, C.; Dong, M.; Li, J.; Cao, Q. A modified kinematic model of shoulder complex based on vicon motion capturing system: Generalized GH joint with floating centre. *Sensors* **2020**, *20*, 3713. [CrossRef]
17. Liu, Y.; Huang, S.; Huang, Y. Motor imagery EEG classification for patients with amy-otrophic lateral sclerosis using fractal dimension and Fisher's criterion-based channel selection. *Sensors* **2017**, *17*, 1557.
18. Gainmann, B.; Allison, B.; Pfurtscheller, G. *Brain-Computer Interface, Revolutionizing Human-Computer Interaction*; Springer: Berlin/Heidelberg, Germany, 2010.
19. Nijholt, A.; Tan, D. Brain-computer interfacing for intelligent system. *IEEE Intell. Syst.* **2008**, *23*, 72–79. [CrossRef]
20. Sajda, P.; Muller, K.-R.; Shenoy, K.V. Brain-computer interfaces. *IEEE Signal Process. Mag.* **2008**, *25*, 16–28. [CrossRef]
21. Asif, S.; Webb, P. Kinematics analysis of 6-DoF articulated robot with spherical wrist. *Math. Probl. Eng.* **2021**, *2021*, 1–11. [CrossRef]
22. Denavit, J.; Hartenberg, R.S. A kinematic notation for lower-pair mechanisms based on matrices. *ASME J. Appl. Mech.* **1995**, *22*, 215–221. [CrossRef]
23. Yoon, K.C.; Cho, S.M.; Kim, K.G. Coupling effect suppressed compact surgical robot with 7-Axis multi-joint using wire-driven method. *Mathematics* **2022**, *10*, 1698. [CrossRef]
24. Ropars, M.; Cretual, A.; Thomazeau, H.; Kaila, R.; Bonan, I. Volumetric definition of shoulder range of motion and its correlation with clinical signs of shoulder hyperlaxity. A motion capture study. *J. Shoulder Elb. Surg.* **2015**, *24*, 310–316. [CrossRef]
25. Bagg, S.D.; Forrest, W.J. A biomechanical analysis of scapular rotation during arm abduction in the scapular plane. *Am. J. Phys. Med. Rehabil.* **1988**, *67*, 238–245. [PubMed]
26. Barnes, C.J.; Van Steyn, S.J.; Fischer, R.A. The effects of age, sex, and shoulder dominance on range of motion of the shoulder. *J. Shoulder Elb. Surg.* **2001**, *10*, 242–246. [CrossRef] [PubMed]

27. Rigoni, M.; Gill, S.; Babazadeh, S.; Elsewaisy, O.; Gillies, H.; Nguyen, N.; Pathirana, P.N.; Page, R. Assessment of Shoulder Range of Motion Using a Wireless Inertial Motion Capture Device-A Validation Study. *Sensors* **2019**, *19*, 1781. [CrossRef]
28. Ahatzitofis, A.; Zarpals, D.; Kollias, S.; Daras, P. DeepmoCap: Deep optical motion capture using multiple depth sensors and retro-reflectors. *Sensors* **2019**, *19*, 282.
29. Cao, Z.; Simon, T.; Wei, S.E.; Sheikh, Y. Realtime multi-person 2D pose estimation using part affinity fields. In Proceedings of the 2017 IEEE Conference on Computer Vision and Pattern Recognition (CVPR), Honolulu, HI, USA, 21–26 July 2017; pp. 7291–7299. [CrossRef]
30. Qiu, S.; Hao, Z.; Wang, Z.; Liu, L.; Liu, J.; Zhao, H.; Fortino, G. Sensor combination selection strategy for kayak cycle phase segmentation based on body sensor networks. *IEEE Internet Things J.* **2022**, *9*, 1–12. [CrossRef]
31. Walha, R.; Lebel, K.; Gaudreault, N.; Dagenais, P.; Cereatti, A.; Croce, U.D. The accuracy and precision of gait spatio-temporal parameters extracted from an instrumented sock during treadmill and overground walking in healthy subjects and patients with a foot impairment secondary to psoriatic arthritis. *Sensors* **2021**, *21*, 6179. [CrossRef]
32. Kim, Y.; Baek, S.; Bae, B.C. Motion capture of the human body using multiple depth sensors. *ETRI J.* **2017**, *39*, 181–190. [CrossRef]
33. Steinebach, T.; Grosse, E.H.; Glock, C.H.; Wakula, J.; Lunin, A. Accuracy evaluation of two markerless motion capture systems for measurement of upper extremities: Kinect V2 and Captiv. *Hum. Factors Ergon. Manuf. Serv. Ind.* **2020**, *30*, 291–302. [CrossRef]

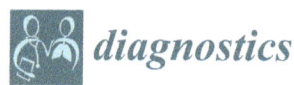

Article

Nonlinear and Linear Measures in the Differentiation of Postural Control in Patients after Total Hip or Knee Replacement and Healthy Controls

Anna Hadamus [1,*], Michalina Błażkiewicz [2], Aleksandra J. Kowalska [3], Kamil T. Wydra [3], Marta Grabowicz [1], Małgorzata Łukowicz [3], Dariusz Białoszewski [1] and Wojciech Marczyński [4]

1. Department of Rehabilitation, Faculty of Medical Sciences, Medical University of Warsaw, 02-091 Warsaw, Poland; marta.grabowicz@wum.edu.pl (M.G.); dariusz.bialoszewski@wum.edu.pl (D.B.)
2. Faculty of Rehabilitation, the Józef Piłsudski University of Physical Education in Warsaw, 00-809 Warsaw, Poland; michalina.blazkiewicz@awf.edu.pl
3. Professor Adam Gruca Independent Public Teaching Hospital in Otwock, Rehabilitation Clinic, 05-400 Otwock, Poland; aleksandra.macheta@wp.pl (A.J.K.); kamil.wydra@interia.eu (K.T.W.); mlukowicz@cmkp.edu.pl (M.Ł.)
4. Medical Centre for Postgraduate Education, 01-813 Warsaw, Poland; wmarczynski@interia.pl
* Correspondence: anna.hadamus@wum.edu.pl

Abstract: Primary osteoarthritis treatments such as a total hip (THR) or knee (TKR) replacement lead to postural control changes reinforced by age. Balance tests such as standing with eyes open (EO) or closed (EC) give a possibility to calculate both linear and nonlinear indicators. This study aimed to find the group of linear and/or nonlinear measures that can differentiate healthy people and patients with TKR or THR from each other. This study enrolled 49 THR patients, 53 TKR patients, and 16 healthy controls. The center of pressure (CoP) path length, sample entropy (SampEn), fractal dimension (FD), and the largest Lyapunov exponent (LyE) were calculated separately for AP and ML directions from standing with EO/EC. Cluster analysis did not result in correct allocation to the groups according to all variables. The discriminant model included LyE (ML-EO, ML-EC, AP-EC), FD (AP-EO, ML-EC, AP-EC), CoP-path AP-EC, and SampEn AP-EC. Regression analysis showed that all nonlinear variables depend on the group. The CoP path length is different only in THR patients. It was concluded that standing with EC is a better way to assess the amount of regularity of CoP movement and attention paid to maintain balance. Nonlinear measures better differentiate TKR and THR patients from healthy controls.

Keywords: hip arthroplasty; knee arthroplasty; older adults; postural control; body balance; osteoarthritis; sample entropy; fractal dimension; Lyapunov exponent

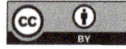

1. Introduction

Osteoarthritis (OA) is a multifactorial disease leading to cartilage degeneration and damage to the surrounding tissues: joint capsule, ligaments, subchondral bone, periarticular muscles, and nerve endings. As a chronic disease, it leads to biomechanical changes in the affected joint as well as burdensome symptoms such as pain, stiffness, swelling, and loss of function. In advanced stages, OA can lead to severe physical impairment [1,2]. Osteoarthritis frequency increases with age and most often involves big joints in the lower limb: hip or knee joint being the dominant source of disability, affecting approximately 776 million people globally [3].

Patients in advanced stages of OA, with persistent pain, loss of function, and advanced radiographic changes are qualified for joint arthroplasty, which is an effective (also cost-effective) procedure, giving much better results than physical therapy programs [4]. Current concepts do not recommend arthroscopic debridement for treating OA. Additionally, arthroscopic partial meniscectomy has a limited role in patients with symptomatic meniscal tear coexisting with knee OA [4]. The number of total hips (THR) and knee replacement (TKR) surgeries has increased rapidly over the last decades [2,3,5]. The incidence rate of TKR in the US population was 272 per 100,000 citizens in 2002, and 429 in 2012, and it is expected to increase by 143% by 2050 [6]. More than 300,000 primary total hip replacements and over 700,000 primary total knee replacements are performed annually in the US, of which more than 90% are due to OA [4]. Symptoms of OA, as well as invasive procedures such as THR or TKR, affect joint function. Due to damaged and/or cut nerve endings and roots, long-lasting pain, and damage to the joints and surrounding tissues, proprioception and motor control in this area are often severely affected. This leads also to postural control changes, which are reinforced by age by impairing the capability of the central nervous system to process signals from somatosensory, visual, and vestibular networks [7]. After both types of surgery—THR, and TKR—leg length discrepancy is often observed [8,9]. Anatomical discrepancies are corrected during the arthroplasty, but functional changes, including movement habits, remain in these groups of patients unchanged. Leg length discrepancy of 2 cm or more is compensated by moving the pelvis to the oblique position and flexing the knee of the longer leg [8,9]. It results in asymmetric loading of the lower limbs [8,10–12]. Effective rehabilitation protocol is needed to change and equalize joint moments and feet loading, both in static and dynamic conditions [13]. In the studies by Heil et al. [9] and Ohlendorf et al. [8] significant differences in postural control were found between the TKR or THR group and healthy controls. The results of the THR group were poorer than those of the TKR group in static conditions [8,9]. Gauchard et al. [11] also reported some postural deficit in balance control during the static test after TKR compared to the control group. They also suggested that knee replacement surgery does not allow accurate orientation of the lower limb and the compensatory role of the knee joint in the regulation of postural control in quiet standing is not restored.

According to Massion [14], postural control depends on several elements. The first is the internal body representation or postural body schema (orientation of body segments and location of the center of mass). The second is multisensory input that regulates the orientation and stabilization of body segments. The third is flexible postural responses or anticipations to recover from a disturbance or postural stabilization during voluntary movement. Small movements accompany the maintenance of any posture. The fact that postural oscillations are small supports the assumption that the system is linear within a limited range of motion [15,16]. While this assumption is correct to some extent, it should be remembered that there is also significant nonlinearity in the postural control system, which tends to be ignored [17].

The most common assessment tool to quantify postural balance is a static standing test with eyes open or closed [1,18]. Center of pressure (CoP) displacements give a possibility to calculate many variables or indicators that can be interpreted as good or poor body balance. Among the most commonly used indicators to assess postural control, some authors [18–20] distinguish between those most commonly called linear and those providing indirect insight into the functioning of the nervous system—called nonlinear. Linear tools, such as the CoP path length, sway velocity, and area, quantify the amount of CoP movement during a specific task, independently of their order in the distribution. The nonlinear system approach helps to evaluate different aspects of the CoP data. Nonlinear measures allow for quantifying the regularity and complexity of the system [21,22]. Nonlinear measures include entropy family, fractal dimension, the largest Lyapunov exponent, Hurst exponent, and recurrence quantification analysis (RQA) [18].

Sample entropy (SampEn) is one of the various types of entropy measures. This coefficient is used to determine the regularity of postural sway [23]. The increased values of SampEn indicate a larger irregularity of the CoP, which is more random and less predictable. Lower SampEn values show that the CoP signal is more regular and predictable, which is associated with less complexity of structure [24]. Fractal dimension (FD) is another measure that indicates the complexity of the CoP signal by describing its shape [25]. It shows the complexity and self-similarity of physiological signals [26]. In the case of the CoP trajectory, a change in FD may indicate a change in control strategies for maintaining a quiet stance. The largest Lyapunov exponent (LyE) is a tool characterizing the chaotic behavior of the signal. The human dynamic stability characterized by LyE measures the resistance of the human locomotor control system to perturbations [18]. It quantifies how well an individual can keep a stable posture under perturbations. A higher LyE points to the capability of a more rapid response of balance control in different body movements [27].

Since there are many linear and nonlinear measures that can be used to quantify balance and postural control, it is often problematic to choose some of them that could be sensitive enough to differentiate patients with various medical conditions. Until now, we found no studies comparing postural control between patients after total hip and knee replacement. There are also no studies analyzing which balance and postural control parameters should be used in these groups of patients as a reliable way to differentiate these groups of patients.

The aim of this study was to find the group of linear and/or nonlinear measures that can differentiate healthy people and patients with total knee or hip replacement from each other. This could help to choose the best set of measures that should be calculated from the static balance test to characterize different clinical conditions. It can also suggest which measures are not necessary.

2. Materials and Methods

2.1. Participants

This study enrolled 49 patients after a total hip replacement (H group) and 53 patients after total knee replacement (K group) due to primary osteoarthritis. All patients were operated on in the Department of Orthopaedics of the Prof. Adam Gruca Independent Public Clinical Hospital in Otwock, Poland. The control group (C group) was 16 healthy persons measured in the Biomechanics Laboratory at the Medical University of Warsaw. None of the measured persons was a professional athlete in the past. The basic data of each group are summarized in Table 1.

Table 1. Mean + standard deviation of anthropometric data of H-, K- and C groups.

	H Group (N = 49)	K Group (N = 53)	C Group (N = 19)
Gender	28 women, 21 men	34 women, 19 men	15 women, 1 man
Age (years)	63.7 ± 8.8 * HKC	68.4 ± 6.3 * HKC	53.0 ± 7.6 * HKC
Bodyweight (kg)	81.5 ± 16.0	85.7 ± 16.1 * KC	74.8 ± 16.3 * KC
Height (cm)	167.5 ± 10.1	166.1 ± 11.5	164.9 ± 4.9
Body Mass Index (kg/m^2)	28.8 ± 4.2 * HK	30.9 ± 3.9 * HK,KC	27.4 ± 5.3 * KC

* $p < 0.01$ in ANOVA test with post hoc Tukey's test; letter (H, K or C) indicates group in Tukey's test.

The inclusion criteria for the control group included: (1) no balance problems (due to neurological, heart, or musculoskeletal disease), (2) no current musculoskeletal complaints, and (3) written consent to participate in the study. The inclusion criteria for the rest two groups comprised: (1) noncomplicated total knee or hip replacement surgery because of primary osteoarthritis, (2) no other balance problems (due to neurological or heart diseases, vertigo, etc.), (3) no current musculoskeletal complaints other than related to the operated joint, and (4) written consent to participate in the study. All patients from H- and K groups were measured within the first 12 weeks (3–11 weeks) after surgery before the rehabilitation program began.

2.2. Ethical Approval

The study protocol was approved by the Bioethics Committee of the Medical University of Warsaw (no. KB/28/2014). The study was conducted according to the ethical guidelines and principles of the Declaration of Helsinki.

2.3. Measurement Methods

The postural stability data for each subject were recorded using an AMTI AccuSway (Advanced Mechanical Technology Inc., Watertown, MA, USA) plate with Balance Clinic software. The sample rate was set at 100 Hz. Each person completed three trials of both legs standing with eyes open and three trials of both legs standing with eyes closed. Each trial lasted thirty seconds with a one-minute rest between trials. The results of the patients' second trials were analyzed. This was performed because patients did not always comply in the first trial and postoperative patients often reported fatigue in the third trial.

2.4. Calculation Methods

The study used the linear parameters of CoP path length and three nonlinear measures, sample entropy, fractal dimension, and the largest Lyapunov exponent to assess CoP dynamics. All coefficients were calculated using MatLab software v. R2018b (MathWorks, Natick, MA, USA), separately for mediolateral (ML) and anterior–posterior (AP) CoP data, according to the rules described below. The data for the 30 s trials included 3000 points in each direction.

The 2D CoP path length was calculated in AP and ML directions using the following formulas:

$$CoP\_ML = \sum_{i=2}^{n} \sqrt{(x_i - x_{i-1})^2} \quad CoP\_AP = \sum_{i=2}^{n} \sqrt{(y_i - y_{i-1})^2} \quad (1)$$

Due to the fact that other commonly used linear parameters (like ellipsis areas, CoP path length) are redundant [28], they were not included in the calculations, as this would distort discrimination analysis and would not give additional information.

SampEn is the negative natural logarithm of the conditional probability that a dataset of length N, having repeated itself within a tolerance r for m points, will also repeat itself for $m + 1$ points, without allowing self-matches:

$$SampEn(m, r, N) = -\ln\left(\frac{A^m(r)}{B^m(r)}\right) \quad (2)$$

B represents the total number of matches of length m while A represents the subset of B that also matches for $m + 1$. For calculating the SampEn, MatLab codes obtained from the Physionet tool [29] were used, with "default" parameter values: $m = 2$ and $r = 0.2 \times$ (standard deviation of the data).

FD was calculated using Higuchi's algorithm [30]. Higher FD values are associated with the greater complexity of a time series.

LyE was calculated to detect chaotic system dynamics, using the following equation:

$$d(t) = Ce^{LyEt} \quad (3)$$

In LyE equation $d(t)$ is the average divergence at time t and C is a constant that normalizes the initial separation [31]. A positive LyE value is often considered a necessary condition for the presence of chaos in a given system. If LyE is zero, it means the system is conservative, (i.e., there is no dissipation). If the system is dissipative, the LyE value is negative.

2.5. Statistical Analysis

Statistical analysis was performed using Statistica v. 13.1 (TIBCO Software, Inc., Palo Alto, CA, USA), PQStat 2021 software v. 1.8.2.238 (PQStat Software, Poznań, Poland), and GRETL software v. 2019a (Free Software Foundation, Boston, MA, USA). The threshold for statistical significance was assumed at $p < 0.05$.

The Shapiro–Wilk test was used to assess the normality of all data distributions. Next, it was checked if variance matrices of variables are homogeneous across groups. For inter group comparison, one-way ANOVA with Tukey's post hoc test was used.

Tree cluster analysis was used for grouping patients according to analyzed linear and nonlinear measures from both tests (EO, EC). The grouping was performed using connectivity-based clustering with a weighted group method with medians with Euclidean distance. There were no assumptions about the number of groups.

Next, discriminant analysis was used to determine which linear and nonlinear parameters discriminate between three groups (K, H, and C). Sixteen variables were included in the analysis: SampEn, FD, LyE, and CoP path from eyes open and eyes closed tests, each calculated separately for AP and ML directions. The forward stepwise analysis was used to build the discriminant model.

In the end, regression analysis with a method of least squares was performed for each balance variable to define what each balance parameter is dependent on. The best model was chosen upon the Akaike information criterion.

3. Results

3.1. Cluster Analysis

Initially, four participants were removed for further analysis, because they did not connect closely with other participants. Then, three groups were extracted (groups no. 1, 2, and 3). None of these groups corresponded to the clinical group (H, K, or C). Patients after hip replacement were classified into groups 2 and 3, patients after knee replacement into groups 1, 2 or 3 (one patient was removed), while controls were included in group no. 3 only (three persons were removed). Then, group no. 3 was divided into three groups according to the tree graph (Figure 1) to analyze the data in detail. Table 2 shows the allocation of participants into five groups.

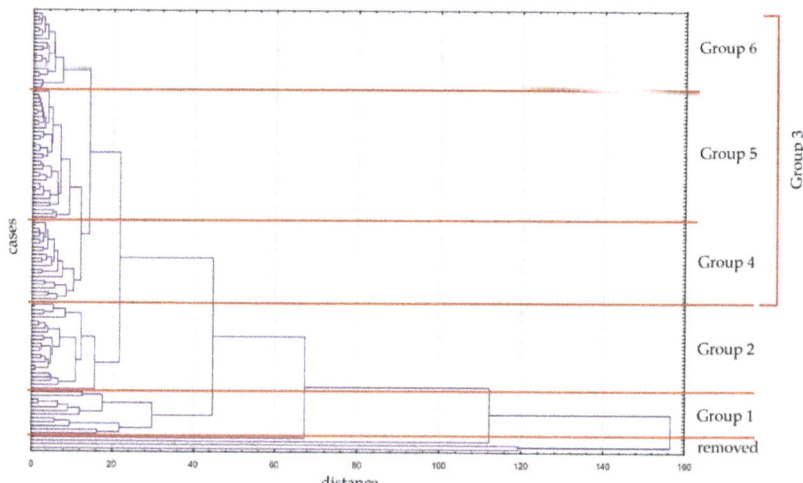

Figure 1. The tree graph from cluster analysis. The *x*-axis presents distance, while the *y*-axis includes participants of the study.

Table 2. Numbers of participants from H, K, and C groups allocated to five groups created based on cluster analysis.

	Group 1	Group 2	Group 3		
			Group 4	Group 5	Group 6
H group	0	8	13	20	8
K group	12	16	4	14	6
C group	0	0	5	1	7

Due to the fact that no person from the C group was allocated to the group no. 1 or 2, we checked the differences between groups no. 1, 2, and 3. No significant differences were found between those groups other than balance parameters.

3.2. Discriminant Analysis

The best model was reached in step eight and included eight variables (Table 3). Overall, the discrimination between three groups (H, K and C) was highly significant (Wilks' Lambda: 0.0354; F (16,216) = 58.247; $p < 0.0001$). The percentage of correctly classified cases is presented in Table 4. Classification functions are presented in Table 5. Model variables are summarized according to test (EO, EC) and direction (ML, AP) in Table 6.

Table 3. Results of the discriminant analysis—model with 8 variables. Non-significant variables are marked with italic.

Variable	Wilks' Lambda	F to Remove (2.108)	p-Value
LyE ML EO	0.042	10.355	< 0.0001
FD AP EO	0.039	5.671	0.0045
CoP path_ML EC	0.045	14.642	< 0.0001
LyE ML EC	0.040	7.254	0.0011
FD ML EC	0.038	3.492	0.0339
LyE AP EC	0.041	8.824	0.0003
FD AP EC	*0.037*	*1.693*	*0.1889*
SampEn AP EC	*0.037*	*2.795*	*0.0656*

LyE—the largest Lyapunov exponent, FD—fractal dimension, SampEn—sample entropy, EO—test with eyes open, EC—test with eyes closed.

Table 4. Results of the discriminant analysis—percentage and number of correctly classified participants.

	% Correctly Classified	H Group (N)	K Group (N)	C Group (N)
H group	73.5	36	13	0
K group	71.7	15	38	0
C group	100	0	0	16
together	76.3	51	51	16

Table 5. Results of the discriminant analysis—classification functions for each group.

Variable	H Group $p = 0.4153$	K Group $p = 0.4492$	C Group $p = 0.1356$
LyE ML EO	53.417	57.047	127.685
FD AP EO	150.088	142.413	102.269
CoP path_ML EC	−0.767	−0.770	−1.746
LyE ML EC	37.833	38.242	99.582
FD ML EC	98.003	98.237	129.198
LyE AP EC	−0.788	3.063	44.772
FD AP EC	257.086	263.192	249.053
SampEn AP EC	−225.615	−220.608	−177.377
const.	−348.296	−348.863	−413.511

LyE—the largest Lyapunov exponent, FD—fractal dimension, SampEn—sample entropy, EO—test with eyes open, EC—test with eyes closed.

Table 6. Discriminant model summarized according to test conditions and direction. Non-significant variables are marked with italic.

	ML	AP
Test with eyes open (EO)	LyE	FD
Test with eyes closed (EC)	LyE, FD	CoP path, LyE, *FD, SampEn*

LyE—the largest Lyapunov exponent, FD—fractal dimension, SampEn—sample entropy.

3.3. Regression Analysis

Analysis of the regression for nonlinear measures showed that sample entropy depends on anthropometrical variables (age, $p = 0.027$ and BMI, $p = 0.021$), test condition (EO/EC, $p = 0.005$), as well as group (H/K/C; $p < 0.001$). Fractal dimension depended only on the group (H/K/C; $p < 0.001$) and gender ($p = 0.043$). The largest Lyapunov exponent depended on gender ($p = 0.045$), BMI ($p = 0.020$), index direction (AP/ML, $p < 0.001$) and group (H/K/C; $p < 0.001$). COP path length depended on belonging to the H group ($p = 0.001$) and the direction (AP/ML; $p < 0.001$). None of the analyzed variables depended on time after surgery.

4. Discussion

The aim of this study was to find the group of linear and/or nonlinear measures that can differentiate healthy people and patients with total knee or hip replacement from each other. Three types of statistical analyses were performed to achieve this goal. Cluster analysis did not result in correct allocation to the groups according to all variables that were calculated from the balance test with eyes open and closed, although all controls were classified into one group in the three-groups model. However, this group also contained patients after THR and TKR. The result of the discriminant analysis was an eight-variables model including the largest Lyapunov exponent (ML EO, ML EC, and AP EC), fractal dimension (AP EO, ML EC, AP EC), CoP path AP EC and SampEn AP EC. The model was correct in 76.3% of cases. Regression analysis showed that all nonlinear variables depend on the group, while CoP path length is different only in the H group. Some influence of anthropometric parameters (gender, BMI, age) as well as direction (AP or ML) was also indicated.

Differences in postural control in patients after total knee or hip replacement and healthy controls were confirmed by Heil et al. [9] and Ohlendorf et al. [8]. In both studies, the CoP path from static measurement was significantly longer in the study group than in the controls. These studies were made by the same research group as well as the same protocol, and therefore, it can be easily seen that patients after TKR reached better results than those after THR. In our study, we did not analyze which group was better, but significant differences can be confirmed by the results of regression analysis. CoP path length was significantly dependent on belonging to the H group, which suggests that results in this group were different from those achieved by participants after TKR and healthy controls.

To the best of our knowledge, no publications are analyzing the ability of a group of linear and/or nonlinear balance measures to different groups with various clinical conditions. However, there are some scientific reports analyzing the usefulness of different variables in discriminating different groups of patients, mostly fallers from non-fallers or older from young adults.

Many publications suggest that nonlinear measures can measure the amount of attention paid to maintaining balance in certain conditions [18,22,32,33]. Introducing mainly nonlinear measures from the eyes-closed test to the discrimination model suggests that this test is more reliable and sensitive than the test with eyes open. For most people standing without visual feedback is a more demanding task and therefore requires more attention, which should decrease the values of nonlinear measures, especially sample entropy [18,32].

This can suggest that standing with eyes closed is a better way to assess the amount of regularity of CoP movement and attention paid to maintain balance.

The largest Lyapunov exponent shows the ability to adapt to the environment by investigating how the musculoskeletal system states change over time in terms of exponential divergence/convergence of initially nearby trajectories [18]. Our results clearly show that this variable has a large impact on the discrimination model, both when calculated from the EO test (LyE ML) and EC test (LyE ML, LyE AP). Additionally, regression analysis confirmed the high dependence of LyE values on the group. This suggests that differences between three clinical groups (THR, TKR, and healthy controls) comprise differences in the ability to adapt to the environment. Higher LyE values suggest a better (faster) response of balance control in different body movements [27]. Significant differences in LyE values between different study groups were confirmed by Ghofrani et al. [34], Huisinga et al. [35], and Liu et al. [36].

Fractal dimension calculates the complexity and irregularity of the signal over time and its values can be interpreted as an ability to synergistically modulate three systems involved in maintaining posture—the somatosensory, visual, and vestibular systems. Kędziorek and Błażkiewicz [18] suggest that the fractal dimension is not sensitive enough to detect an age group difference. Results of the discriminant analysis showed that FD can be useful in determining group classification, while calculated from the EC test. Regression analysis also confirmed that this variable is group dependent. FD also depended on gender, but the direction (AP/ML) did not influence the result. The latter fact was confirmed by Szafraniec et al. [37] by comparing results of FD in AP and ML directions.

Montesinos et al. [38] showed that sample entropy can discriminate fallers from non-fallers and younger from older adults for AP direction and a specific combination of calculating parameters (m, r) only. Borg and Laxaback [39] also found significant differences between young and older adults in SampEn AP. Regression analysis in our study showed that SampEn depends, among others, on age. Raffalt et al. [40] found a group (ankle instability/controls) significant effect on sample entropy values. This can be partially confirmed in our study, where sample entropy for AP direction from the EC test was included in the discriminant function, although it was not statistically significant. In the studies of Szafraniec et al. [37] and Raffalt et al. [40] the influence of direction (AP/ML) on SampEn values was demonstrated. In our study, regression analysis did not confirm this, but on the other hand, only SampEn AP values were included in the discrimination model.

Linear measures are more often used to assess balance in clinical practice, than nonlinear measures. Borg and Laxaback [39] found out that CoP ML amplitude can discriminate between elderly fallers and non-fallers, but only for foam and head extension conditions. Other differences (between young and older adults) were not significant. Our study was performed only in static conditions and the influence of CoP path in AP direction in EC-test in discriminating patients after THR, TKR, and healthy controls were confirmed, although it should be pointed out that regression analysis showed only the H group influence on CoP path values.

Analysis of classification functions clearly shows that coefficients for healthy controls are significantly different from those for H and K groups. Additionally, the percentage of correctly classified participants from the C group is 100%, which confirms that this group reached completely different results from those of patients after joint replacement, and therefore, it was easier to build the discrimination model that correctly classified healthy controls. Differentiation between THR and TKR groups is less effective, reaching above 70% of correctly classified cases and coefficient values show that these two groups are more similar to each other.

Cluster analysis showed that some patients from THR and TKR groups are similar regarding all analyzed variables together to healthy controls and these were classified together to group no. 3. However, some of them (eight patients from the H group and twenty-eight patients from the K group) were classified into other two groups that included no healthy controls. Probably, there are other clinical, anthropometrical, or psychological factors that were not analyzed in this study and which influence the results of balance tests.

Some limitations of this study have to be acknowledged. First of all, significant differences in age between the three groups could have contributed to worse classifications of the groups. However, this was not confirmed in post hoc calculations. Secondly, the analyzed groups differ also in BMI, but this is hard to avoid, as obese and overweight people are more likely to have knee or hip osteoarthritis [4]. Thirdly, it seems to be clear that there are some other factors that can influence the classification of the groups that were not included in this study. Probably, including the results of physical examination, additional measurements such as body composition or densitometric tests, clinical assessment scales, or gait analysis in future studies are needed. It would be also worthwhile to analyze the medical history of the patients in a more detailed way.

5. Conclusions

Inclusion of the variables calculated from the standing with eyes closed test into the discrimination model suggests that standing with eyes closed is a better way to assess the amount of regularity of CoP movement and attention paid to maintain balance. The obtained results also suggest that nonlinear measures better differentiate TKR and THR patients from healthy controls than linear variables and therefore, it is worthwhile to include nonlinear measures in patient balance analysis, especially the largest Lyapunov exponent and fractal dimension. This study did not conclude with a clear result and the set of parameters found in discriminant analysis is probably not the best one, although it can easily differentiate healthy controls of patients after joint replacement in the lower limb. In further studies, it is recommended to include the results of physical examination, clinical assessment scales, or gait analysis for more satisfying results.

Author Contributions: Conceptualization, A.H., D.D. and W.M; methodology A.H., D.B., A.J.K., and K.T.W.; formal analysis, A.H. and M.B.; investigation, A.J.K., K.T.W., M.G.; resources, A.H. and M.Ł.; data curation, A.H., A.J.K., K.T.W. and M.G.; writing—original draft preparation, A.H., M.B.; writing—review and editing, A.H.; supervision, D.B., M.Ł. and W.M.; project administration, A.H. and D.B.; funding acquisition, D.B. and W.M. All authors have read and agreed to the published version of the manuscript.

Funding: This research was funded by a National Centre for Research and Development Grant under the program Strategmed III as part of the "VB-Clinic" project (no. STRATEGMED3/306011/1/NCBR/2017), statutory funds of the Medical University of Warsaw (grant no. 2F1/N/22), statutory funds of the Medical Centre for Postgraduate Education in Warsaw, and by the Ministry of Science and Higher Education in the year 2020–2022 under Research Group no 3 at the Józef Piłsudski University of Physical Education in Warsaw "Motor system diagnostics in selected dysfunctions as a basis for planning the rehabilitation process".

Institutional Review Board Statement: The study was conducted in accordance with the Declaration of Helsinki, and approved by the Bioethics Committee of the Medical University of Warsaw (no. KB/28/2014), approval date 18 February 2014).

Informed Consent Statement: Informed consent was obtained from all subjects involved in the study.

Data Availability Statement: The measurement data used to support the findings of this study are available from the corresponding author upon request.

Acknowledgments: The authors would like to acknowledge Edyta Urbaniak, Agnieszka Kobza, and Rafał Boratyński for their support in data collection and Małgorzata Syczewska for her comments on the final version of the manuscript.

Conflicts of Interest: The authors declare no conflict of interest. The funders had no role in the design of the study; in the collection, analyses, or interpretation of data; in the writing of the manuscript, or in the decision to publish the results.

References

1. de Lima, F.; Melo, G.; Fernandes, D.A.; Santos, G.M.; Rosa Neto, F. Effects of total knee arthroplasty for primary knee osteoarthritis on postural balance: A systematic review. *Gait Posture* **2021**, *89*, 139–160. [CrossRef] [PubMed]
2. Gianola, S.; Stucovitz, E.; Castellini, G.; Mascali, M.; Vanni, F.; Tramacere, I.; Banfi, G.; Tornese, D. Effects of early virtual reality-based rehabilitation in patients with total knee arthroplasty: A randomized controlled trial. *Medicine* **2020**, *99*, e19136. [CrossRef] [PubMed]
3. Wang, X.; Hunter, D.J.; Vesentini, G.; Pozzobon, D.; Ferreira, M.L. Technology-assisted rehabilitation following total knee or hip replacement for people with osteoarthritis: A systematic review and meta-analysis. *BMC Musculoskelet. Disord.* **2019**, *20*, 506. [CrossRef] [PubMed]
4. Katz, J.N.; Arant, K.R.; Loeser, R.F. Diagnosis and Treatment of Hip and Knee Osteoarthritis: A Review. *JAMA* **2021**, *325*, 568–578. [CrossRef]
5. Prvu Bettger, J.; Green, C.L.; Holmes, D.N.; Chokshi, A.; Mather, R.C., III; Hoch, B.T.; de Leon, A.J.; Aluisio, F.; Seyler, T.M.; Del Gaizo, D.J.; et al. Effects of Virtual Exercise Rehabilitation In-Home Therapy Compared with Traditional Care After Total Knee Arthroplasty: VERITAS, a Randomized Controlled Trial. *JBJS* **2020**, *102*, 101–109. [CrossRef]
6. Inacio, M.C.S.; Paxton, E.W.; Graves, S.E.; Namba, R.S.; Nemes, S. Projected increase in total knee arthroplasty in the United States—An alternative projection model. *Osteoarthr. Cartil.* **2017**, *25*, 1797–1803. [CrossRef]
7. Hadamus, A.; Białoszewski, D.; Błażkiewicz, M.; Kowalska, A.J.; Urbaniak, E.; Wydra, K.T.; Wiaderna, K.; Boratyński, R.; Kobza, A.; Marczyński, W. Assessment of the Effectiveness of Rehabilitation after Total Knee Replacement Surgery Using Sample Entropy and Classical Measures of Body Balance. *Entropy* **2021**, *23*, 164. [CrossRef]
8. Ohlendorf, D.; Lehmann, C.; Heil, D.; Hörzer, S.; Kopp, S. The impact of a total hip replacement on jaw position, upper body posture and body sway. *Cranio J. Craniomandib. Pract.* **2015**, *33*, 107–114. [CrossRef]
9. Heil, L.; Maltry, L.; Lehmann, S.; Heil, D.; Lehmann, C.; Kopp, S.; Wanke, E.M.; Bendels, M.H.K.; Groneberg, D.A.; Ohlendorf, D. The impact of a total knee arthroplasty on jaw movements, upper body posture, plantar pressure distribution, and postural control. *Cranio J. Craniomandib. Pract.* **2021**, *39*, 35–46. [CrossRef]
10. Truszczyńska-Baszak, A.; Dadura, E.; Drzał-Grabiec, J.; Tarnowski, A. Static balance assessment in patients with severe osteoarthritis of the knee. *Knee* **2020**, *27*, 1349–1356. [CrossRef]
11. Gauchard, G.C.; Vançon, G.; Meyer, P.; Mainard, D.; Perrin, P.P. On the role of knee joint in balance control and postural strategies: Effects of total knee replacement in elderly subjects with knee osteoarthritis. *Gait Posture* **2010**, *32*, 155–160. [CrossRef] [PubMed]
12. de Lima, F.; Fernandes, D.A.; Melo, G.; de Roesler, C.R.M.; Neves, F.D.S.; Neto, F.R. Effects of total hip arthroplasty for primary hip osteoarthritis on postural balance: A systematic review. *Gait Posture* **2019**, *73*, 52–64. [CrossRef] [PubMed]
13. Domínguez-Navarro, F.; Igual-Camacho, C.; Silvestre-Muñoz, A.; Roig-Casasús, S.; Blasco, J.M. Effects of balance and proprioceptive training on total hip and knee replacement rehabilitation: A systematic review and meta-analysis. *Gait Posture* **2018**, *62*, 68–74. [CrossRef] [PubMed]
14. Massion, J. Postural control system. *Curr. Opin. Neurobiol.* **1994**, *4*, 877–887. [CrossRef]
15. Kiemel, T.; Elahi, A.J.; Jeka, J.J. Identification of the plant for upright stance in humans: Multiple movement patterns from a single neural strategy. *J. Neurophysiol.* **2008**, *100*, 3394–3406. [CrossRef]
16. Assländer, L.; Peterka, R.J. Sensory reweighting dynamics in human postural control. *J. Neurophysiol.* **2014**, *111*, 1852–1864. [CrossRef]
17. Ivanenko, Y.; Gurfinkel, V.S. Human Postural Control. *Front. Neurosci.* **2018**, *12*, 171. [CrossRef]
18. Kedziorek, J.; Błażkiewicz, M. Nonlinear Measures to Evaluate Upright Postural Stability: A Systematic Review. *Entropy* **2020**, *22*, 1357. [CrossRef]
19. Horak, F.B. Postural orientation and equilibrium: What do we need to know about neural control of balance to prevent falls? *Age Ageing* **2006**, *35* (Suppl. 2), ii7–ii11. [CrossRef]
20. Stergiou, N. *Nonlinear Analysis for Human Movement Variability*; CRC Press: Boca Raton, FL, USA, 2016; pp. 1–388.
21. Roerdink, M.; Hlavackova, P.; Vuillerme, N. Center-of-pressure regularity as a marker for attentional investment in postural control: A comparison between sitting and standing postures. *Hum. Mov. Sci.* **2011**, *30*, 203–212. [CrossRef]
22. Donker, S.F.; Roerdink, M.; Greven, A.J.; Beek, P.J. Regularity of center-of-pressure trajectories depends on the amount of attention invested in postural control. *Exp. Brain Res.* **2007**, *181*, 1–11. [CrossRef] [PubMed]
23. Potvin-Desrochers, A.R.; Lajoie, Y.N. Cognitive task promote automatization of postural control in young and older adults. *Gait Posture* **2017**, *57*, 40–45. [CrossRef] [PubMed]
24. Hansen, C.; Wei, Q.; Shieh, J.-S.; Fourcade, P.; Isableu, B.; Majed, L. Sample Entropy, Univariate, and Multivariate Multi-Scale Entropy in Comparison with Classical Postural Sway Parameters in Young Healthy Adults. *Front. Hum. Neurosci.* **2017**, *11*, 206. [CrossRef] [PubMed]
25. Doherty, C.; Bleakley, C.; Hertel, J.; Caulfield, B.; Ryan, J.; Delahunt, E. Postural control strategies during single limb stance following acute lateral ankle sprain. *Clin. Biomech.* **2014**, *29*, 643–649. [CrossRef]
26. Doherty, C.; Bleakley, C.; Hertel, J.; Caulfield, B.; Ryan, J.; Delahunt, E. Balance failure in single limb stance due to ankle sprain injury: An analysis of center of pressure using the fractal dimension method. *Gait Posture* **2014**, *40*, 172–176. [CrossRef]
27. Rosenstein, M.T.; Collins, J.J.; De Luca, C.J. A practical method for calculating largest Lyapunov exponents from small data sets. *Phys. D Nonlinear Phenom.* **1993**, *65*, 117–134. [CrossRef]

28. Nagymate, G.; Kiss, R. Parameter Reduction in the Frequency Analysis of Center of Pressure in Stabilometry. *Period. Polytech. Mech. Eng.* **2016**, *60*, 238–246. [CrossRef]
29. Goldberger, A.L.; Amaral, L.A.; Glass, L.; Hausdorff, J.M.; Ivanov, P.C.; Mark, R.G.; Mietus, J.E.; Moody, G.B.; Peng, C.K.; Stanley, H.E. PhysioBank, PhysioToolkit, and PhysioNet: Components of a new research resource for complex physiologic signals. *Circulation* **2000**, *101*, E215–E220. [CrossRef]
30. Higuchi, T. Approach to an irregular time series on the basis of the fractal theory. *Phys. D Nonlinear Phenom.* **1988**, *31*, 277–283. [CrossRef]
31. Razjouyan, J.; Shahriar, G.; Fallah, A.; Khayat, O.; Ghergherehchi, M.; Afarideh, H.; Moghaddasi, M. A neuro-fuzzy based model for accurate estimation of the Lyapunov exponents of an unknown dynamical system. *Int. J. Bifurc. Chaos Appl. Sci. Eng.* **2012**, *22*, 1250043. [CrossRef]
32. Rigoldi, C.; Cimolin, V.; Camerota, F.; Celletti, C.; Albertini, G.; Mainardi, L.; Galli, M. Measuring regularity of human postural sway using approximate entropy and sample entropy in patients with Ehlers-Danlos syndrome hypermobility type. *Res. Dev. Disabil.* **2013**, *34*, 840–846. [CrossRef] [PubMed]
33. Błażkiewicz, M. Nonlinear measures in posturography compared to linear measures based on yoga poses performance. *Acta Bioeng. Biomech.* **2020**, *22*, 15–21. [CrossRef] [PubMed]
34. Ghofrani, M.; Olyaei, G.; Talebian, S.; Bagheri, H.; Malmir, K. Test-retest reliability of linear and nonlinear measures of postural stability during visual deprivation in healthy subjects. *J. Phys. Ther. Sci.* **2017**, *29*, 1766–1771. [CrossRef] [PubMed]
35. Huisinga, J.M.; Yentes, J.M.; Filipi, M.L.; Stergiou, N. Postural control strategy during standing is altered in patients with multiple sclerosis. *Neurosci. Lett.* **2012**, *524*, 124–128. [CrossRef] [PubMed]
36. Liu, J.; Zhang, X.; Lockhart, T.E. Fall risk assessments based on postural and dynamic stability using inertial measurement unit. *Saf. Health Work* **2012**, *3*, 192–198. [CrossRef]
37. Szafraniec, R.; Barańska, J.; Kuczyński, M. Acute effects of core stability exercises on balance control. *Acta Bioeng. Biomech.* **2018**, *20*, 145–151.
38. Montesinos, L.; Castaldo, R.; Pecchia, L. On the use of approximate entropy and sample entropy with centre of pressure time-series. *J. Neuroeng. Rehabil.* **2018**, *15*, 116. [CrossRef]
39. Borg, F.G.; Laxaback, G. Entropy of balance—Some recent results. *J. Neuroeng. Rehabil.* **2010**, *7*, 38. [CrossRef]
40. Raffalt, P.C.; Spedden, M.E.; Geertsen, S.S. Dynamics of postural control during bilateral stance—Effect of support area, visual input and age. *Hum. Mov. Sci.* **2019**, *67*, 102462. [CrossRef]

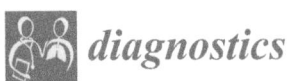

Article

Can We Use the Oculus Quest VR Headset and Controllers to Reliably Assess Balance Stability?

Cathy M. Craig [1,*], James Stafford [2], Anastasiia Egorova [3], Carla McCabe [4] and Mark Matthews [4]

1. School of Psychology, Ulster University, Coleraine BT52 1SL, UK
2. School of Psychology, Queen's University Belfast, Belfast BT7 1NN, UK; j.stafford@incisiv.tech
3. School of Maths & Physics, Queen's University Belfast, Belfast BT7 1NN, UK; aegorova01@qub.ac.uk
4. School of Sport, Ulster University, Belfast BT15 1ED, UK; c.mccabe@ulster.ac.uk (C.M.); m.matthews@ulster.ac.uk (M.M.)
* Correspondence: c.craig1@ulster.ac.uk

Abstract: Balance is the foundation upon which all other motor skills are built. Indeed, many neurological diseases and injuries often present clinically with deficits in balance control. With recent advances in virtual reality (VR) hardware bringing low-cost headsets into the mainstream market, the question remains as to whether this technology could be used in a clinical context to assess balance. We compared the head tracking performance of a low-cost VR headset (Oculus Quest) with a gold standard motion tracking system (Qualisys). We then compared the recorded head sway with the center of pressure (COP) measures collected from a force platform in different stances and different visual field manipulations. Firstly, our analysis showed that there was an excellent correspondence between the two different head movement signals (ICCs > 0.99) with minimal differences in terms of accuracy (<5 mm error). Secondly, we found that head sway mapped onto COP measures more strongly when the participant adopted a Tandem stance during balance assessment. Finally, using the power of virtual reality to manipulate the visual input to the brain, we showed how the Oculus Quest can reliably detect changes in postural control as a result of different types of visual field manipulations. Given the high levels of accuracy of the motion tracking of the Oculus Quest headset, along with the strong relationship with the COP and ability to manipulate the visual field, the Oculus Quest makes an exciting alternative to traditional lab-based balance assessments.

Keywords: balance assessment; VR; postural control; low-cost; visual field manipulation

Citation: Craig, C.M.; Stafford, J.; Egorova, A.; McCabe, C.; Matthews, M. Can We Use the Oculus Quest VR Headset and Controllers to Reliably Assess Balance Stability? *Diagnostics* **2022**, *12*, 1409. https://doi.org/10.3390/diagnostics12061409

Academic Editors: Carlo Ricciardi, Francesco Amato and Mario Cesarelli

Received: 17 May 2022
Accepted: 31 May 2022
Published: 7 June 2022

Publisher's Note: MDPI stays neutral with regard to jurisdictional claims in published maps and institutional affiliations.

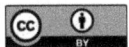

Copyright: © 2022 by the authors. Licensee MDPI, Basel, Switzerland. This article is an open access article distributed under the terms and conditions of the Creative Commons Attribution (CC BY) license (https://creativecommons.org/licenses/by/4.0/).

1. Introduction

Maintaining balance is a complex process that requires sensory inputs from the visual, vestibular, and proprioceptive sensory systems of the body. All these systems work seamlessly together to give us our sense of balance [1,2]. To maintain balance, a person must continually monitor multiple sources of information coming from different sensory inputs and continually perform the necessary adjustments to position the body and limbs, so the center of mass is in a position of equilibrium. In fact, good control of the balance system is the foundation upon which other movements are built. For instance, standing on our tip toes to place a book on a high shelf or running to intercept an opponent's pass in sport, not only involves the control of the movement of limbs but also the control of the center of mass as the limbs move.

This ability to maintain good balance (postural control) is vital for simple everyday actions, but also for the fluid, dynamic movements needed for any type of skillful action [1,2]. Indeed, difficulties in being able to control posture appropriately are often indicative of an underlying medical condition. As a result, it has become common for scientists and clinical experts to want to assess balance abilities to determine the extent of any underlying neurological problems post head injury [3], identify opportunities for motor development [4], but also profile a person's susceptibility to future risk (e.g., falls in older adults) [5].

Given the importance of identifying deficiencies in balance, there is a strong need to develop accessible, low-cost, valid ways of assessing postural stability. The Balance Error Scoring System (BESS) is an example of a simple balance test that is widely used in professional sport and clinical settings [6]. It uses four different types of stances (double, single dominant, single non-dominant, tandem) to modify the base of support and challenge a participant's postural stability as they try to stand as still as possible for a fixed period (usually 20 s). During that time, a clinician/experimenter observes the participant's posture with errors being counted (i.e., losing balance, use of arms, stepping out, etc.) and scored (maximum 10 allowed). To further assess balance, modifying visual input (i.e., eyes open, eyes closed) can be added to the BESS to increase the difficulty and complexity of balance assessment. Although the test is quick and easy to administer, it has been criticized for its lack of reliability due to the subjectivity of human raters in counting errors [7]. Furthermore, the magnitude of the error (or loss of balance) cannot be quantified, meaning the extent of the balance deficits are not measured with any level of granularity.

Another limitation of observational balance tests such as the BESS is that they lack the required sensitivity for long-term monitoring of postural control. For instance, it is thought that balance disturbances following a neurological event, such as a concussion, typically resolve within 72 h of initial injury when assessed through observation alone. However, when the same participants are assessed using objective data collection methods such as motion capture and force plates, balance disturbances can be observed up to 30 days after the initial injury [8]. The inability of the BESS to pick up these residual balance deficits following head injury may put the player at increased risk of other injuries further down the line.

Full-body motion tracking, using optical-based camera systems, has also been extensively used in postural studies when the experimental protocol makes the use of force plates impossible or inconvenient (for example when the movement area was greater than the force plate's dimensions). In such cases, motion tracking several joints is used to accurately estimate the position of the body's Center of Gravity (CoG). This kinematic method of measuring balance is based on the definition of the CoG, which is the imaginary point around which the force of gravity appears to act, and the combined mass of the body is concentrated. From this definition, the position of a body's CoG can be computed as the weighted average of the position of the Center of Mass of all body segments [9]. This requires accurate anthropometric and kinematic data from all body segments and is very labor intensive [10].

Several different full-body kinematic models have been used by research teams to measure CoG movement [11,12]. While the Ground Reaction Force (GRF) double-integration method and the segmental kinematic method are the gold standard for accurate measurements of human body CoG movement, more accessible measurement methods have been shown to be viable for research too. Studies have shown that measuring the movement of the sacrum, through optical tracking or inertial sensors, also provides a usable approximation of participants' CoG [13].

Although this method is useful, another more widely adopted approach is to measure the position and displacement of the center of pressure (COP) as a person stands still on a force platform [1,2,14]. The force platform provides a point projection of the vertical reaction forces that are represented in the anterior–posterior (AP) and medial–lateral (ML) axes of movement. Although the person may be standing still, the position of the COP will change over time as the person controls their balance through micromovements of the body that are inherent in this closed-loop feedback system (predominantly ankles (AP axis) and adductors/abductors (ML axis)).

The problem with these methods is that they often involve expensive, lab-based equipment that lacks portability and applicability to more general settings. Other alternatives that use more simple methods are now being explored. For example, a recent study showed that different visual images invoked similar changes in postural control when head position (measured using an overhead webcam) and COP measures were recorded at the same time [15]. Although the purpose of this study was to measure behavioral responses to different emotive images, the strong link between head sway and COP (correlations of 0.82 AP axis and 0.73 ML axis) means that tracking head movement could offer a promising alternative to force platforms when assessing changes in postural control. Given these findings, it is possible that a new way of assessing balance in a low-cost, reliable way could be provided by a virtual reality (VR) head mounted display (HMD). This technology would not only track head movements to capture changes in postural control but would also provide the option of manipulating a participant's visual field using a "swinging room" style protocol that in turn would invoke change in balance stability [16]. This moving room simulation is important in balance assessment [17], as it allows the clinician to go beyond a binary eyes-open and eyes-closed manipulation and probe possible causes of balance deficits in more depth.

This study will investigate the usability of head sway measures, recorded from a low-cost, consumer-based VR headset (Oculus Quest) [18] as a means of assessing changes in postural stability. The first two parts of the study focus on the technical validation of the technology, while the third part examines its use as a means of capturing changes in postural control, induced by visual field manipulations, in a group of young, healthy adult males. The aims of the study were threefold:

(1) Measure the technical reliability of the Oculus Quest to track head movement (sway) by comparing it to a gold standard motion tracking system (Qualisys, Göteborg, Sweden).
(2) Measure the strength of the relationship between head sway (head movements captured by both the Oculus and the Qualisys motion capture system) and Centre of Pressure (force platform, Kistler Instruments, Winterthur, Switzerland) when performing a modified version of a balance test (BESS).
(3) Determine the responsiveness of a low-cost VR headset (i) to presentation of different visual field manipulations (static and dynamic) that invoke changes in postural control when a person is in a dominant and a non-dominant stance and (ii) for measuring the resulting postural adjustments (head and hand movement) in a group of healthy adults and measure their reliability across two different testing sessions.

2. Materials and Methods

2.1. Technical Validation—Balance Tracking Hardware

A passive, reflective marker was attached in the center of a VR headset (Oculus Quest, Facebook Technologies Ltd., Menlo Park, CA, USA). Fifteen Qualisys infrared motion capture cameras (Oqus 100, Qualisys, Göteborg, Sweden) recorded the movement (x, y, z) of the marker attached to the VR headset at 50 Hz. Centre of Pressure was also recorded at 50 Hz using the force plate Kistler 9260 AA force platform (Kistler Instruments, Winterthur, Switzerland). Both the Qualisys and Kistler data were recorded using the same software and synchronized using the same time stamp. The Oculus Quest head movement data (x, y, z) were also captured at 50 Hz using a data collector function in Unity game design software (MOViR, INCISIV Ltd., Belfast, UK). This data collector also collected the visual field data that indicated the transition from one visual field to another. This was important for the analysis of visual field induced differences in postural control which represented the third part of the experiment.

2.2. Data Collection

The data for the technical validation were obtained using a single subject design in which the female volunteer (height 1.68 m; mass 59 kg) provided informed consent and was noted as right foot dominant. The participant was asked to remove her shoes and stand on the force platform wearing the Oculus HMD and hold the two hand controllers. For all conditions, the participant was immersed in a virtual gym where two red spheres were positioned in front of the participant at elbow height. The participant was asked to place the controllers inside the spheres, so they turned green. This was to encourage the participant to keep the arms as still as possible while performing the balance tests. The Oculus Quest was calibrated using its own built-in "Guardian setup" procedure so that the Anterior/Posterior (AP, X axis) and Medial Lateral (ML, Y axis) axes were aligned with those of the force plate. The Z axis for all systems represented the vertical axis. The Qualisys system was also calibrated in alignment to the Oculus Quest defined axes and the calibration residual was deemed acceptable (<0.80 mm). Data collected from the Oculus and the Qualisys motion capture system were synchronized using two easily recognizable events (small vertical jump and oscillatory head movements) that were performed by the participant at the start of each trial. These two discrete events were used in the analysis to temporally align the Qualisys and Oculus head movement time series data.

2.3. Technical Validation—Testing Conditions

The participant performed a modified version of the BESS test that involved standing as still as possible in three different stances—double, tandem, and single leg dominant (30 s each stance). If the participant lost balance or moved out of the instructed stance, she was told to regain her balance and assume the instructed stance as soon as possible. The 3 stances were presented in the following order:

1. Double: Standing with both feet side by side.
2. Tandem: Standing with the heel of the right foot just in front of the toe of the left foot (non-dominant foot at the back).
3. Single leg dominant: Standing on her right foot, hip flexed to approximately 30° and left knee bent upwards to approximately 45°.

The participant performed 3 consecutive sets of testing for each of the stances giving 13,500 data points per signal for analysis.

2.4. Behavioural Validation—Visual Field Manipulation

To see if virtual reality can also be used to reliably manipulate the visual field and induce measurable changes in postural control, a group of 30 healthy adult males (mean age = 26.3 ± 5 years; mean height = 1.82 ± 0.06 m); mean weight = 85.1 ± 7.6 kg; right foot dominant n = 23) gave informed consent and agreed to participate in the experiment.

Testing took place in a room with a solid floor and participants were asked to remove their footwear. The Oculus Quest was placed on the participant's head and participants were asked to hold the hand controllers in their hands. The environment presented in the headset was a virtual gym. Once the participant was familiar with the environment and comfortable, they were asked to adopt a tandem stance with their left foot in front of their right foot (see Figure 1). A tandem stance was selected as it demonstrated the best relationship between the measures of COP and head sway in the technical validation study (see Section 3). Participants were asked to place the hand controllers in a standardized position (virtual spheres at elbow height in the virtual gym) and stand as still as possible until the trial ended. Each trial lasted 40 s with participants given a short break before performing the trial again with the opposite leg forward. During each trial the visual field was manipulated to create different sensory processing demands to challenge postural control. These visual field manipulations were created using off the shelf VR software (MOViR; INCISIV Ltd.) programmed using Unity3D and presented inside the headset at 2880 × 1600 pixel resolution (1440 × 1600 pixels per eye) with a 90° field of view and a refresh rate of 90 Hz.

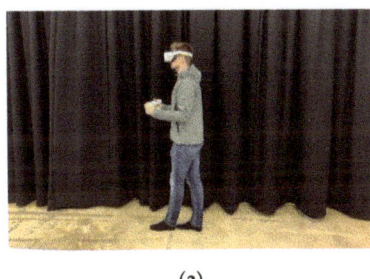
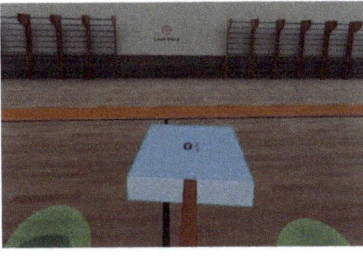

(a)   (b)

Figure 1. (**a**) A participant wearing the Oculus Quest headset and holding the two hand controllers. Any movements of the head and hands are captured by the motion controllers at 50 Hz. (**b**) An image showing what the participant saw inside the Oculus Quest headset when they were subjected to the 'tilt' visual field manipulation. Note the virtual green spheres at the bottom of the image which acted as a standardized visual reference for the hand position.

The changes in the visual field were classed as either static or dynamic and lasted for 10 s. The static visual field had two conditions: (i) Static Light—a stationary well-lit virtual gym, and (ii) Static Dark—a stationary dark virtual gym. These two static visual fields replicated the traditional 'eyes open' or 'eyes closed' balance tests, respectively. The dynamic visual field had two conditions: (i) Dynamic Forward/Back—a virtual gym that simulated forward-backwards room motion (in the anterior posterior axis), and (ii) Dynamic Tilt—a virtual gym with rotational (tilt) movement around the anterior posterior axis. The forward–backwards manipulation involved the virtual gym moving away from the participant (2 cm/s) for 5 s, and then back towards the participant at 2 cm/s for 5 s. The rotation ('tilt') of the anterior–posterior axis consisted of positive roll for the 1st 5 s and negative roll for the last 5 s at a rate of 5 degrees/second. Participants completed all 4 conditions, for tandem stance with one trial for the left and one trial for the right foot forward, on two separate occasions (4 days apart to test reliability of measures).

2.5. Technical Validation—Data Analysis

Both the head movement captured using Qualisys motion capture technology and the Oculus Quest were recorded at 50 Hz in three axes of motion (x, y, z). The total distance travelled (head sway) was calculated in all three axes, whereas the distance covered by the COP was calculated only in the anterior posterior (y) and medial lateral (x) axes, as per the recognized method [10]. Intraclass correlations (ICC) were used to determine the level of correspondence between the different signals. ICCs were calculated using the standard method and values interpreted as follows: <0.4 = poor; 0.4–0.59 = moderate; 0.6–0.79 = good; >0.8 = excellent [19]. Root Mean Square Errors (RMSE) were calculated in millimeters to determine the level of precision of head movement captured using the Qualisys motion capture system and the Oculus Quest.

2.6. Behavioral Validation—Data Analysis

The postural changes induced by the visual field manipulations were measured using the head and hand controllers of the Oculus Quest. The head and hand controller data were captured with the same time stamp as the visual field manipulations so that the total sway for each visual field manipulation could be analyzed separately. The test was repeated 4 days later so that the reliability of the measures could also be tested using an analysis of measurement variance.

3. Results

3.1. Technical Validation Part 1—Reliability of Head Movement Captured Using the Oculus Quest

The first part of the analysis aimed to see how closely the head movement captured using the Qualisys motion capture system corresponded to the data captured from the Oculus Quest's proprietary in built motion sensing system. Head movement data captured using the Qualisys system were directly compared with that obtained using the Oculus Quest HMD. The graphs in Figure 2 show how closely the two signals correspond when the participant adopted three different stances (Double, Tandem and Single). As expected, the most sway (movement) took place in the Single leg stance with the least in the Double leg stance condition and the Tandem stance in between.

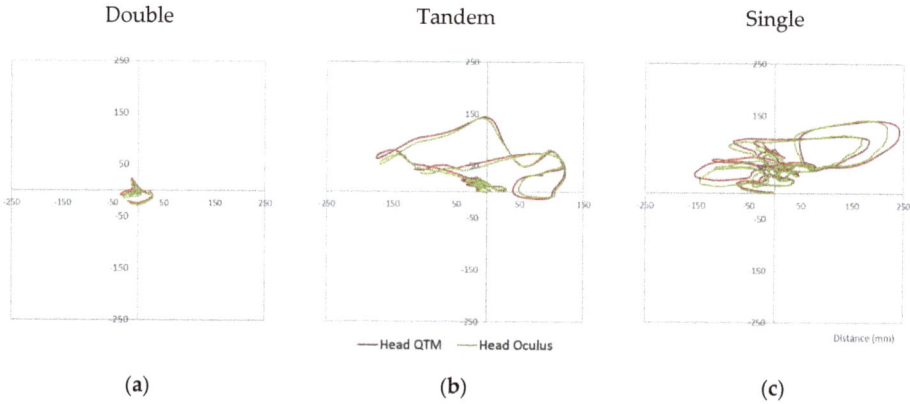

Figure 2. Three stabilogram plots representing the head sway (distance in mm) captured by the Oculus Quest (green) and the Qualisys motion capture cameras (red) in the three different stances (Double (**a**), Tandem (**b**), Single (**c**)) in two different axes (AP and ML).

In terms of the similarity of the signals, both the Intraclass Correlation Coefficients (ICC) and Root Mean Square Errors (RMSE) were calculated for the head movement data. As can be seen from Table 1 the Tandem and the Single leg stances had the highest ICC values (≥ 0.99) whereas the Double leg stance was slightly lower (0.936) for the distance (sway) calculations. In terms of the RMSE values, both the Double and Tandem stances had the lowest RMSEs (3.8 mm and 3.9 mm, respectively) with the Single leg stance being slightly higher (4.7 mm). Overall, these values indicate a very strong correspondence between the two signals and a very high level of accuracy for the Oculus Quest head movement data.

Table 1. The average ICC and RMSE values for the Head movements recorded from the Qualisys and the Oculus Quest systems. The values are for the three axes (ML, AP and Vertical) and the calculated distance (sway) are presented for the three different stances (Double, Tandem, Single). ICC values can be interpreted as follows: ICC > 0.8 is excellent; ICC < 0.8 > 0.6 is good; ICC < 0.6 > 0.4 is moderate, while ICC < 0.4 is poor [19]. RMSE values are measured in mm with values closest to 0.0 indicating the highest levels of precision.

Stance	Oculus vs. Qualisys Head Movement							
	ICC				RMSE (mm)			
	ML	AP	Vertical	Distance	ML	AP	Vertical	Distance
Double	0.877	0.983	0.978	0.936	4.2	1.3	3.3	3.8
Tandem	0.994	0.996	0.937	0.994	3.4	4.2	1.6	3.9
Single	0.990	0.998	0.994	0.998	3.9	4.3	4.4	4.7

3.2. Technical Validation Part 2—Comparing COP and Head Sway as Measures of Postural Control

The second part of the analysis aimed to see if head sway (distance), recorded from the Qualisys and the Oculus Quest, can be compared to the COP measured using a Kistler force platform. In this analysis the three different stances (Double, Tandem, Single) were analyzed separately. The Intraclass Correlation Coefficients (ICC) were calculated for each data set ($n = 1500$ per set, and three sets per stance) to determine the degree of similarity between the measures of COP and head movement. Figure 3 shows that although the COP and head movement are capturing data at extreme ends of the body, both measures appear to reflect similar changes in postural control.

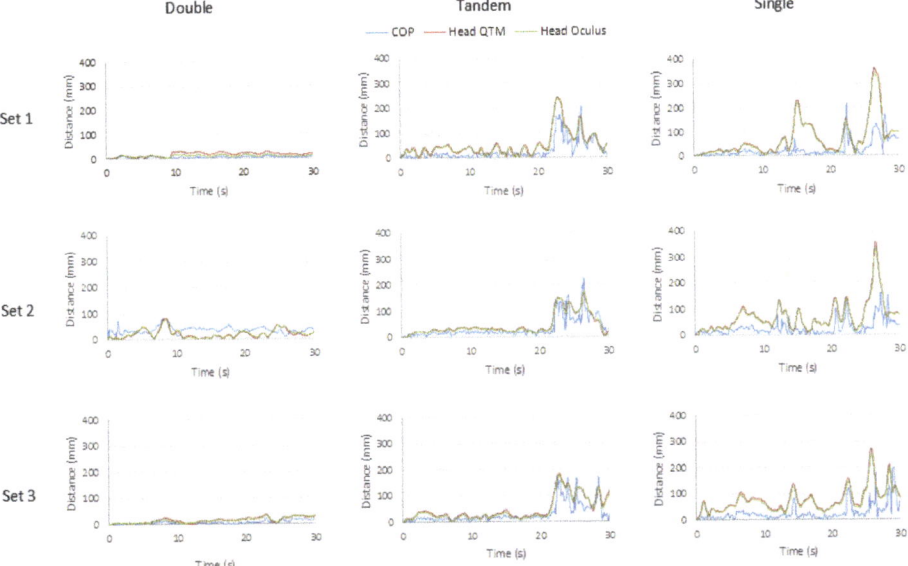

Figure 3. Graphs showing the distance covered by each of the three signals calculated in all three data sets for the COP (blue), Head Sway Qualisys (red) and Head Sway Oculus (green) measures. Notice how the correspondence is closest for all 3 signals in the Tandem stance data. This is also reflected in the ICC values presented in Table 2.

Table 2. The ICC values for head sway and CoP data in the ML, AP axes of motion for each of the three stances (Double, Tandem, Single). The ICC values for COP excursion and Head Sway (distance column) combine movement in both axes.

Stance	Oculus Head vs. COP (ICC)			Qualisys Head vs. COP (ICC)		
	ML	AP	Distance	ML	AP	Distance
Double	0.875	0.765	0.546	0.782	0.720	0.451
Tandem	0.687	0.858	0.888	0.697	0.850	0.879
Single	0.667	0.658	0.654	0.685	0.642	0.643

The Intraclass Correlation Coefficients showing the relationship between Head Sway (Oculus and Qualisys) and COP excursion in each of the axes (ML and AP) for the three different stances can be found in Table 2. Very strong ICC values were found for the Tandem stance when head sway distance was calculated using the Oculus (0.888) and the Qualisys (0.879) motion capture data. The values for Double (0.546 and 0.451) and Single leg stances

(0.654 and 0.643) were considerably lower, indicating a less strong relationship between the two measurements.

3.3. Measuring the Effects of Visual Field Manipulation on Postural Control

The final part of the study looked to (i) measure the effects of four visual field conditions and two types of tandem stance (dominant vs. non-dominant) on postural control in a group of 30 healthy, adult males' and (ii) check to see if the measures of postural control were reliable over two different testing sessions. The similarity between the sway measures captured 4 days apart using the Oculus Quest was found to be very strong ($r = 0.84$; $p < 0.0001$). This affirmed that the balance measures were reliable across testing sessions. As a consequence, the average of the sway measures from the two sessions were used for all subsequent analyses. A two-way ANCOVA showed that there was indeed a significant main effect of visual field manipulation ($F_{(3,499)} = 73.7$; $p < 0.0001$) on mean total sway (across the two sessions) that was moderated by stance type (dominant vs. non-dominant) ($F_{(1,499)} = 9.6$; $p = 0.002$). Post hoc analysis showed how the Static Light condition had significantly less sway than the Static Dark but also than the Dynamic Tilt conditions (see Figure 4) ($p < 0.001$). Although the Dynamic Forward-Back condition (mean = 31.4 cm) was marginally better than the Static Light condition (mean = 34.0 cm) this difference was not significant ($p = 0.685$). It was, however, significantly better than both the Static Dark (mean = 61.7 cm; $p < 0.001$) and the Dynamic Tilt conditions (mean = 82.8 cm; $p < 0.001$). These differences can be explained by the Dynamic Tilt manipulation forcing postural corrections in the medial lateral axes, the axis that is least stable when a participant adopts a Tandem stance where the base of support is at its narrowest in the medial lateral axis.

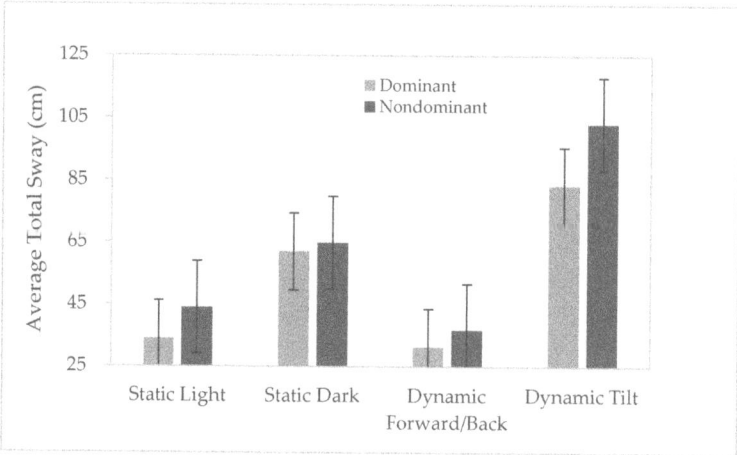

Figure 4. A graph showing the differences in mean total sway for the four different visual field conditions and for the dominant (light grey) and non-dominant (dark grey) stances. The error bars represent the standard deviations for the two different stance conditions.

In terms of effects of stance on postural control, Figure 4 shows the mean average total sway when the visual manipulations occurred in the dominant stance compared to the non-dominant stance.

4. Discussion

This study aimed to see if a low-cost Virtual Reality technology (Oculus Quest) could reliably assess balance. The first part looked at the technical aspects of the technology and assessed how accurately the Oculus Quest could track head movements during a simple balance task (modified version of the BESS) compared to the Qualisys motion capture system. The data clearly showed that the level of correspondence between the Oculus

Quest head movement recordings and that of the Qualisys motion capture system were almost perfect (ICC > 0.99) with less than 5 mm error difference between the two signals (n = 4500). This was in line with a similar study that showed the Oculus Quest was able to track a user's head movement with a mean positional accuracy of 6.86 mm [20,21].

Although this high degree of accuracy and reliability supports the potential use of VR as a viable head tracking technology, it was important to see if head movement (head sway) captures changes in postural control in a similar way to other balance measurement systems. The second technical part of the study looked at the correspondence between balance control measured using head sway (measured by the Oculus Quest and the Qualisys motion capture system) and balance control measured simultaneously using the Centre of Pressure data captured using a Kistler force platform. Although a perfect relationship is not expected as the COP is measuring what is happening between the feet and the ground and head sway is capturing head adjustments, it was predicted that both signals are capturing essential elements of postural control that will be strongly related.

The data showed that the type of stance influenced the ICC values (comparisons between COP measures and head sway measures), with the Double stance showing a moderate relationship (0.55 (Oculus); 0.45 (Qualisys)), Single stance showing a good relationship (0.65 (Oculus) and 0.64 (Qualisys) and Tandem stance showing an excellent relationship (0.89 (Oculus) and 0.88 (Qualisys) when it comes to comparing head movement distance and COP excursion. The lower correspondence between the Double stance can be explained by the fact subtle micromovements can be made between the feet and the ground to change the distribution of weight across this wider base of support. In this case, movements of the head to adjust postural imbalance is likely to be minimal. The opposite is true for the Single stance condition where there is only one foot in contact with the ground and the registration of postural adjustments through the COP are less obvious as the other limbs and the head will be used to control balance. Tandem stance, however, is still a double support stance meaning more force will be exerted through the ground giving more credence to the COP measure. Importantly, however, in a Tandem stance (see Figure 1), the base of support is narrowed in the medial-lateral axis meaning any movements to adjust posture will be in the medial–lateral axis and will be accentuated through movements of the head. This makes head sway an ideal candidate for measuring changes in postural control in Tandem stance. Furthermore, the Oculus head measurements were ever so marginally stronger than Qualisys, again offering support for low-cost VR head tracking as an alternative to more expensive balance measurement systems.

The final part of the study introduced factors that are known to challenge the balance system, namely the type of support (dominant versus non-dominant) and visual field manipulations (similar to the 'moving room' paradigm [17]) and tested the effects on postural control at two different time points (4 days apart). The predictions were that postural control would be best (minimal total sway) for the Tandem balance dominant foot conditions compared to the non-dominant conditions, and in the Static Light and Dynamic Forward/back conditions compared to the Static Dark and Dynamic Tilt conditions [20]. We also predicted that the measures would be stable over time with a strong relationship between the measures when participants were re-tested using the same stances and visual field manipulations 4 days later. Our analysis of the balance control exhibited by a group of thirty healthy adult males showed that there was excellent reliability in the measures of sway across two different testing sessions (r = 0.84), which affirmed that the test–retest reliability of these types of balance tests was excellent. The analysis of the sway in the different visual field conditions showed that the Static Light and Dynamic Forward/Back conditions yielded the least amount of postural adjustment. On the other hand, Static Dark and Dynamic Tilt both induced significant postural adjustments that were captured by the measures of sway ($p < 0.001$). This was in line with previous literature that showed that eyes closed and tilt conditions [20] perturb balance the most. The effect of the Dynamic Tilt condition on sway are more pronounced in Tandem stance as corrective postural movement adjustments are mainly in the medial lateral axis where the base of support was narrowest.

The effect of stance, dominant versus non-dominant, also significantly affected postural control, with sway being significantly less in the dominant stance condition.

In short, this study provides strong evidence that VR technology can be used as an accurate, reliable, low-cost alternative to COP for balance assessment, particularly for Tandem stance. Furthermore, it provides the opportunity to take balance assessment further by providing the option of manipulating the visual field to induce changes in postural stability. This means balance assessments can probe more deeply the origins of any postural control deficits that may have been observed.

In terms of limitations, it is important to note that the VR technology can only measure movement of the head and hand controllers. This means using it to assess postural control during Single leg stance is limited as the sway data would not capture any balance errors associated with dropping the position of the non-supporting leg. New peripheral sensors that can be attached to the feet, but that are compatible with the Oculus Quest, will help overcome this problem in the future. Another limitation of this study is that special software is required to capture the movement data from the three controllers in real time to calculate total sway. The software used in this study (MOViR, INCISIV Ltd.) also generated the changes in visual field allowing for an accurate calculation of sway with respect to the visual condition experienced. Going forward it will be important that appropriate software for capturing movement data and manipulating the visual field is readily available to maximize the potential of using the Oculus Quest VR technology to assess balance.

In terms of applications, one of the other most striking areas where this type of assessment could have a large impact is on concussion detection and management. Current protocols rely heavily on human observation, meaning the subtle changes in balance that occur following a head injury may be missed. As Santos and colleagues [??] pointed out, using technology that is precise and reliable means concussion management can now be taken out of the lab and brought to the pitch. Having access to this type of technology and standardized tests would revolutionize the management of concussed players, allowing subtle changes in balance to be spotted, reducing the risk of having players return to play too quickly and putting themselves at increased risk of another injury. In fact, previous research has shown how balance abnormalities can be indicative of future risk of injury [23], but also a way to spot weaknesses that may directly impact on a player's ability to execute a skill and perform effectively [4].

Like research a decade ago that showed how the Nintendo Wii balance board could be used to measure and train balance [5], this study shows how the Oculus Quest, a low-cost VR gaming headset can also be used to measure and train balance in older adults [24]. Previous research has shown how lab-based VR is well tolerated by more vulnerable groups, with studies showing how VR can be effectively used to cue gait in people with Parkinson's [25,26], but also understand older adults' decisions about when and how to cross a virtual road [27]. Given the power of this technology, creating VR balance games that use AI to adapt to the user's abilities, opens a whole new vista in terms of balance rehabilitation and training possibilities [28,29]. Unlike the Nintendo Wii, where the parent company disinvested in the technology, multinational companies like Meta (Oculus Quest) and Bytedance (Pico Neo) are investing heavily in low-cost virtual reality hardware and relevant applications that will transform how we live our lives.

5. Conclusions

In conclusion, this study demonstrates how the Oculus Quest, a low-cost VR headset, can be used to reliably measure, but also challenge, a person's ability to maintain their balance. Given the importance of postural control for a wide range of clinical applications, this technology offers promising new possibilities for not only balance assessment but also balance training.

Author Contributions: Conceptualization, C.M.C. and M.M.; methodology, C.M.C., M.M. and C.M.; software, A.E. and C.M.C.; validation, A.E., C.M.C., J.S. and C.M.; formal analysis, A.E. and C.M.C.; investigation, C.M. and C.M.C.; resources, C.M.; data curation, A.E.; writing—original draft preparation, J.S. and C.M.C.; writing—review and editing, C.M. and M.M.; visualization, A.E.; supervision, C.M.C. All authors have read and agreed to the published version of the manuscript.

Funding: This research received no external funding.

Institutional Review Board Statement: The study was conducted in accordance with the Declara-tion of Helsinki and approved by the Institutional Review Board (or Ethics Committee) of Ulster University.

Informed Consent Statement: Informed consent was obtained from all subjects involved in the study.

Data Availability Statement: Data are available at the following GitHub repository.

Acknowledgments: The authors would like to thank Mathias Debrabant for his assistance with the initial data collection.

Conflicts of Interest: The authors declare no conflict of interest.

References

1. Asseman, F.B.; Caron, O.; Crémieux, J. Are there specific conditions for which expertise in gymnastics could have an effect on postural control and performance? *Gait Posture* **2008**, *27*, 76–81. [CrossRef]
2. Aalto, H.; Pyykkö, I.; Ilmarinen, R.; Kähkönen, E.; Starck, J. Postural stability in shooters. *ORL* **1990**, *52*, 232–238. [CrossRef] [PubMed]
3. Bell, D.R.; Guskiewicz, K.M.; Clark, M.A.; Padua, D.A. Systematic review of the balance error scoring system. *Sport Health* **2011**, *3*, 287–295. [CrossRef]
4. Hrysomallis, C. Balance ability and athletic performance. *Sports Med.* **2011**, *41*, 221–232. [CrossRef]
5. Young, W.; Ferguson, S.; Brault, S.; Craig, C.M. Assessing and training standing balance in older adults: A novel approach using the 'Nintendo Wii' Balance Board. *Gait Posture* **2011**, *33*, 303–308. [CrossRef] [PubMed]
6. Rahn, C.; Munkasy, B.A.; Joyner, A.B.; Buckley, T.A. Sideline performance of the balance error scoring system during a live sporting event. *Clin. J. Sport Med.* **2015**, *25*, 248. [CrossRef]
7. Donahue, C.C.; Marshall, A.N.; Eddy, R.M.; Feng, X.; Saliba, S.A.; Resch, J.E. The Reliability and Concurrent Validity of the kBESS. *J. Athl. Train.* **2017**, *52*, S240.
8. Slobounov, S.; Slobounov, E.; Sebastianelli, W.; Cao, C.; Newell, K. Differential rate of recovery in athletes after first and second concussion episodes. *Neurosurgery* **2007**, *61*, 338–344. [CrossRef]
9. Lafond, D.; Duarte, M.; Prince, F. Comparison of three methods to estimate the center of mass during balance assessment. *J. Biomech.* **2004**, *37*, 1421–1426. [CrossRef]
10. Winter, D.A. *Biomechanics and Motor Control of Human Movement*; John Wiley & Sons: Hoboken, NJ, USA, 2009.
11. Gutierrez-Farewik, E.M.; Bartonek, Å.; Saraste, H. Comparison and evaluation of two common methods to measure center of mass displacement in three dimensions during gait. *Hum. Mov. Sci.* **2006**, *25*, 238–256. [CrossRef]
12. Xiao, J.Z.; Yang, Z.F.; Wang, H.R.; Yang, X.C. Detection method of human three-dimensional body center of gravity based on inclinometer network. *Sens. Mater.* **2007**, *29*, 1081–1087.
13. Floor-Westerdijk, M.J.; Schepers, H.M.; Veltink, P.H.; van Asseldonk, E.H.; Buurke, J.H. Use of inertial sensors for ambulatory assessment of center-of-mass displacements during walking. *IEEE Trans. Biomed. Eng.* **2012**, *59*, 2080–2084. [CrossRef] [PubMed]
14. Paillard, T.; Costes-Salon, C.; Lafont, C.; Dupui, P. Are there differences in postural regulation according to the level of competition in judoists? *Br. J. Sport Med.* **2002**, *36*, 304–305. [CrossRef]
15. Ciria, L.F.; Muñoz, M.A.; Gea, J.; Peña, N.; Miranda, J.G.V.; Montoya, P.; Vila, J. Head movement measurement: An alternative method for posturography studies. *Gait Posture* **2017**, *52*, 100–106. [CrossRef]
16. Lopez, C.; Blanke, O. The thalamocortical vestibular system in animals and humans. *Brain Res. Rev.* **2011**, *67*, 119–146. [CrossRef]
17. Lee, D.N.; Aronson, E. Visual proprioceptive control of standing in human infants. *Percept. Psychophys.* **1974**, *15*, 529–532. [CrossRef]
18. Facebook Inc. *Powered by AI: Oculus Insight*; Facebook Inc.: Menlo Park, CA, USA, 2019. Available online: https://ai.facebook.com/blog/powered-by-ai-oculus-insight (accessed on 5 June 2022).
19. Cicchetti, D.V. Guidelines, criteria, and rules of thumb for evaluating normed and standardized assessment instruments in psychology. *Psychol. Assess.* **1994**, *6*, 284–290. [CrossRef]
20. Teel, E.F.; Slobounov, S.M. Validation of a virtual reality balance module for use in clinical concussion assessment and management. *Clin. J. Sport Med.* **2015**, *25*, 144–148. [CrossRef] [PubMed]
21. Eger Passos, D.; Jung, B. Measuring the accuracy of inside-out tracking in XR devices using a high-precision robotic arm. In Proceedings of the International Conference on Human-Computer Interaction, Copenhagen, Denmark, 19–24 July 2020; Springer: Cham, Switzerland, 2020; pp. 19–26.
22. Santos, F.V.; Yamaguchi, F.; Buckley, T.A.; Caccese, J.B. Virtual reality in concussion management: From lab to clinic. *J. Clin. Transl. Res.* **2020**, *5*, 148–154.
23. Hrysomallis, C. Relationship between balance ability, training and sports injury risk. *Sports Med.* **2007**, *37*, 547–556. [CrossRef]

24. Whyatt, C.; Merriman, N.S.; Young, W.R.; Newell, F.N.; Craig, C. A Wii bit of fun: A novel platform to deliver effective training to older adults. *J. Games Health* **2015**, *4*, 423–433. [CrossRef] [PubMed]
25. Gomez-Jordana, L.; Stafford, J.; Peper, C.E.; Craig, C.M. Crossing virtual doors: A new method to study gait impairments and freezing of gait in Parkinson's Disease. *Parkinsons Dis.* **2018**, *2018*, 2957427. [CrossRef] [PubMed]
26. Gomez-Jordana, L.; Stafford, J.; Peper, C.E.; Craig, C.M. Virtual Footprints can improve walking in people with Parkinson's Disease. *Front. Neurol.* **2018**, *9*, 681. [CrossRef] [PubMed]
27. Stafford, J.; Rodger, M.; Gómez-Jordana, L.I.; Whyatt, C.; Craig, C.M. Developmental differences across the lifespan in the use of perceptual information to guide action-based decisions. *Psychol. Res.* **2022**, *86*, 268–283. [CrossRef] [PubMed]
28. Paraskevopoulos, I.; Tsekleves, E.; Craig, C.M.; Whyatt, C.P.; Cosmas, J.P. Design guidelines for developing customised serious games for Parkinson's disease rehabilitation using bespoke game sensors. *Lect. Notes Comput. Sci.* **2014**, *5*, 413–424. [CrossRef]
29. Awad, M.; Ferguson, S.; Craig, C. Designing games for older adults an affordance-based approach. In Proceedings of the IEEE SeGAH, Rio de Janeiro, Brazil, 14–16 May 2014; pp. 1–7.

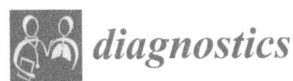

Article

Sleep Position Detection with a Wireless Audio-Motion Sensor—A Validation Study

Wojciech Kukwa [1,*], Tomasz Lis [2], Jonasz Łaba [3], Ron B. Mitchell [4] and Marcel Młyńczak [3]

1. Faculty of Dental Medicine, Medical University of Warsaw, 02-091 Warsaw, Poland
2. Department of Pediatric ENT, Medical University of Warsaw, 02-091 Warsaw, Poland; lis.tomasz.lis@gmail.com
3. Institute of Metrology and Biomedical Engineering, Faculty of Mechatronics, Warsaw University of Technology, 02-525 Warsaw, Poland; jonasz.laba.dokt@pw.edu.pl (J.Ł.); marcel.mlynczak@pw.edu.pl (M.M.)
4. Department of Otolaryngology, UT Southwestern Medical Center, Dallas, TX 75390, USA; ron.mitchell@utsouthwestern.edu
* Correspondence: wojciechkukwa@gmail.com

Abstract: It is well documented that body position significantly affects breathing indices during sleep in patients with obstructive sleep apnea. They usually worsen while changing from a non-supine to a supine position. Therefore, body position should be an accurately measured and credible parameter in all types of sleep studies. The aim of this study was to specify the accuracy of a neck-based monitoring device (Clebre, Olsztyn, Poland) mounted at the suprasternal notch, in determining a supine and non-supine sleeping position, as well as specific body positions during sleep, in comparison to polysomnography (PSG). A sleep study (PSG along with a neck-based audio-motion sensor) was performed on 89 consecutive patients. The accuracy in determining supine and non-supine positions was 96.9% ± 3.9% and 97.0% ± 3.6%, respectively. For lateral positions, the accuracy was 98.6% ± 2% and 97.4% ± 4.5% for the right and left side, respectively. The prone position was detected with an accuracy of 97.3% ± 5.6%. The study showed a high accuracy in detecting supine, as well as other gross positions, during sleep based on a sensor attached to the suprasternal notch, compared to the PSG study. We feel that the suprasternal notch is a promising area for placing wireless sleep study devices.

Keywords: home sleep study; polysomnography; actigraphy; positional sleep apnea

Citation: Kukwa, W.; Lis, T.; Łaba, J.; Mitchell, R.B.; Młyńczak, M. Sleep Position Detection with a Wireless Audio-Motion Sensor—A Validation Study. *Diagnostics* **2022**, *12*, 1195. https://doi.org/10.3390/diagnostics12051195

Academic Editors: Carlo Ricciardi, Francesco Amato and Mario Cesarelli

Received: 25 March 2022
Accepted: 9 May 2022
Published: 11 May 2022

Publisher's Note: MDPI stays neutral with regard to jurisdictional claims in published maps and institutional affiliations.

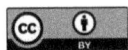

Copyright: © 2022 by the authors. Licensee MDPI, Basel, Switzerland. This article is an open access article distributed under the terms and conditions of the Creative Commons Attribution (CC BY) license (https://creativecommons.org/licenses/by/4.0/).

1. Introduction

Obstructive sleep apnea (OSA) is the most common form of sleep-disordered breathing (SDB), characterized by repeated episodes of absent (apnea) or reduced (hypopnea) airflow in the upper airway during sleep. Airway obstruction is associated with either oxygen desaturation or frequent brain arousal and is linked to increased incidence of hypertension, type 2 diabetes, atrial fibrillation, heart failure, coronary artery disease, stroke, and death [1,2].

The gold standard test for diagnosis of OSA is a laboratory-based attended polysomnography (PSG) during which multiple data channels are recorded, including sleep and respiratory parameters, muscle activity, heart rhythm, snoring, and body position. The presence and severity of OSA are typically determined by the apnea–hypopnea index (AHI), defined as the number of apneas and hypopneas per hour of sleep. It is generally accepted that AHI $\geq$ 5 events/h defines OSA.

It is well documented that body position significantly affects breathing indices, expressed among others by the AHI, which usually worsens while changing from a non-supine to a supine position [3]. Therefore, body position should be an accurately measured and credible parameter. Positional obstructive sleep apnea (POSA), first described by Cartwright in 1984 [3], is defined as an AHI at least twice as high in the supine position as in the lateral (non-supine) position [4]. According to Cartwright's criteria, two subtypes of POSA were defined: supine-isolated OSA (siOSA; non-supine AHI < 5 with at least 15 min of sleep in both positions) and supine-predominant OSA (spOSA; non-supine AHI ⩾ 5) [5–7]. In selected patients with POSA, positional therapy (PT), which is based on preventing patients from sleeping in a supine position, may be an effective treatment option [8,9]. Ravesloot et. al. provided an overview of 16 articles, examining the impact of PT on OSA, showing that all included studies reported a positive effect of PT on AHI reduction in POSA patients [9].

As mentioned before, for the clinical needs of sleep study analysis, body position can be divided into supine and non-supine, which consists of prone and both lateral positions. Body position sensors are usually attached to either the chest or abdomen, which does not always reflect the actual orientation of the upper airways. Furthermore, current American Academy of Sleep Medicine (AASM) guidelines, except for frequency of measurement, do not provide recommendations concerning the recording of body position during sleep. To our knowledge, there is also a lack of comparison studies between different PSG systems, moreso regarding the accuracy of detecting body position.

Furthermore, full PSG is a very uncomfortable, expensive, and availability-limited study. Lately, multiple sensors have been introduced into sleep medicine studies with a promise to diagnose sleep disordered breathing in the home environment. These cheaper and more comfortable than in-lab PSG devices belong mostly to home sleep apnea tests (HSATs). Here we used a small audio-motion wireless sensor (Clebre, Olsztyn, Poland). Clebre is attached to the skin at the suprasternal notch on the neck with a double-sided medical patch (see Section 2), allowing detection of the patient's position and activity. Previously we showed a very high accuracy in detecting a supine and non-supine sleep position in comparison to PSG on a group of 30 patients [10].

The aim of this study was to validate the accuracy of a neck-based Clebre device in determining a supine and non-supine sleeping position, as well as specific body positions during sleep, in comparison to the NOX A1 PSG system (Nox Medical Inc., Reykjavik, Iceland) in a large cohort of patients.

2. Materials and Methods

2.1. Participants

The study included 89 consecutive adult patients who underwent PSG and Clebre examinations. The inclusion criteria were: 18 years of age or older, PSG for suspected OSA, at least 6 h of simultaneously recorded PSG and Clebre. The exclusion criteria were a previous history of OSA treatment such as positive airway pressure (PAP) therapy and class III and IV heart failure according to the classification of the New York Heart Association (NYHA) [11].

All participants signed an informed consent. The study was approved by the Ethics Committee of Medical University of Warsaw (KB/14/2018).

Demographic information, including age, sex, height, and weight, was collected. The body mass index (BMI) was calculated for each patient.

2.2. Protocol and Devices

Each subject underwent a full-night attended PSG in the sleep laboratory of the Otorhinolaryngology Department at Czerniakowski Hospital, Warsaw, Poland. PSGs were recorded with the Nox A1 PSG System [12,13]. The recording montage comprised a 6-channel encephalogram (EEG), a 3-channel submental electromyogram (EMG), a left and right electrooculogram (EOG), an electrocardiogram (ECG), airflow recording through the nose and mouth by a nasal air pressure transducer and oronasal thermistor, thoracic and abdominal effort measurement by inductance plethysmography, and arterial oxygen saturation using a Nonin 3150 WristOx2™ wireless oximeter (Nonin Medical, Plymouth, MN, USA) [14]. An in-built microphone was used to record snoring. Body positions, differentiated between upright, right side, left side, prone, and supine, were determined by a 3-axis, ±2 g accelerometer with 20 Hz sampling frequency, incorporated in the PSG headbox. The video was recorded throughout the night using AXIS M3106-LVE [15] and AXIS M3116-LVE [16] network cameras (Axis Communications AB, Lund, Sweden) with 1024 × 768 resolution and a frame rate of 30.

For each patient, sleep and respiratory events were scored by an experienced sleep physician using the AASM Manual for the Scoring of Sleep and Associated Events v.2.6 [17]. The sleep position was obtained from the PSG's raw data acquired from European Data Format (EDF) files, exported from the Noxturnal software (Nox Medical Inc., Reykjavik, Iceland). Sleep parameters calculated by the software were obtained from PSG sleep reports.

Simultaneously, subjects underwent full night examination with a Clebre audio and motion sensor. The sensor was placed by the technician in the suprasternal notch on the neck and attached using a medical double-sided patch. The way the sensor was placed is presented in Figure 1. The dimensions of the sensor were 33 × 39 × 13 mm, and it weighed 18 g. The battery allowed for at least 14 h of operation. The memory capacity was defined internally by a 2 GB FLASH chip. Motion accelerometry based signals (3-axis, with a 52 Hz sampling frequency) were used to estimate sleep body position characteristics, using the algorithms presented in a previous study, which reported 97% accuracy in supine versus non-supine body position differentiation compared to the simultaneously acquired PSG [18]. The sleep studies in which there were differences in estimation of body position between PSG and Clebre were visually inspected by two PSG technicians, using video monitoring. To synchronize the devices, both the Clebre and PSG had an internal clock. It ran parallel to the connected computer (PSG) or was synchronized at the beginning of the study using a dedicated smartphone app (Clebre).

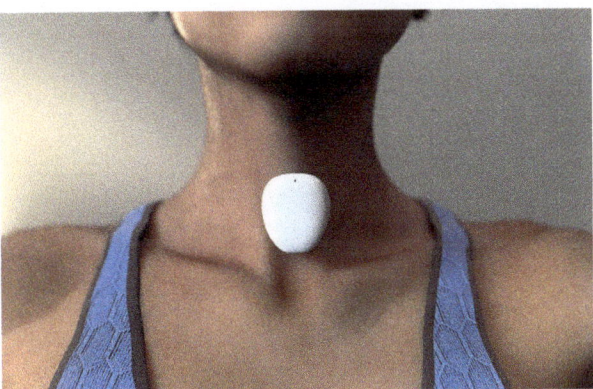

Figure 1. The placement of the Clebre audio and motion sensor.

2.3. Data Analysis and Statistics

For each patient the percentage of supine/non-supine body position was recorded. Among POSA patients, subjects who spent less than 15 min of sleep in either supine or non-supine sleeping positions were excluded [7]. We analyzed differences between PSG and Clebre using paired t tests. Furthermore, Lin's Concordance Coefficients [19] were estimated for each body position, and Bland–Altman analyses [20] were performed. All calculations were performed using Python 3.9.7 (default, 16 September 2021, 13:09:58), graphs were created using matplotlib package [21]. The significance level was established at the level of 0.05.

3. Results

Demographics of the study population are presented in Table 1 and OSA data in Table 2. There were 89 participants in the study, including 21 females. Their average age was around 50 and average BMI around 30. Almost all (95.5%) were considered OSA patients, from which 52.8% were POSA ones.

Table 1. Baseline characteristics of study participants and polysomnography data.

Characteristic	Males	Females	Total Patients
N	68	21	89
Age (years)	50.15 ± 11.78	53.62 ± 11.93	50.97 ± 11.91
BMI (kg/m^2)	30.09 ± 4.91	29.35 ± 6.04	29.91 ± 5.21
TST (min)	386.21 ± 49.09	399.66 ± 50.54	389.38 ± 49.76
Sleep efficiency * (%)	91.58 ± 41.49	87.45 ± 6.76	90.60 ± 36.45
AHI (events/h)	37.12 ± 24.12	28.45 ± 17.06	35.08 ± 22.95
AHI supine (events/h)	50.03 ± 25.47	45.42 ± 28.72	48.94 ± 26.34
AHI non-supine (events/h)	25.78 ± 26.17	14.82 ± 14.77	23.19 ± 24.42
Supine position in TST (min)	166.31 ± 107.02	194.84 ± 100.21	173.04 ± 106.15
Supine position in TST (%)	43.70 ± 27.79	48.82 ± 24.26	44.91 ± 27.08
Non-supine position in TST (min)	212.08 ± 109.67	199.40 ± 99.01	209.09 ± 107.38
Non-supine position in TST (%)	55.35 ± 27.52	50.29 ± 24.78	54.16 ± 26.98

Values were presented as mean ± standard deviation. BMI = body mass index, TST = total sleep time, TRT = total recording time, AHI = apnea–hypopnea index; * Calculated as (TST/TRT × 100%).

Table 2. Characterictics of OSA patients.

Characteristic	Males	Females	Total Patients
OSA patients *; n (% from specific group)	67 (98.5)	18 (85.7)	85 (95.5)
Supine OSA patients **; n (%)	34 (38.2)	13 (14.6)	47 (52.8)
Supine-isolated OSA patients ***; n (%)	5 (5.6)	6 (6.7)	11 (12.4)
Supine-predominant OSA patients ****; n (%)	29 (32.6)	7 (7.9)	36 (40.5)

* Patients with AHI ⩾ 5; ** OSA patients with supine to non-supine sleep ratio of more than 2; *** positional OSA patients with non-supine AHI < 5, who slept at least 15 min both supine and non-supine; **** positional OSA patients with non-supine AHI ⩾ 5; OSA—Obstructive sleep apnea.

The accuracy in determining supine and non-supine positions was 96.9% ± 3.9% and 97.0% ± 3.6%, respectively. For lateral positions, the accuracy was 98.6% ± 2.0% and 97.4% ± 4.5% for the right and left side, respectively. Paired t tests suggested no basis to reject the null hypothesis (equal means) for left and right side body positions. The prone position was detected with an accuracy of 97.3% ± 5.6% (p-value = 0.0009). The p-value for supine (0.016) showed a statistically significant difference; however, their absolute values were relatively small.

The sample actigraphy curves for three patients were presented comparatively in Figure 2. Those were selected to show examples with almost identical signals, with a small level of error, and with a moderate level of error, respectively.

The Lin's Concordance Coefficients and Bland–Altman curves were also prepared to compare PSG and Clebre percentages of each lying body position in relation to sleep time and are presented in Figures 3 and 4, respectively.

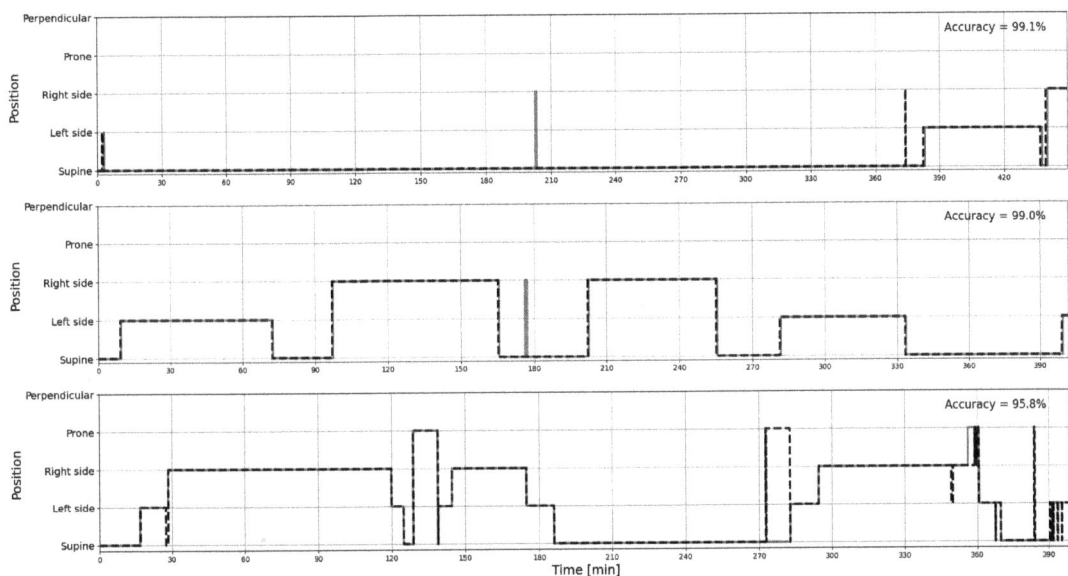

Figure 2. The sample curves of actigraphy signals recorded by PSG (solid line) and estimated from Clebre (dashed line), selected to show an almost perfect match (**top**), a small level of error (**middle**), and a moderate level of error (**bottom**), respectively.

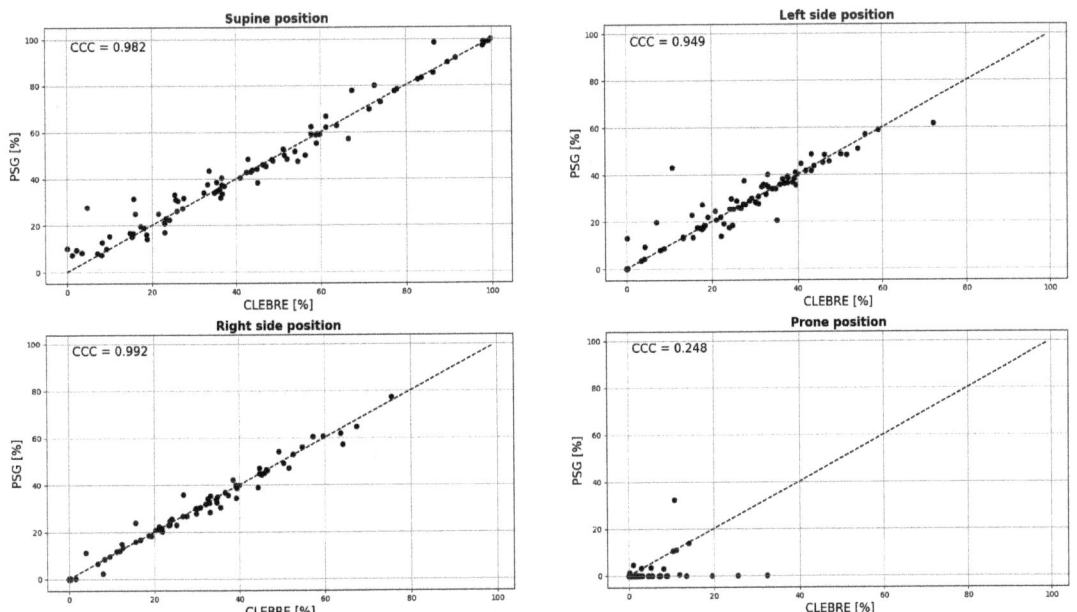

Figure 3. The PSG versus Clebre plots for percentages of each lying body position in relation to sleep time, along with the estimation of Lin's Concordance Coefficients (CCC).

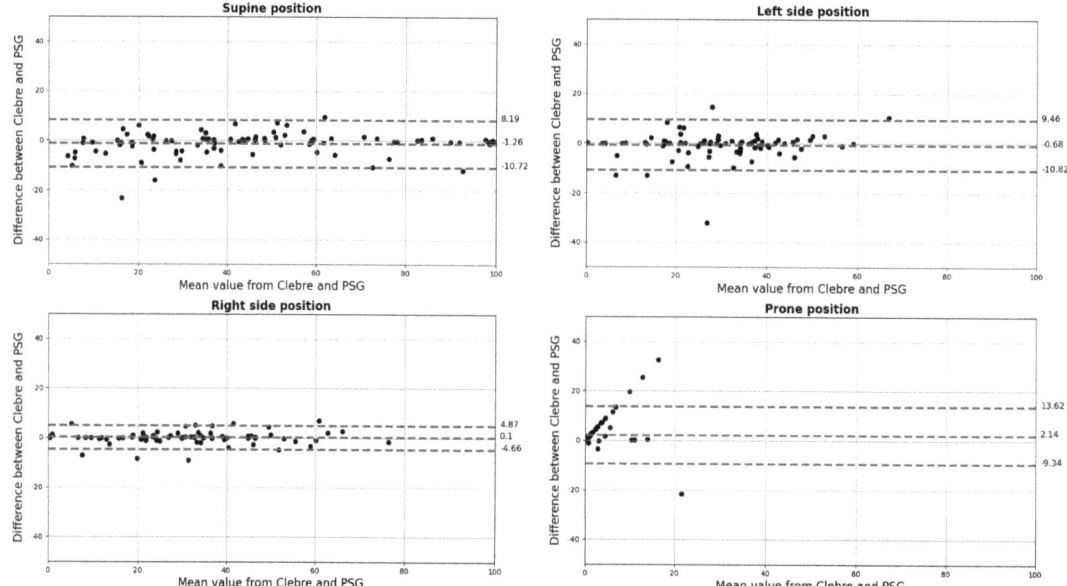

Figure 4. The Bland–Altman plots for percentages of each lying body position in relation to sleep time; percentages on both axes.

4. Discussion

To our knowledge, this is the first study validating sleep position detection of any wireless HSAT sensor in a large cohort of patients against in-lab PSG, as such reports are scarce and all prepared on very limited number of patients [22–24].

According to a paper recently published by Ravesloot and colleagues, a standardized framework emphasizing the role of the sleeping position should be an important dataset in every sleep report [18,25]. This is because sleep position may significantly influence sleep study results, as well as the fact that a large group of OSA patients can benefit largely from PT. Therefore, accurate sleep position detection should be a crucial part of every sleep study.

Our study showed high accuracy in detecting both supine vs. non-supine and specific sleep positions with a wireless sensor attached to the skin at the suprasternal notch, in comparison to PSG, in a large cohort of patients. In terms of sleep study results, the binary division into supine and non-supine is of most importance. Here, the accuracy equaled 96.9% ± 3.9% and 97.0% ± 3.6%, respectively. In some patients where differences were noticed, they resulted mostly from discrepancies between head versus thorax orientation.

Every PSG system (type 1 and type 2 devices; the full classification is provided in [26,27]) measures and analyzes sleep position. According to AASM, the required sampling rate for body position measurement is 1 Hz [28]. Aside from that, there is no information regarding accuracy of measurement or angle-limit values in each axis for classification of body positions while asleep (supine, prone, and lateral positions). Interestingly, a study by Ferrer-Lluis et al. showed on 19 OSA patients that automatic sleep position determination in PSG agreed, on average, only in 83.1% with video-validated positions [23].

Unlike PSG, home sleep apnea testing (HSAT) which typically uses type 3 devices, are not required to record the sleep position [29,30], only "conventional" type 3 devices do measure these parameters [31]—for sensors without the measurement of sleep position it is impossible to confirm POSA and to implement PT. As there are on average 56% of patients with POSA [32–35] when using the most commonly used Cartwright's definition, this parameter is absolutely crucial to include in the sleep study. Type 4 devices measure one or two variables: oxygen saturation, airflow, and chest movement, and in most cases they do not take body position into account, therefore their use in determining POSA is very limited.

There are many different new technologies that are being introduced in sleep medicine to assess body position. The devices in which these are introduced belong largely to HSAT. Among them, there are both contact and non-contact technologies. Non-contact technologies are bed mattresses and radar sensors. In terms of bed mattresses, the Sonomat is the most validated in sleep medicine [36,37]. No data regarding sleep position recognition are available in the published papers. For other mattress systems, there are studies showing a potentially high accuracy in detecting all four major sleep positions. The accuracy of a system described by Liu et al., based on a piezo-electric polymer film sensor applied in a form of a mattress, showed a 97% accuracy in detecting four major positions during sleep on a group of 11 healthy participants [38] Few radar systems have been described in the literature. No data regarding the feasibility of automatic sleep position detection were found in these papers [39–42].

Contact sensors are ones attached to a patient's body, and the placement of the sensor on the body is crucial to what signals could be detected. Contact sensors can be wrist or finger, chest, neck, or forehead devices. The most common contact sensors currently used in sleep evaluation are wrist/finger wearables. Most of these measure heart rate, heart rate variability, SaO2, and accelerometric signals. It has to be emphasized that this placement of the accelerometer does not allow accurate evaluation of the sleep position, as the trunk orientation does not depend on the forearm orientation. Current commercial wristband products, such as MI Band, Garmin Smartwatch, and Apple Watch, cannot recognize sleep positions [43]. A study by Yeng and colleagues showed that correct classification of sleep position was achieved in up to 85% of recording time with a wrist sensor, but the study was performed only on two participants. When placing an accelerometer on the chest, the accuracy in detecting sleep positions is very high. This was also shown in studies with the use of smartphone accelerometry. Two such studies showed accuracy in detecting sleep position as high as 97% and 95.9% on 6 and 19 subjects, respectively, [22,23].

Our previous study showed a 97.3% accuracy in distinguishing between supine and non-supine positions on 30 patients. Here, we confirmed about 97% in supine and non-supine position accuracies and at least 97.3% in other body position detection. We suggest the suprasternal notch is a perfect candidate to mount a small wireless sensor for sleep study purposes, as this place enables perfect detection of the acoustic signal related to breathing and a heart rhythm. Furthermore, as was shown in this study, sleep position can be accurately detected from this location. Moreover, this location of the sensor should not discourage patients from adopting a prone sleep position as this might be a problem with mounting the sensor on the chest.

5. Conclusions

Our study showed that placing the position sensor on the neck, at the suprasternal notch, may be highly effective in detecting sleep positions. We showed an accuracy above 97% for detecting each of four gross positions in a large cohort of patients. As this placement of the sensor might be less inconvenient than the chest placement, we feel the suprasternal notch is a good candidate for a single sensor placement in sleep studies.

Author Contributions: Conceptualization, W.K. and M.M.; methodology, W.K., T.Ł., J.Ł. and M.M.; software, J.Ł. and M.M.; validation, W.K. and M.M.; formal analysis, W.K., T.Ł., J.Ł. and M.M.; investigation, W.K. and T.Ł.; resources, W.K. and M.M.; data curation, T.Ł. and J.Ł.; writing—original draft preparation, W.K., T.Ł., J.Ł. and M.M.; writing—review and editing, W.K., R.B.M. and M.M.; visualization, J.Ł. and M.M.; supervision, W.K.; project administration, W.K. and M.M.; funding acquisition, W.K. and M.M. All authors have read and agreed to the published version of the manuscript.

Funding: This research was performed as project number POIR.01.01.01-00-0212/19 titled: "Wireless sensor and telemedical system for the diagnosis of sleep disordered breathing" co-financed by European Union from the European Regional Development Fund, Smart Growth 2014-2020 Operational

Program. The Project is implementing under competition of the Polish National Center for Research and Development (2/1.1.1/2019 Szybka ścieżka).

 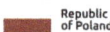 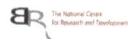

Institutional Review Board Statement: The study was conducted according to the guidelines of the Declaration of Helsinki and approved by the Ethics Committee of Medical University of Warsaw (KB/14/2018) on 6 February 2018.

Informed Consent Statement: Informed consent was obtained from all subjects involved in the study.

Data Availability Statement: Data supporting the reported results are available from the corresponding author on reasonable request.

Conflicts of Interest: W.K. and M.M. are shareholders of Clebre but received no remuneration on performing this study. T.L. is an employee of Clebre. The funders had no role in the design of the study; in the collection, analyses, or interpretation of data; in the writing of the manuscript, or in the decision to publish the results.

References

1. Strollo, P.J., Jr.; Rogers, R.M. Obstructive sleep apnea. *N. Engl. J. Med.* **1996**, *334*, 99–104. [CrossRef] [PubMed]
2. Dempsey, J.A.; Veasey, S.C.; Morgan, B.J.; O'Donnell, C.P. Pathophysiology of sleep apnea. *Physiol. Rev.* **2010**, *90*, 47–112. [CrossRef] [PubMed]
3. Cartwright, R.D.; Diaz, F.; Lloyd, S. The effects of sleep posture and sleep stage on apnea frequency. *Sleep* **1991**, *14*, 351–353. [CrossRef] [PubMed]
4. Quan, S.; Gillin, J.C.; Littner, M.; Shepard, J. Sleep-related breathing disorders in adults: Recommendations for syndrome definition and measurement techniques in clinical research. *Sleep* **1999**, *22*, 662–689. [CrossRef]
5. Lee, S.A.; Paek, J.H.; Chung, Y.S.; Kim, W.S. Clinical features in patients with positional obstructive sleep apnea according to its subtypes. *Sleep Breath.* **2017**, *21*, 109–117. [CrossRef]
6. Kim, K.T.; Cho, Y.W.; Kim, D.E.; Hwang, S.H.; Song, M.L.; Motamedi, G.K. Two subtypes of positional obstructive sleep apnea: Supine-predominant and supine-isolated. *Clin. Neurophysiol.* **2016**, *127*, 565–570. [CrossRef]
7. Mador, M.J.; Kufel, T.J.; Magalang, U.J.; Rajesh, S.; Watwe, V.; Grant, B.J. Prevalence of positional sleep apnea in patients undergoing polysomnography. *Chest* **2005**, *128*, 2130–2137. [CrossRef]
8. Oksenberg, A.; Gadoth, N. Are we missing a simple treatment for most adult sleep apnea patients? The avoidance of the supine sleep position. *J. Sleep Res.* **2014**, *23*, 204–210. [CrossRef]
9. Ravesloot, M.; Van Maanen, J.; Dun, L.; De Vries, N. The undervalued potential of positional therapy in position-dependent snoring and obstructive sleep apnea—A review of the literature. *Sleep Breath.* **2013**, *17*, 39–49. [CrossRef]
10. Młyńczak, M.; Valdez, T.A.; Kukwa, W. Joint Apnea and Body Position Analysis for Home Sleep Studies Using a Wireless Audio and Motion Sensor. *IEEE Access* **2020**, *8*, 170579–170587. [CrossRef]
11. New York Heart Association (NYHA). *Functional Classification: The Criteria Committee of the New York Heart Association. Nomenclature and Criteria for Diagnosis of Diseases of the Heart and Great Vessels*; NYHA: New York, NY, USA, 1994.
12. Nox A1 Manual. Available online: https://noxmedical.com/wp-content/uploads/2021/01/Nox-A1-US-Manual.pdf (accessed on 4 May 2022).
13. Nox A1 Brochure. Available online: https://noxmedical.com/wp-content/uploads/2021/11/A1_brochure_US_adress.pdf (accessed on 4 May 2022).
14. Nonin 3150 WristOx2 Operator's Manual. Available online: https://www.nonin.com/wp-content/uploads/2018/10/3150-BLE-USB-Operators-Manual.pdf (accessed on 4 May 2022).
15. AXIS M3106-LVE Datasheet. Available online: https://www.axis.com/dam/public/ed/2b/8a/datasheet-axis-m3106-lve-network-camera-en-US-278038.pdf (accessed on 4 May 2022).
16. AXIS M3116-LVE Datasheet. Available online: https://www.axis.com/dam/public/d2/ca/50/datasheet-axis-m3116%E2%80%93lve-network-camera-en-US-353775.pdf (accessed on 4 May 2022).
17. AASM Scoring Manual—American Academy of Sleep Medicine. Available online: http://www.aasmnet.org/scoringmanual/ (accessed on 4 May 2022).
18. Kukwa, W.; Łaba, J.; Lis, T.; Sobczyk, K.; Mitchell, R.B.; Młyńczak, M. Supine sleep patterns as a part of phenotyping patients with sleep apnea—A pilot study. *Sleep Breath.* **2022**. [CrossRef]
19. Lin's Concordance Correlation Coefficient. Available online: https://ncss-wpengine.netdna-ssl.com/wp-content/themes/ncss/pdf/Procedures/PASS/Lins_Concordance_Correlation_Coefficient.pdf (accessed on 4 May 2022).
20. Giavarina, D. Understanding bland altman analysis. *Biochem. Med.* **2015**, *25*, 141–151. [CrossRef]
21. Hunter, J.D. Matplotlib: A 2D graphics environment. *Comput. Sci. Eng.* **2007**, *9*, 90–95. [CrossRef]

22. Ferrer-Lluis, I.; Castillo-Escario, Y.; Montserrat, J.M.; Jané, R. Analysis of Smartphone Triaxial Accelerometry for Monitoring Sleep-Disordered Breathing and Sleep Position at Home. *IEEE Access* **2020**, *8*, 71231–71244. [CrossRef]
23. Ferrer-Lluis, I.; Castillo-Escario, Y.; Montserrat, J.M.; Jané, R. Enhanced Monitoring of Sleep Position in Sleep Apnea Patients: Smartphone Triaxial Accelerometry Compared with Video-Validated Position from Polysomnography. *Sensors* **2021**, *21*, 3689. [CrossRef]
24. Bignold, J.J.; Mercer, J.D.; Antic, N.A.; McEvoy, R.D.; Catcheside, P.G. Accurate position monitoring and improved supine-dependent obstructive sleep apnea with a new position recording and supine avoidance device. *J. Clin. Sleep Med.* **2011**, *7*, 376–383. [CrossRef]
25. Ravesloot, M.; Vonk, P.; Maurer, J.; Oksenberg, A.; De Vries, N. Standardized framework to report on the role of sleeping position in sleep apnea patients. *Sleep Breath.* **2021**, *25*, 1717–1728. [CrossRef]
26. Standards of Practice Committee of the American Sleep Disorders Association. Practice parameters for the use of portable recording in the assessment of obstructive sleep apnea. *Sleep* **1994**, *17*, 372–377.
27. Collop, N.A.; Anderson, W.M.; Boehlecke, B.; Claman, D.; Goldberg, R.; Gottlieb, D.J.; Hudgel, D.; Sateia, M.; Schwab, R. Clinical guidelines for the use of unattended portable monitors in the diagnosis of obstructive sleep apnea in adult patients. *J. Clin. Sleep Med.* **2007**, *3*, 737–747.
28. Berry, R.B.; Brooks, R.; Gamaldo, C.E.; Harding, S.M.; Marcus, C.; Vaughn, B.V. *The AASM Manual for the Scoring of Sleep and Associated Events. Rules, Terminology and Technical Specifications*; American Academy of Sleep Medicine: Darien, IL, USA, 2012; Volume 176.
29. Ferber, R.; Millman, R.; Coppola, M.; Fleetham, J.; Murray, C.F.; Iber, C.; McCall, W.V.; Nino-Murcia, G.; Pressman, M.; Sanders, M.; et al. Portable recording in the assessment of obstructive sleep apnea. *Sleep* **1994**, *17*, 378–392. [CrossRef]
30. Littner, M.R. Portable monitoring in the diagnosis of the obstructive sleep apnea syndrome. *Semin. Respir. Crit. Care Med.* **2005**, *26*, 56–67. [CrossRef] [PubMed]
31. Kapur, V.K.; Auckley, D.H.; Chowdhuri, S.; Kuhlmann, D.C.; Mehra, R.; Ramar, K.; Harrod, C.G. Clinical practice guideline for diagnostic testing for adult obstructive sleep apnea: An American Academy of Sleep Medicine clinical practice guideline. *J. Clin. Sleep Med.* **2017**, *13*, 479–504. [CrossRef] [PubMed]
32. Oksenberg, A.; Arons, E.; Radwan, H.; Silverberg, D.S. Positional vs. nonpositional obstructive sleep apnea patients: Anthropomorphic, nocturnal polysomnographic and multiple sleep latency test data. *Chest* **1997**, *112*, 629–639. [CrossRef] [PubMed]
33. Oksenberg, A.; Khamaysi, I.; Silverberg, D.S.; Tarasiuk, A. Association of body position with severity of apneic events in patients with severe nonpositional obstructive sleep apnea. *Chest* **2000**, *118*, 1018–1024. [CrossRef]
34. Oksenberg, A.; Arons, E.; Greenberg-Dotan, S.; Nasser, K.; Radwan, H. The significance of body posture on breathing abnormalities during sleep: Data analysis of 2077 obstructive sleep apnea patients. *Harefuah* **2009**, *148*, 304–309.
35. Richard, W.; Kox, D.; den Herder, C.; Laman, M.; van Tinteren, H.; de Vries, N. The role of sleep position in obstructive sleep apnea syndrome. *Eur. Arch. Oto-Rhino-Laryngol. Head Neck* **2006**, *263*, 946–950. [CrossRef]
36. Norman, M.B.; Middleton, S.; Erskine, O.; Middleton, P.G.; Wheatley, J.R.; Sullivan, C.E. Validation of the Sonomat: A contactless monitoring system used for the diagnosis of sleep disordered breathing. *Sleep* **2014**, *37*, 1477–1487. [CrossRef]
37. Norman, M.B.; Pithers, S.M.; Teng, A.Y.; Waters, K.A.; Sullivan, C.E. Validation of the Sonomat Against PSG and Quantitative Measurement of Partial Upper Airway Obstruction in Children with Sleep-Disordered Breathing. *Sleep* **2017**, *40*, zsx017. [CrossRef]
38. Liu, M.; Qin, L.; Ye, S. A Mattress System of Recognizing Sleep Postures Based on BCG Signal. *Zhongguo Liao Xie Zhi Chin. J. Med. Instrum.* **2019**, *43*, 243–247.
39. Zhou, Y.; Shu, D.; Xu, H.; Qiu, Y.; Zhou, P.; Ruan, W.; Qin, G.; Jin, J.; Zhu, H.; Ying, K.; et al. Validation of novel automatic ultra-wideband radar for sleep apnea detection. *J. Thorac. Dis.* **2020**, *12*, 1286. [CrossRef]
40. Kang, S.; Kim, D.K.; Lee, Y.; Lim, Y.H.; Park, H.K.; Cho, S.H.; Cho, S.H. Non-contact diagnosis of obstructive sleep apnea using impulse-radio ultra-wideband radar. *Sci. Rep.* **2020**, *10*, 5261. [CrossRef]
41. Zhao, R.; Xue, J.; Dong, X.S.; Zhi, H.; Chen, J.; Zhao, L.; Zhang, X.; Li, J.; Penzel, T.; Han, F. Screening for obstructive sleep apnea using a contact-free system compared with polysomnography. *J. Clin. Sleep Med.* **2021**, *17*, 1075–1082. [CrossRef]
42. Weinreich, G.; Terjung, S.; Wang, Y.; Werther, S.; Zaffaroni, A.; Teschler, H. Validation of a non-contact screening device for the combination of sleep-disordered breathing and periodic limb movements in sleep. *Sleep Breath.* **2018**, *22*, 131–138. [CrossRef]
43. Jeng, P.Y.; Wang, L.C.; Hu, C.J.; Wu, D. A wrist sensor sleep posture monitoring system: An automatic labeling approach. *Sensors* **2021**, *21*, 258. [CrossRef]

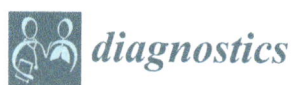

Article

Effect of Plano-Valgus Foot on Lower-Extremity Kinematics and Spatiotemporal Gait Parameters in Children of Age 5–9

Anna Boryczka-Trefler, Małgorzata Kalinowska, Ewa Szczerbik, Jolanta Stępowska, Anna Łukaszewska and Małgorzata Syczewska *

Department Rehabilitation, The Children's Memorial Health Institute, Al. Dzieci Polskich 20, 04-730 Warszawa, Poland; a.boryczka-trefler@ipczd.pl (A.B.-T.); m.kalinowska@ipczd.pl (M.K.); e.szczerbik@ipczd.pl (E.S.); jolanta@stepowscy.pl (J.S.); a.lukaszewska@ipczd.pl (A.Ł.)
* Correspondence: m.syczewska@ipczd.pl

Abstract: Aim of the study was to see how a definition of the flexible flat foot (FFF) influences the results of gait evaluation in a group of 49 children with clinically established FFF. Objective gait analysis was performed using VICON system with Kistler force platforms. The gait parameters were compared between healthy feet and FFF using two classifications: in static and dynamic conditions. In static condition, the ink footprints with Clarke's graphics were used for classification, and in dynamic condition, the Arch Index from Emed pedobarograph while walking was used for classification. When the type of the foot was based on Clarke's graphics, no statistically significant differences were found. When the division was done according to the Arch Index, statistically significant differences between flat feet and normal feet groups were found for normalized gait speed, normalized cadence, pelvic rotation, ankle range of motion in sagittal plane, range of motion of foot progression, and two parameters of a vertical component of the ground reaction force: FZ2 (middle of stance phase) and FZ3 (push-off). Some statically flat feet function well during walking due to dynamic correction mechanisms.

Keywords: children; flat foot; gait; classification; statics vs. dynamics

1. Introduction

A plano-valgus foot is the most common posture deformity among children [1–3]. Despite this fact, there are still neither unambiguous diagnostic criteria of pediatric plano-valgus foot nor commonly agreed foot assessment methods. That is why the prevalence of pediatric flexible flat foot in the literature is rated from a few to ten per cent, and it depends very much on diagnostic methods used, their accuracy, evaluation criteria, children's age, their gender, and weight [4–8]. Assessment methods used by clinicians vary from clinical observation to measurements and imaging techniques both in weight-bearing and no weight-bearing positions or in static and dynamic conditions. Still, the reliability, validity, and accuracy of all these methods are unproven [9–11]. In our previous study [12], when the same feet were assessed using two different methods, one in static condition and one while walking, we found out the significant difference between the classification outcome: 35 feet (out of 100) classified as flat by static method were not flat according to dynamic classification method, and four feet classified as normal according to static method were flat according to the dynamic method.

Nowadays, the plano-valgus foot kinematics assessment methods are gaining importance because they can be used not only for the evaluation of the flat foot posture but also for the assessment of the flat foot performance during walking. Additionally, the influence of the flat foot on the overall gait pattern can be assessed. They seem to be more objective and their results more compatible among researchers. Twomey et al. [13] found increased forefoot supination and medial longitudinal arch (MLA) collapse during walking in children with a flat foot; Caravaggi et al. [14] reported greater hindfoot eversion and its plantarflexion relatively to the tibia, larger MLA collapse, and hallux dorsiflexion throughout most of the stance phase, dorsiflexion, eversion, and abduction of the midtarsal joint and plantarflexion and adduction of the tarso-metatarsal joint. He did not observe any significant forefoot abduction relatively to the hindfoot. Similar to Caravaggi, Saraswat et al. [15] also observed larger hindfoot eversion and plantarflexion together with increased midfoot pronation and dorsiflexion in plano-valgus foot. Similar observation concerning plano-valgus foot during gait was also made by Kerr et al. [16], Kothari et al. [17], and others [18,19].

The human musculoskeletal system is a biomechanical chain; therefore, a pertinent question is whether the plano-valgus foot deformity affects not only foot joints but also upper joints of the lower extremities, pelvis. and lower back [19]. Duval et al. [20] observed that placing a foot in eversion caused subtalar pronation and this resulted in the increased internal knee and hip rotation, while placing a foot in inversion resulted in subtalar supination and increased external knee and hip rotation. However, he did not find any evidence of dependence between increased foot pronation or supination and pelvic anterior or posterior tilt. Opposite results were obtained by Pinto et al. [21]. He stated that both unilateral and bilateral calcaneal eversion obtained using medially tilted wedges resulted in pelvic anteversion. Additionally, unilateral calcaneal eversion caused a lateral pelvic tilt. Svoboda et al. [19] also reported an increase in pelvic anteversion as a result of unilateral and bilateral hindfoot eversion and additionally a significantly higher hip external rotation during the first half of the stance phase with bilateral everted hindfoot. Additionally, a study of Lopez and co-workers [22] found that the foot arch height has a global, negative impact on the quality of life of the schoolchildren, proving the importance of the foot deformities on the overall wellbeing. The similar study done under the same leadership [23] in the adults did not show any dependence between the height of the foot arch and quality of life although another study performed in the adults with foot pathologies showed that they have a worse quality of life than the general population [24].

Taking into consideration the wide range of clinical diagnostic tools and findings concerning the influence of the flat foot on gait pattern, the aim of this study was to see how a definition of the flexible flat foot (FFF) influences gait parameters in children five to nine years of age and if the choice of a diagnostic method of FFF used in the study (in static vs. dynamic conditions) affects its results. The definitions of FFF used in practice differ from each other, which means that the applied method of foot classification influences the assessment of the patient's gait stereotype and the resulting therapeutic management. The importance of the research undertaken is due to the potentially negative impact of foot deformation on the quality of life in adulthood.

2. Materials and Methods

2.1. Patients

Forty-nine children (37 boys and 12 girls) were recruited to the study. Recruitment was carried out in the period of two years during the clinical examination at The Children's Memorial Health Institute in Warsaw, Dept. Rehabilitation, at the Outpatient Clinic. All children fulfilling the criteria were invited to participate. The inclusion criteria were as follows: age from 5 to 9 years and flexible flat foot, clinically established. The exclusion criteria were: rigid flat foot, secondary flat foot caused by the damaged central nervous system (CNS), neuromuscular diseases, lower-limb injury, or surgical intervention in the lower legs in the past. The demographic characteristic of the group is presented in Table 1. The study was approved by the Local Ethical Committee. It was a prospective cohort type study.

Table 1. Demographic characteristics of the group.

	No of Subjects	Median	Minimum	Maximum	10th Percentile	90th Percentile
Height	49	124.5	109.5	140.0	113.0	135.0
Body mass	49	24.0	18.7	39.0	20.5	34.6
BMI	49	16.23	12.62	21.73	14.22	19.19
Age	49	6.41	5.04	10.37	5.24	8.20

Informed consent was obtained from the parents of all children taking part in the study before their enrolment.

2.2. Methods

Figure 1 presents the flow chart of the study.

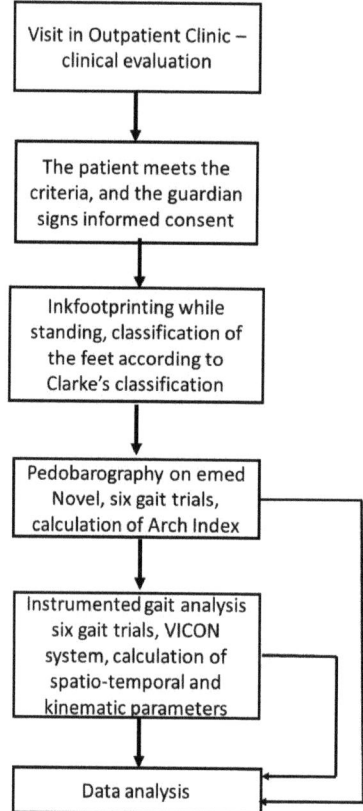

Figure 1. Flow chart of the study.

2.3. Clinical Feet Assessment

Preliminary diagnose of the flexible flat foot was based on a clinical examination conducted independently by an experienced physician and physiotherapist. A foot was defined as flat when, during the examination while standing, the MLA was collapsed, and/or the medial side of the foot was bulging because of the talus head protruding just under the medial malleolus. The heel valgus angle was measured with a goniometer during standing on both feet. It was measured three times, and then, an averaged result was calculated. Flexible flat foot was identified when the MLA rebuilt in non-weight-bearing position and while tiptoe standing.

2.4. Ink Footprints

After the preliminary examination, ink footprints from the Harris and Beath pedograph were obtained, and they were further compared with Clarke's footprinting graphics. A foot was diagnosed as flat if the ink footprint from the Harris and Beath pedograph matched Clarke's footprinting graphics types between 7 and 10. The matching of footprints was performed independently by two experienced examiners, and no discrepancy between their results occurred. The complete description of the examination methodology on the Harris and Beath pedograph is included in the previous study [12].

2.5. Pedobarography

Next, plantar loads during gait were evaluated (Figure 2A). Plantar loads were captured using the emed system (Novel Company) [25]. The complete description of the examination methodology on the emed platform is included in a previous study [12].

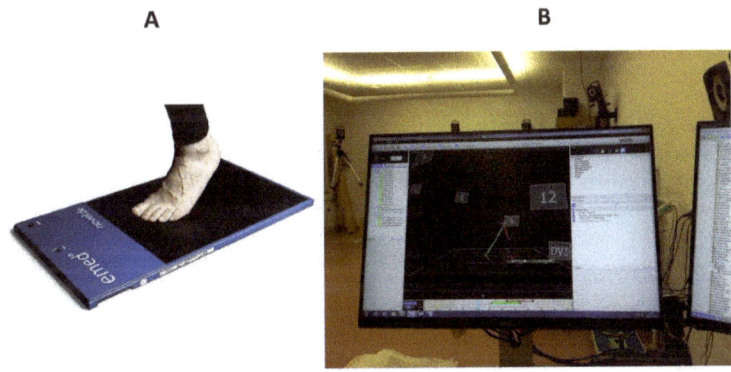

Figure 2. (**A**) Gait trial during pedobarography (photo from Novel's web page www.novel.de, accessed on 28 November 2021). (**B**) Instrumented gait analysis.

Data from three plantar loads of left and three plantar loads of right foot of each child were averaged and taken for further analysis. Geometric measures of the feet (midfoot width, instep width, instep, foot width) were calculated by Novel software. The Arch Index was calculated based on the definition introduced by Cavanagh and Rodgers. The value of Arch Index equal to 0.27 was taken as cut-off value between normal and flat foot.

2.6. Instrumented Gait Analysis

Objective gait analysis was performed using a 12 camera VICON MX System (Figure 2B). The Plug-In-Gait marker set and lower-body model were used. Patients walked with their preferred, self-selected speed several times along the walkway to obtain six technically correct trials, which were later imported to the Polygon software and averaged. The data extracted from the averaged reports were later analysed. Spatio-temporal data were expressed as per cent of the age- and sex-matched reference data [26]. The following parameters were taken into the analysis: gait speed, cadence, step length, step width, stance phase, single-stance phase, pelvic tilt, pelvic range of motion (ROM) in sagittal plane, pelvic obliquity, pelvic range of motion in frontal plane, pelvic rotation, pelvic range of motion in transversal plane, hip flexion at initial contact, hip flexion in terminal stance, hip flexion in swing, pass retract, hip range of motion, hip abduction, hip range of motion in frontal plane, hip rotation in swing, hip range of motion in transversal plane, knee flexion at initial contact, knee flexion in weight acceptance, knee flexion in standing, maximal knee flexion in

Table 2. The gait parameters when the feet were divided according to the ink footprinting. The parameters were summarized by medians and 10th and 90th percentiles. Z—the results of the Mann-Whitney U test, p-level—probability value.

Parameter	Flat Foot Group	Normal Foot Group	Z	p-Level
Normalized gait speed (%) *	75.0 <56.0–100.0>	74.5 <61.5–104.0>	−0.333	0.739
Cadence (%) *	79.0 <68.0–92.0>	81.0 <71.0–94.5>	−0.369	0.711
Step width (m)	0.16 <0.12–0.2>	0.155 <0.13–0.235>	−0.454	0.649
Normalized step length (%) *	93.0 <79.0–115.0>	95.5 <84.0–115.0>	−0.916	0.360
Stance phase (%)	60.6 <58.8–63.2>	61.7 <58.3–64.1>	−0.734	0.463
Single stance phase (%)	39.5 <35.0–43.0>	39.2 <36.6–44.4>	0.006	0.995
Pelvic tilt (deg)	8.0 <2.0–15.0>	10.0 <−0.5–15.5>	−0.340	0.734
Pelvic range in sagittal plane (deg)	3.0 <2.0–5.0>	3.0 <2.0–5.0>	−0.261	0.794
Pelvic obliquity (deg)	0.0 <−3.0–2.0>	0.0 <−3.5–3.0>	0.024	0.981
Pelvic range in frontal plane (deg)	6.0 <5.0–10.0>	6.0 <5.5–8.5>	−0.455	0.649
Pelvic rotation (deg)	0.0 <−2.0–5.0>	0.0 <0.0–4.0>	−0.366	0.714
Pelvic range in transverse plane (deg)	9.0 <5.0–14.0>	8.5 <4.5–12.5>	0.540	0.589
Hip flexion at initial contact (deg)	24.0 <15.0–34.0>	26.5 <16.5–36.5>	−0.309	0.757
Hip flexion at terminal stance (deg)	−13.0 <−22.0–−3.0>	−11.0 <−25.5–−5.5>	−0.170	0.865
Hip flexion in swing (deg)	26.0 <17.0–36.0>	28.0 <18.5–40.5>	−0.449	0.654
Pass retract (deg)	0.0 <0.0–5.0>	3.0 <0.0–5.0>	−0.914	0.361
Hip range in sagittal plane (deg)	38.0 <31.0–46.0>	38.5 <33.5–49.0>	−0.285	0.776
Hip range in sagittal plane (%)	90.0 <76.0–105.0>	92.0 <77.5–116.5>	−0.358	0.721
Hip abduction (deg)	0.0 <−5.0–5.0>	−1.0 <−5.0–4.5>	0.667	0.505
Hip range in frontal plane (deg)	10.0 <6.0–13.0>	10.0 <7.0–13.5>	−0.164	0.870
Hip rotation (deg)	−8.0 <−22.0–14.0>	−7.5 <−15.0–13.5>	−1.644	0.100
Hip range in transverse plane (deg)	20.0 <14.0–35.0>	19.0 <13.5–34.0>	0.434	0.664
Knee flexion at initial contact (deg)	0.0 <−4.0–5.0>	1.0 <−2.5–8.0>	−0.819	0.413
Knee flexion at weight acceptance (deg)	11.0 <5.0–17.0>	11.5 <5.5–21.0>	−0.400	0.689
Knee flexion at midstance (deg)	1.0 <−4.0–5.0>	0.5 <−4.5–7.0>	−0.182	0.856
Max knee flexion at swing (deg)	53.0 <46.0–58.0>	54.0 <48.5–60.0>	−0.673	0.501
Knee flexion in terminal swing (deg)	−5.0 <−11.0–−2.0>	−5.0 <−6.0–−3.0>	−0.772	0.440
Knee range in sagittal plane (deg)	55.0 <47.0–62.0>	55.0 <47.0–64.0>	−0.461	0.645
Ankle flexion at initial contact (deg)	−5.0 <−10.0–0.0>	−4.5 <−9.0–2.0>	0.018	0.985
Max dorsiflexion in swing (deg)	14.0 <8.0–17.0>	14.5 <9.5–18.5>	−0.606	0.544
Max plantarflexion (deg)	−13.0 <−28.0–−2.0>	−17.0 <−20.0–−2.0>	0.434	0.664
Ankle range in sagittal plane (deg)	27.0 <22.0–39.0>	29.0 <21.0–33.5>	−0.109	0.914
Foot progression (deg)	−3.0 <−15.0–8.0>	0.0 <−8.0–13.5>	−0.806	0.420
Range of foot progression (deg)	13.0 <9.0–22.0>	12.5 <9.5–17.0>	0.327	0.743
FZ1 **	104.0 <94.0–120.0>	101.0 <93.5–114.5>	0.891	0.373
FZ2 **	85.0 <71.0–94.0>	82.5 <66.5–94.0>	0.509	0.611
FZ3 **	102.0 <95.0–110.0>	103.0 <98.5–115.5>	−0.685	0.493
FX1 **	9.0 <7.0–13.0>	9.0 <8.0–11.0>	−0.200	0.841
FX2 **	0.0 <0.0–2.5>	0.3 <0.0–3.8>	−0.382	0.702
FY1 **	18.0 <12.0–23.0>	16.5 <11.0–26.0>	0.315	0.753
FY2 **	18.0 <12.0–24.0>	18.0 <14.5–25.0>	−0.806	0.420

* normalized to age matched reference data of healthy children; ** normalized to body weight.

Table 3. The gait parameters when the feet were divided according to the Arch Index from pedobarograhy. The parameters were summarized by medians and 10th and 90th percentiles. The statistically significant differences were marked by bolded font. **Z—the results of the Mann-Whitney U test,** *p*-level—probability value.

Parameter	Flat Foot Group	Normal Foot Group	Z	p-Level
Normalized gait speed (%) *	72.0 <56.0–102.0>	84.0 <61.0–100.0>	2.112	0.035
Cadence (%) *	78.0 <68.0–92.0>	83.0 <72.0–94.0>	2.243	0.025
Step width	0.16 <0.12–0.22>	0.15 <0.13–0.19>	−1.373	0.170
Normalized step length (%) *	90.0 <77.0–113.0>	96.0 <80.0–116.0>	−1.699	0.089
Stance phase (%)	61.0 <59.0–63.8>	60.4 <58.7–62.9>	−0.701	0.483
Single stance phase (%)	39.2 <35.0–43.4>	39.8 <35.5–43.0>	0.430	0.667
Pelvic tilt (deg)	9.0 <2.0–15.0>	6.0 <−2.0–12.5>	−1.756	0.079
Pelvic range in sagittal plane (deg)	3.0 <2.0–5.0>	3.0 <2.0–5.0>	0.653	0.514
Pelvic obliquity (deg)	0.0 <−3.0–2.0>	0.0 <−3.0–3.5>	0.637	0.524
Pelvic range in frontal plane (deg)	6.5 <5.0–10.0>	6.0 <5.0–9.0>	−0.499	0.618
Pelvic rotation (deg)	**0.0 <−2.0–4.0>**	**2.0 <−2.0–5.0>**	**2.128**	**0.033**
Pelvic range in transverse plane (deg)	9.0 <6.0–14.0>	9.0 <5.0–14.5>	0.523	0.601
Hip flexion at initial contact (deg)	26.0 <16.0–35.0>	21.0 <15.0–33.5>	−1.269	0.204
Hip flexion at terminal stance (deg)	−13.0 <−20.0–−5.0>	−14.5 <−27.0–−3.5>	−0.556	0.578
Hip flexion in swing (deg)	28.0 <17.0–37.0>	25.5 <16.5–35.5>	−1.313	0.189
Pass retract (deg)	2.0 <0.0–5.0>	0.0 <0.0–5.0>	−0.241	0.810
Hip range in sagittal plane (deg)	37.5 <32.0–46.0>	38.0 <30.5–45.5>	0.227	0.820
Hip range in sagittal plane (%)	88.0 <76.0–105.0>	90.0 <77.5–108.5>	0.706	0.480
Hip abduction (deg)	0.0 <−5.0–5.0>	0.0 <−5.0–5.0>	−0.726	0.468
Hip range in frontal plane (deg)	10.0 <6.0–14.0>	10.0 <8.0–13.0>	0.819	0.413
Hip rotation (deg)	−8.5 <−30.0–12.0>	−5.0 <−15.0–15.0>	−0.608	0.543
Hip range in transverse plane (deg)	20.0 <14.0–30.0>	21.5 <12.5–43.0>	0.722	0.470
Knee flexion at initial contact (deg)	0.0 <−3.0–5.0>	1.0 <−5.0–5.0>	0.260	0.795
Knee flexion at weight acceptance (deg)	11.5 <5.0–20.0>	11.0 <5.0–16.5>	−0.268	0.789
Knee flexion at midstance (deg)	0.0 <−4.0–7.0>	2.0 <−4.5–9.0>	1.095	0.274
Max knee flexion at swing (deg)	53.0 <46.0–59.0>	53.0 <47.5–59.0>	0.053	0.958
Knee flexion in terminal swing (deg)	−5.0 <−10.0–−2.0>	−5.0 <−13.0–−3.0>	−1.323	0.186
Knee range in sagittal plane (deg)	55.5 <45.0–62.0>	54.0 <46.5–67.5>	0.016	0.987
Ankle flexion at initial contact (deg)	−5.0 <−10.0–0.0>	−3.0 <−12.0–0.0>	0.811	0.417
Max dorsiflexion in swing (deg)	14.0 <9.0–17.0>	13.0 <7.0–18.0>	−0.118	0.906
Max plantarflexion (deg)	−13.0 <−22.0–−2.0>	−17.0 <−28.5–−5.0>	−1.837	0.067
Ankle range in sagittal plane (deg)	**26.0 <21.0–35.0>**	**32.5 <24.0–39.5>**	**3.265**	**0.001**
Foot progression (deg)	−3.0 <−17.0–8.0>	−1.0 <−8.0–11.5>	1.099	0.272
Range of foot progression (deg)	**12.0 <8.0–19.0>**	**15.0 <10.0–25.5>**	**3.265**	**0.001**
FZ1 **	103.0 <93.0–117.0>	104.5 <95.0–122.0>	0.754	0.451
FZ2 **	85.0 <71.0–94.0>	81.5 <68.0–90.0>	−2.101	0.036
FZ3 **	101.5 <94.0–101.0>	105.0 <97.5–116.0>	2.295	0.022
FX1 **	10.0 <7.0–13.0>	9.0 <6.5–10.5>	−1.387	0.165
FX2 **	0.0 <0.0–2.5>	1.0 <0.0–3.8>	1.095	0.274
FY1 **	17.5 <12.0–22.0>	17.5 <11.5–24.0>	0.466	0.641
FY2 **	17.0 <12.0–23.0>	20.5 <12.0–25.0>	1.926	0.054

* normalized to age matched reference data of healthy children; ** normalized to body weight.

4. Discussion

It is commonly believed that flat foot affects walking pattern [14,27]. Although some tests involving children's sport performance showed no difference between children with and without flat foot, the clinical observations show that a great part of flat feet are symptomatic, and more and more researchers find proof that not just symptomatic, but also asymptomatic flat feet do affect function [14,19,28,29]. Such discrepancies between the researchers may be a consequence of different diagnostic methods they use to classify a flat foot for their research. That is why it is also so difficult to compare different study results.

The aim of this study was to investigate how, if at all, a FFF influences gait parameters in children and if a choice of a diagnostic method used to identify FFF affects the results of the gait pattern assessment. We examined spatio-temporal, kinematic, and kinetic parameters of the flat feet and healthy feet in a group of children, using two different classification methods. The main result is the finding that a diagnostic method according to which the flat foot is established has an important impact on the results. The statistically significant differences of gait parameters between healthy and flat feet were found only when the classification was based on the Arch Index in dynamic condition. We decided to use two classification methods because defects in foot posture in static conditions are not always seen in dynamic conditions: in fact, flat foot posture is not always accompanied by the impaired function [12,18,30,31]. In our previous study, it was proven that there is a significant difference between the outcome when classifying the feet in static and dynamic conditions [12]. A great number of feet classified in static conditions as flat feet according to the classification executed in dynamic conditions turned out to be not flat.

Examining the spatio-temporal parameters, we found, as observed also by Carravaggi et al., Lin et al., and Hösl et al. [7,14,18] a statistically significant decrease in walking speed and cadence in children with flat feet in comparison to healthy feet. Lin and co-authors additionally observed a reduction in stride length, which was not the case in our study [7]. Similar results but in adults were found by Levinger et al. [31]. He found a reduction in cadence but, contrary to Lin's study, an increase in stride length.

From other researchers' studies, it is already known that speed is a factor that significantly affects both kinematic and kinetic parameters, such as joint ROM, joints moments, the ground reaction forces [32]. Stansfield et al. in his longitudinal study of gait of healthy children (5–12 years old) stated that walking speed has a greater impact on gait parameters than age [33,34]. He found that a decreased walking speed can cause the decrease in the peak plantar flexion angle.

Regarding the kinematic parameters in this study, a statistically significant decrease in ankle ROM in sagittal plane was observed in children with FFF in comparison to healthy feet. The decrease in the ankle range of motion in a sagittal plane means a weaker push-off during gait and relates to a lower FZ3—a parameter of the vertical component (second maximum) of the ground reaction force during this phase of gait. Similar results were obtained by other researchers [18,31]. Hösl et al. [18] observed a limited hindfoot motion in the sagittal plane, which was probably compensated by increased midfoot dorsiflexion and an excessively mobile hallux during the push-off phase. He also noticed a trend towards lower FZ3 in the symptomatic flat foot together with a reduced gait speed. Remarkably similar results were obtained by Saraswat et al. [15] He observed a reduced ROM in the sagittal plane of an ankle joint in children with flat feet, accompanied by its eversion and plantarflexion. Regarding kinetic parameters, the smaller plantarflexion and outward rotation moment peaks together with smaller power generated by an ankle joint of the FFF were found.

Recently more proofs were found to support the hypothesis that morphology of the flat foot is not always accompanied by its abnormal function [31]. Therefore, maybe we should differentiate between morphological features of flat foot and its influence on the function, i.e., walking. That is why, in our study, we used two methods of flat foot classifications: in static and in dynamic conditions. Using the classification in static conditions, we did not find any statistically significant differences between flat and healthy feet in any functional parameters, i.e., spatio-temporal, kinematic, and kinetics parameters. This finding can lead to the conclusion that examining foot posture in static conditions does not help a clinician to find patients who have real functional walking problems. Sometimes statically flat feet function well during walking because they have the potential of dynamic correction of themselves. Thus, maybe a clinical examination in static conditions should not be the only one while deciding on the treatment. It seems that the dynamic tests, which identify individuals with functional problems, should be the basis for planning the treatment. Children with FFF identified in static conditions who do not have gait impairments should probably be put under observation and not immediately under treatment. A classification done in dynamic conditions identifies children with FF who have walking impairments and really need treatment.

The main limitation of the present study is the relatively low number of patients and the imbalance between female and male participants. This resulted from the fact that the patients were recruited from the outpatient clinic, and all patients who fulfilled the criteria were invited to participate.

In conclusion, the diagnosis of the flat foot based on the evaluation in the static condition and during the clinical assessment seems not be sufficient for decision making about the treatment of pediatric patients with flexible flat foot. One of the main findings from our study is that the gait pattern pathology seen in the gait parameters can depend on the classification method within the same group of patients with clinical problem.

Author Contributions: Conceptualization, A.B.-T., J.S., A.Ł. and M.S.; methodology, A.B.-T., J.S., A.Ł. and M.S.; formal analysis, A.B.-T., E.S., M.K. and M.S.; investigation, A.B.-T., M.K., E.S., J.S. and A.Ł.; data curation, A.B.-T., M.K. and M.S.; writing—original draft preparation, A.B.-T. and M.S.; writing—review and editing, A.B.-T., M.K., E.S., J.S., A.Ł. and M.S.; visualization, M.S.; supervision, M.S.; project administration, A.B.-T. and M.K. All authors have read and agreed to the published version of the manuscript.

Funding: This research received no external funding.

Institutional Review Board Statement: The protocol and the study was approved by Bioethical Committee of The Children's Memorial Health Institute, Warsaw, Poland, agreement 196/KBE/2015.

Informed Consent Statement: Informed consent was obtained from all subjects involved in the study.

Data Availability Statement: The data presented in this study are available in anonymized form on request from the corresponding author. The data are not publicly available due to ethical reasons.

Acknowledgments: The authors would like to thank all the patients and their parents for the agreement to participate in this study.

Conflicts of Interest: The authors declare no conflict of interest.

References

1. Gawron, A.; Janiszewski, M. Płaskostopie u dzieci—Częstość występowania wady a wartości masy i wzrostu odniesione do siatki centylowej. *Med. Sport* **2005**, *21*, 99–110.
2. Puzder, A.; Gworys, K. Ocena występowania zaburzeń statyki kończyn dolnych wśród dzieci z regionu miejskiego i wiejskiego badania pilotażowe. *Kwart Ortop.* **2011**, *4*, 377–385.
3. Radzimińska, A.; Bułatowicz, I.; Strojek, K.; Struensee, M.; Lakomski, M.; Klimczak, K.; Dzierzanowski, M.; Zukow, W. Analysis of the occurrence of foot defects among children grades 1–3 elementary school. *J. Health Sci.* **2014**, *4*, 197–208.
4. Halabchi, F.; Mazaheri, R.; Mirshahi, M.; Abbasian, L. Pediatric Flexible Flatfoot; Clinical Aspects and Algorithmic Approach. *Iran. J. Pediatr.* **2013**, *23*, 247–260.
5. Harris, E.J.; Vanore, J.V.; Thomas, J.L.; Kravitz, S.R.; Mendelson, S.A.; Mendicino, R.W.; Silvani, S.H.; Gassen, S.C. Clinical Practice Guideline Pediatric Flatfoot Panel of the American College of Foot and Ankle Surgeons. Diagnosis and treatment of pediatric flatfoot. *J. Foot Ankle Surg.* **2004**, *43*, 341–373. [CrossRef]
6. Labovitz, J.M. The algorithmic approach to pediatric flexible pes planovalgus. *Clin. Podiatr. Med. Surg.* **2006**, *23*, 57–76. [CrossRef]
7. Chii-Jeng, L.; Kuo-An, L.; Ta-Shen, K.; You-Li, C. Correlating Factors and Clinical Significance of Flexible Flatfoot in Preschool Children. *J. Pediatr. Orthop.* **2001**, *21*, 378–382.
8. Groner, C. Numbers Needed to Treat? The Pediatric Flexible Flatfoot Debate. Available online: https://lermagazine.com/cover_story/numbers-needed-to-treat-thepediatric-flexible-flatfoot-debate (accessed on 20 January 2021).
9. Kerr, C.; Stebbins, J.; Theologis, T.; Zavatsky, A. Static postural differences between neutral and flat feet in children with and without symptoms. *Clin. Biomech.* **2015**, *30*, 314–317. [CrossRef] [PubMed]
10. Evans, A.M. The flat-footed child—to treat or not to treat: What is the clinician to do? *J. Am. Podiatr. Med. Assoc.* **2008**, *98*, 386–393. [CrossRef]
11. Uden, H.; Scharfbillig, R.; Causby, R. The typically developing paediatric foot: How flat should it be? A systematic review. *J. Foot Ankle Res.* **2017**, *10*, 37. [CrossRef]
12. Boryczka-Trefler, A.; Kalinowska, M.; Szczerbik, E.; Stępowska, J.; Łukaszewska, A.; Syczewska, M. How to Define Pediatric Flatfoot: Comparison of 2 Methods: Foot Posture in Static and Dynamic Conditions in Children 5 to 9 Years Old. *Foot Ankle Spec.* **2021**, 1938640021991345. [CrossRef] [PubMed]

13. Twomey, D.; McIntosh, A.S.; Simon, J.; Lowe, K.; Wolf, S.I. Kinematic differences between normal and low arched feet in children using the Heidelberg foot measurement method. *Gait Posture* **2010**, *32*, 1–5. [CrossRef] [PubMed]
14. Caravaggi, P.; Sforza, C.; Leardini, A.; Portinaro, N.; Panou, A. Effect of plano-valgus foot posture on midfoot kinematics during barefoot walking in an adolescent population. *J. Foot Ankle Res.* **2018**, *11*, 55. [CrossRef] [PubMed]
15. Saraswat, P.; MacWilliams, B.A.; Davis, R.B.; D'Astous, J.L. Kinematics and kinetics of normal and planovalgus feet during walking. *Gait Posture* **2014**, *39*, 339–345. [CrossRef]
16. Kothari, A.; Dixon, P.; Stebbins, J.; Zavatsky, A.; Theologis, T. The relationship between quality of life and foot function in children with flexible flatfeet. *Gait Posture* **2015**, *41*, 786–790. [CrossRef] [PubMed]
17. Hösl, M.; Böhm, H.; Multerer, C.; Döderlein, L. Does excessive flatfoot deformity affect function? A comparison between symptomatic and asymptomatic flatfeet using the Oxford foot model. *Gait Posture* **2014**, *39*, 23–28. [CrossRef] [PubMed]
18. Shih, Y.; Chen, C.; Chen, W.; Lin, H. Lower extremity kinematics in children with and without flexible flatfoot: A comparative study. *BMC Musculoskelet. Disord.* **2012**, *13*, 31. [CrossRef] [PubMed]
19. Svoboda, Z.; Honzikova, L.; Janura, M.; Vidal, T.; Martinaskova, E. Kinematic gait analysis in children with valgus deformity of the hindfoot. *Acta Bioeng. Biomech.* **2014**, *16*, 89–93. [PubMed]
20. Duval, K.; Lam, T.; Sanderson, D. The mechanical relationship between the rearfoot, pelvis and low-back. *Gait Posture* **2010**, *32*, 637–640. [CrossRef] [PubMed]
21. Pinto, R.; Souza, T.; Trede, R.; Kirkwood, R.; Eigueiredo, E.; Fonseca, S. Bilateral and unilateral increases in calcaneal eversion affect pelvic alignment in standing position. *Man. J. Ther.* **2008**, *13*, 513–519. [CrossRef]
22. Lopez, D.L.; de Los Prego, M.A.B.; Constenla, A.R.; Saleta Canosa, J.L.; Bautista Casasnovas, A.; Tajes, F.A. The impact of foot arch height on quality of life in 6–12 years old. *Colomb. Med.* **2014**, *45*, 168–172. [CrossRef]
23. Lopez, D.L.; Vilar-Fernandez, J.M.; Barros-Garcia, G.; Palomo-López, P.; Becerro-de-Bengoa-Vallejo, R.; Calvo-Lobo, C. Foot arch height and quality of life in adults: A Stobe Observational Study. *Int. J. Environ. Res. Public Health* **2018**, *15*, 1555. [CrossRef] [PubMed]
24. Lopez, D.L.; Peres-Rios, M.; Ruano-Ravina, A.; Losa-Iglesias, M.E.; Becerro-de-Bengoa-Vallejo, R.; Romero-Morales, C.; Calvo-Lobo, C.; Navarro-Flores, E. Impact of quality of life related to foot problems: A case-control study. *Sci. Rep.* **2021**, *11*, 14515. [CrossRef]
25. Novel Scientific Medical Manual V.2.3. Novel Gmbh. 2012. Available online: https://www.novel.de/products/emed/ (accessed on 28 November 2021).
26. Dusing, S.C.; Thorpe, D.E. A normative sample of temporal and spatial gait parameters in children using the GAITRite electronic walkway. *Gait Posture* **2007**, *25*, 135–139. [CrossRef]
27. Rodriguez, N.; Volpe, R.G. Clinical diagnosis and assessment of the pediatric pes planovalgus deformity. *Clin. Podiatr. Med. Surg.* **2010**, *27*, 43–58. [CrossRef]
28. Tudor, A.; Ruzic, L.; Sestan, B.; Sirola, L.; Prpic, T. Flat-footedness is not a disadvan-tage for athletic performance in children aged 11–15 years. *Pediatrics* **2009**, *123*, e386–e392. [CrossRef]
29. Benedetti, M.G.; Ceccarelli, F.; Berti, L.; Luciani, D.; Catani, F.; Boschi, M.; Giannini, S. Diagnosis of flexible flatfoot in children: A systematic clinical approach. *Orthopedics* **2011**, *34*, 94. [CrossRef] [PubMed]
30. Bertani, A.; Cappello, A.; Benedetti, M.G.; Simoncini, L.; Catani, F. Flat foot functional evaluation using pattern recognition of ground reaction data. *Clin. Biomech.* **1999**, *14*, 484–493. [CrossRef]
31. Levinger, P.; Murley, G.S.; Barton, C.J.; Cotchett, M.P. A comparison of foot kinematics in people with normal- and flat-arched feet using the Oxford Foot Model. *Gait Posture* **2010**, *32*, 519–523. [CrossRef]
32. Van der Linden, M.L.; Kerr, A.M.; Hazlewood, M.E.; Hillman, S.J.; Robb, J.E. Kinematic and Kinetic Gait Characteristics of Normal Children Walking at a Range of Clinically Relevant Speeds. *J. Pediatr. Orthop.* **2002**, *22*, 800–806. [CrossRef]
33. Stansfield, B.W.; Hillman, S.J.; Hazlewood, M.E.; Lawson, A.A.; Mann, A.M.; Loudon, I.R.; Robb, J.E. Normalized speed, not age, characterizes ground reaction force patterns in 5- to 12-year-old children walking at self-selected speeds. *J. Pediatr. Orthop.* **2001**, *21*, 395–402. [CrossRef] [PubMed]
34. Stansfield, B.W.; Hillman, S.J.; Hazlewood, M.E.; Lawson, A.A.; Mann, A.M.; Loudon, I.R.; Robb, J.E. Sagittal joint kinematics, moments, and powers are predominantly characterized by speed of progression, not age, in normal children. *J. Pediatr. Orthop.* **2001**, *21*, 403–411. [CrossRef] [PubMed]

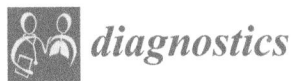

Article

Low-Dose PET Imaging of Tumors in Lung and Liver Regions Using Internal Motion Estimation

Sang-Keun Woo [1,*,†], Byung-Chul Kim [1,†], Eun Kyoung Ryu [2], In Ok Ko [1] and Yong Jin Lee [1]

1. Division of RI-Convergence Research, Korea Institute of Radiology and Medical Sciences, Seoul 01812, Korea; xikian@kirams.re.kr (B.-C.K.); inogi99@kirams.re.kr (I.O.K.); yjlee@kirams.re.kr (Y.J.L.)
2. Center of Magnetic Resonance Research, Korea Basic Science Institute, Ochang 28119, Korea; ekryu@kbsi.re.kr
* Correspondence: skwoo@kirams.re.kr; Tel.: +82-2-970-1659
† These authors contributed equally to this work.

Abstract: Motion estimation and compensation are necessary for improvement of tumor quantification analysis in positron emission tomography (PET) images. The aim of this study was to propose adaptive PET imaging with internal motion estimation and correction using regional artificial evaluation of tumors injected with low-dose and high-dose radiopharmaceuticals. In order to assess internal motion, molecular sieves imitating tumors were loaded with ^{18}F and inserted into the lung and liver regions in rats. All models were classified into two groups, based on the injected radiopharmaceutical activity, to compare the effect of tumor intensity. The PET study was performed with injection of F-18 fluorodeoxyglucose (^{18}F-FDG). Respiratory gating was carried out by external trigger device. Count, signal to noise ratio (SNR), contrast and full width at half maximum (FWHM) were measured in artificial tumors in gated images. Motion correction was executed by affine transformation with estimated internal motion data. Monitoring data were different from estimated motion. Contrast in the low-activity group was 3.57, 4.08 and 6.19, while in the high-activity group it was 10.01, 8.36 and 6.97 for static, 4 bin and 8 bin images, respectively. The results of the lung target in 4 bin and the liver target in 8 bin showed improvement in FWHM and contrast with sufficient SNR. After motion correction, FWHM was improved in both regions (lung: 24.56%, liver: 10.77%). Moreover, with the low dose of radiopharmaceuticals the PET image visualized specific accumulated radiopharmaceutical areas in the liver. Therefore, low activity in PET images should undergo motion correction before quantification analysis using PET data. We could improve quantitative tumor evaluation by considering organ region and tumor intensity.

Keywords: animal model; imaging; rat; radioisotope; respiratory organ

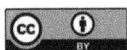

1. Introduction

Positron emission tomography (PET) provides functional images, including biological information, using radiopharmaceuticals emitting positrons. PET system allows imaging of biochemical changes in tumors before morphological changes, unlike anatomical imaging diagnostic methods, such as computed tomography (CT) or magnetic resonance imaging (MRI). The small animal PET scanner is widely used in noninvasive molecular imaging research in the preclinical stage because of its high sensitivity and spatial resolution. However, when the injected radiopharmaceutical activity was low, the PET image quality was also quite low, and was insufficient for detecting specific areas in small animals. However, when performing the clinical study, high injected doses of radiopharmaceuticals were harmful to subjects.

Respiration and cardiac motion induce degradation of image quality and quantity by causing deficiency of count and blurring of lesions during PET acquisition [1]. Accordingly, motion correction is necessary for the improvement of quantitative tumor evaluation and for preventing decline in image quality while acquiring PET images [2]. In order to minimize these repercussions, various motion estimation methods measuring external motion have been introduced. These methods include the detection of pressure variations using pressure sensors, and optical motion tracking systems, such as POLARIS (Northern Digital, Inc., Waterloo, Canada) and the charge-coupled device (CCD) camera [3–5].

Various techniques have been researched to correct for motion due to the cardiac and respiratory cycle. Methods using image registration [1,6,7] and optical flow algorithms [8,9] have been applied to reconstructed images as post-processing stages. Among preprocessing methods, some approaches used system matrix in the image reconstruction period [10–12], and some used rigid or affine algorithms in sinogram correction [13,14]. All the abovementioned methods require estimates of organ motion. Currently, the respiratory gating method is most commonly used for motion correction, and the electrocardiogram (ECG) gating method is used for cardiovascular disease study [14,15].

Previous studies have shown that the gated PET method using an external monitoring device provides motion-corrected images. When the number of gates increases, the acquired image becomes similar to the real shape; but the contrast in the image is reduced by noise increase due to loss of count [16]. The monitoring data do not accurately represent the real organ motion [17]. The lungs and liver are among the organs most influenced by respiration and heartbeat; therefore, motion compensation is important for tumors located near the thoracic abdomen [17].

In this study, we designed the lung and liver motion model imaging with dual cardiac-respiratory gating for regional tumor quantification [18]. We tried to ascertain acute internal motion in PET images with 2-deoxy-2-[^{18}F] fluoro-D-glucose (^{18}F-FDG) by insertion of artificial tumors containing radioactive substances [19]. The purpose of this study was the improvement of quantitative tumor evaluation, depending on the target organ region and tumor intensity, through internal motion estimation and correction using thoracic artificial tumors.

2. Materials and Methods

2.1. Motion Model Preparation

All protocols of this study were approved by the Institutional Animal Care and Use Committee of the Korea Institute of Radiological and Medical Science (KIRAMS 2012-13). This study was performed in accordance with the guidelines of the KIRAMS and the Guide for the Care and use of Laboratory Animals [6]. Eight female Sprague-Dawley (SD) strain rats, aged 6 weeks and weighing approximately 300 g, were employed in these experiments. They were purchased from Harlan Laboratories (Indianapolis, IN, USA). They were quarantined 6 days before surgical procedure. All rats were considered to be in good health on the basis of physical examinations. The rats were housed in a facility approved by KIRAMS and were fed a standard diet. Rats were anesthetized by isoflurane inhalation anesthesia (2% mixed with 100% oxygen by the endotracheal catheter; Foran®, Choongwae Pharma Co., Suwon, Korea) [20]. In order to supply oxygen during open chest surgery, we disinfected the neck region of the rats by povidone—iodine and ethanol. The dedicated small animal ventilator (DJI-101, Daejong Instrument Industry Co., Seoul, Korea) was connected and the catheter was inserted. Temperature was achieved at 30 °C using a plastic pad with a water-filled chamber and an infrared ramp during injection and uptake time.

Rats were divided into 2 groups according to the region planted with the molecular sieve containing radioactive material; one was the lung region group and the other the liver region group. As shown in Figure 1a, the planting surgeries in the lung region were performed inside the opened thorax region. Skin and intercostalis muscle were incised at the right 8th intercostal region, then the incised thoracic wall was expanded using surgical retractor. The molecular sieve was attached on the sternal surface of the right caudal lung lobe. In the liver region group, skin and abdominal muscles were incised at the left cranial abdominal region following the rib line and expanded by retractor. The molecular sieve was inserted into the left medial lobe of the liver. After attachment and insertion of the molecular sieve, incision sites were closed with 4-0 silk suture. The experimental conditions, including warming and anesthesia, were maintained during the entire study period.

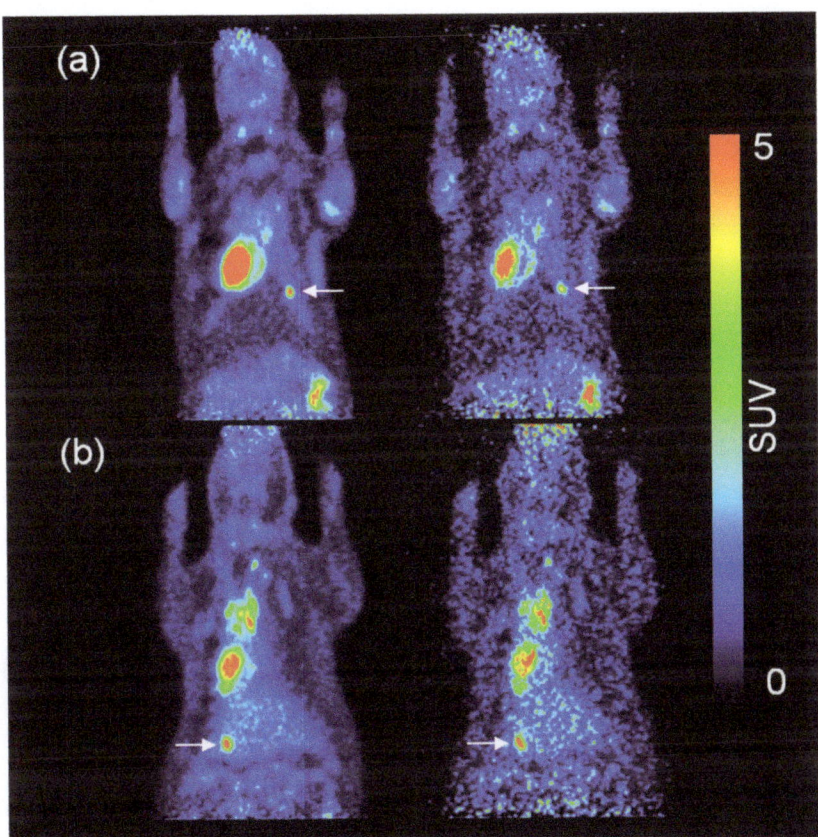

Figure 1. The results of motion correction PET image. (**a**) The left side image represents no motion correction, and the right side is a motion correction image of the lung. (**b**) The left side of the PET image represents no motion correction in liver, and right side represents a motion correction image.

Molecular sieves were immersed in 70% ethanol for one whole day before study and were allowed to absorb ^{18}F on the verge of surgery. We adjusted the absorbed activity level of molecular sieves, and thus classified them into two groups: the high-activity group (about 0.67 MBq) and the low-activity group (about 0.37 MBq). All the molecular sieves were coated with thermoreversible gel (Pluronic® 127F hydrogel) for quantitative estimation [21]. We excluded the models with poor vital conditions, such as respiratory, anesthesia, suture, and ^{18}F-FDG uptake, from the experimental group.

2.2. PET Image Acquisition

All PET images in each region were acquired on a dedicated small animal PET scanner (Inveon™, Siemens Preclinical Solutions, Knoxville, TN, USA), as shown in Figure 1b, after radioactive molecular sieve insertion under anesthesia maintenance. This PET scanner had Lutetium oxyorthosilicate (LSO) with 1.6 mm × 1.6 mm detector pixel spacing. The rats were injected with ^{18}F-FDG (37 MBq in 0.2 mL) via the tail vein. For sufficient FDG distribution in the body, a 60 min uptake period was required following the injection. PET images were obtained as list-mode data for 20 min. Breathing signals were collected from pneumatic sensors attached to the thorax of the rat [22]. Cardiac signals were obtained from

ECG by standard limb lead method. These signals were converted into trigger signals by the external motion monitoring system (BioVet, m2m Imag. Corp., Newark, NJ, USA). The threshold value of the trigger event was determined at systole by R-wave from ECG and inhale state of respiration cycle. The trigger signals simultaneously reflected the motion of the heart and breathing using the dual-trigger method [23]. Each line of response in the list-mode data was converted into sinogram gated various frames (2~16 bin) by a respiratory trigger event and an ECG trigger event, simultaneously. The acquired emission data were reconstructed using Fourier rebinning and ordered subsets expectation maximization 2D (OSEM 2D) algorithm with 4 iterations.

2.3. MRI Data Acquisition

MRI studies were performed using a 3T clinical MRI system (Magnetom Tim Trio, Siemens Medical Solutions, Erlangen, Bavaria, Germany) with a human wrist coil. Coronal 2D MR images were acquired using a T1-FLASH sequence with respiratory triggering and integrated parallel acquisition techniques (iPAT). The parameters were as follows: repetition time = 65.25 ms, echo time = 3.58 ms, flip angle = 12°, slice thickness = 2.5 mm, filter = distortion correction, phase oversampling = 10%, and field of view = 150 mm.

Coronal 3D MRI were acquired using a T1-VIBE sequence with generalized auto-calibrating partially parallel acquisitions (GRAPPA). The parameters were as follows: repetition time = 5.67 ms, echo time = 1.42 ms, flip angle = 10°, slice thickness = 2.11 mm, filter = elliptical filter, phase oversampling = 1%, field of view = 200 mm, and slices per slab = 12.

A tagged MRI study was performed using a 4.7 T MRI system (BioSpec, Bruker Corp., Billerica, MA, USA) with a horizontal bore magnet and a 72-mm birdcage coil. 2D tagged images were acquired at 10 frames per cardiac cycle using a FLASH-cine-tagging sequence with ECG and respiration triggering. The parameters were as follows: repetition time = 115 ms, echo time = 6 ms, flip angle = 20°, slice thickness = 0.8 mm, filter = distortion correction, phase oversampling = 10%, field of view = 150 mm, and matrix = 256 × 256. acquisition time for tagged MRI was 58 min and coronal 3D MRI was 30 min.

2.4. Motion Data Extraction from PET, 2D MRI, and 3D MRI

We analyzed the movement patterns and variations in movement during the respiratory cycle in the thoracic–abdominal region on both PET and MRI. Motion extraction was performed using a mutual information algorithm to register the mean image calculated from the whole image set after the first realignment. A 7-mm Gaussian kernel filter was applied to the PET images for smoothing prior to realignment. For the MRI, we used a 5-mm Gaussian kernel. Motion fields, which were used in motion correction, were estimated from the acquired PET image's in vivo fiducial marker, 3D MRI, and 2D MRI. A 7th degree B-spline interpolation method was implemented to estimate the optimal transformation.

2.5. Motion Correction with PET, 2D MRI, and 3D MRI

We performed an image transformation for the motion correction of the PET data. An affine transformation was performed based on the matrix generated from the motion data [12]. The first frame of the gated PET image was set as the reference, and the other frames were co-registered to it using a transformation derived from the sieve images, 3D MRI, and 2D MRI. These transformations were used to correct the identical PET data in the image space.

A PET image acquired by measured optimal gate number was separated by each bin from the respiratory phase, and each frame of the image was adjusted by the coordinate information based on a mid-exhalation image and a rotation about an axis. A motion-corrected image was acquired from the sum of all transformed phase images.

2.6. PET Image Analysis

All the data were converted into standardized uptake value (SUV) for quantitative analysis [11]. The SUV PET image was visualized using trilinear interpolation. The sensitivity of the image was evaluated on count and signal-to-noise ratio (SNR) by drawn volume of interest (VOI). The VOI for measuring target count was spherical with a diameter of approximately 2 mm^3, and was drawn on the target in the lung and liver region of each image. Background for calculating SNR and contrast was measured from VOI drawn on the surround of target region. SNR and contrast were calculated using the following equation: SNR = (Target count/Background standard deviation) × 100; Contrast = (Target count − Background)/Background.

The spatial resolution was evaluated on a full width at half maximum (FWHM) line profile. The line profile was drawn through the target region in both the horizontal and vertical directions on each image. The FWHMs were measured by Gaussian fitting from line profile. PET image analysis was performed using the Amide's a medical image data examiner software. The results are presented as the mean ± SD (standard deviation).

2.7. Motion Compensation

We performed image transformation for motion correction of the PET data. Affine transformation was operated by matrix generated from motion data [24]. The acquired PET image by measured optimal gate number was separated by each bin from the respiratory phase. Each frame of the image was adjusted by the information of the coordinates, based on the mid-exhale image and the rotation of the axis. The motion-corrected image was acquired from the sum of all transformed phase images.

3. Results

3.1. Small Animal Molecular Sieve PET Imaging

The horizontal and vertical length of the molecular sieve as motion target was 1.50 × 2.50 mm^2. Figure 2 demonstrates the molecular sieve in each region in the obtained static and gated PET images. The SUV of molecular sieves in the high-activity group was more than 7, and in the low-activity group was less than 4. The horizontal and vertical FWHMs of the reference molecular sieve PET image were 1.43 mm and 2.91 mm, respectively.

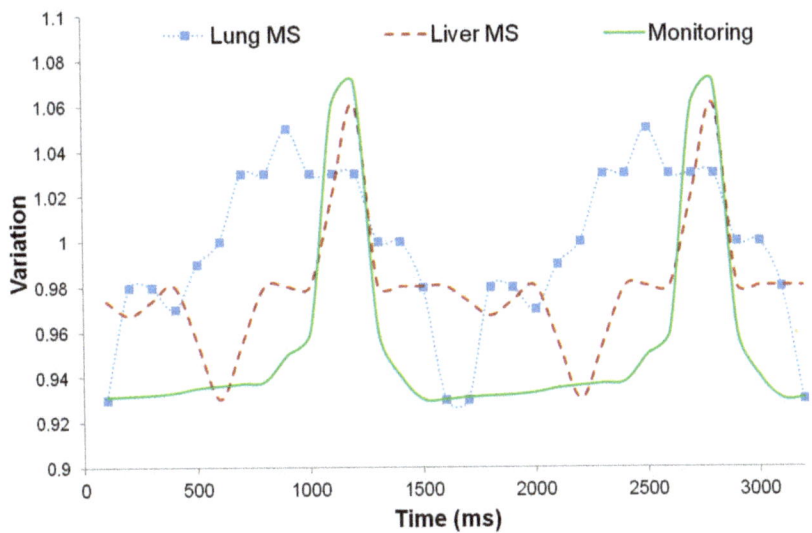

Figure 2. Results of detected motion variation in lung and liver during the PET image acquisition.

The ECG and respiratory phases were simultaneously measured with PET image acquisition. ECG pulse signals of SD-Rats using three electrodes were approximately 200~350 bpm under 2% isoflurane anesthesia after surgery. Respiration signals of SD-Rats using a pneumatic sensor were approximately 25~40 bpm under 2% isoflurane anesthesia after surgery.

3.2. PET, 2D MRI, 3D MRI, and Tagged MRI

The horizontal and vertical lengths of the molecular sieve were 1.50 mm × 2.50 mm. The horizontal and vertical FWHM values of a reference molecular sieve image as a fiducial marker were 1.43 mm and 2.91 mm, respectively. Figure 1 presents images from static PET, gated PET, 3D VIBE MRI, 2D FLASH MRI, and 2D tagged MRI.

3.3. Motion Estimation from PET and MRI Images

Internal and external motion was measured in the lung region. The lung motion data are presented as they varied over the time interval in Figure 2. The internal motion data were measured from a gated PET image of a molecular sieve inserted into the body of a small animal, and the external motion data were measured from a molecular sieve adhered to the skin. Monitoring data measured with an external monitoring device are also presented in Figure 2. The motion data were normalized based on the monitoring data. The results showed that the internal variation in the lung region was on average 30–40% higher than the external variation. On the other hand, the results from the liver region revealed that the internal variation was lower than the external variation. In both regions of the small animals, the monitoring data were different from the internal motion measured directly from the molecular sieve.

The estimated variations in the translations (X, Y, and Z axes) of the lung sieve in the PET image were 2.98, 0.71, and 1.42 mm, respectively. The estimated rotation degrees according to each axis were 0.02, 0.05, and 0.13, respectively. After motion correction using the sieve motion data, the estimated variation in the translations was 0.25, 0.29, and 0.32 mm, respectively. The estimated rotation degrees were 0.01, 0.01, and 0.01, respectively. After motion correction was performed by applying the motion data derived from the 3D MRI, the estimated variations in the translations in the lung PET image were 0.11, 0.08, and 0.21 mm, respectively. The estimated rotation degrees were 0.0051, 0.0012, and 0.0047, respectively. The estimated variations in translations in the lung region using a 2D MRI FLASH sequence were 2.6 and 1.3 mm for the X and Z axes, respectively. The estimated variations using a 2D tagged MRI were 1.9 and 2.3 mm for the X and Z axes, respectively. The results described above are shown as a graph in Figure 3.

3.4. Regional Motion Estimation

We measured internal motion in the thorax abdomen region. The lung and liver motion data are demonstrated through the variation with time intervals in Figure 3. Internal motion data were measured from inserted molecular sieve in small animal body of gated PET image. Monitoring data measured from external monitoring device are also presented in the graph. In both the regions of small animals, monitoring data were different from the internal motion measured directly from molecular sieve.

3.5. Count, SNR, Contrast and FWHM Assessment in PET Image

We performed analysis of PET images by comparison of count, SNR, contrast and FWHM for determining gating effect regarding the organ region and tumor intensity. Figure 4 shows the estimated values of count, SNR and contrast in both the high-activity group and low-activity group in the lung region. Estimated counts (counts/s) in the lung target of the high-activity group were 9.31 ± 0.36, 8.12 ± 0.06, and 7.72 ± 0.09, and in the low-activity group were 3.49 ± 0.32, 3.57 ± 0.45, and 3.27 ± 0.52 for static, 4 bin and 8 bin images, respectively. Evaluated SNRs in the lung target of the high-activity group were 108.07 ± 11.01, 51.69 ± 2.90, and 28.79 ± 0.61, and in the low-activity group were

32.57 ± 1.44, 11.01 ± 2.87, and 8.96 ± 3.75 for the static, 4 bin and 8 bin images, respectively. Evaluated contrasts in the lung target of the high-activity group were 10.01, 8.36 and 6.97, and in the low-activity group were 3.57, 4.08 and 6.19, for static, 4 bin and 8 bin images, respectively (Table 1). Horizontal and vertical FWHMs in the lung target were 1.91 ± 0.17 and 3.11 ± 0.01 in the static image, 1.85 ± 0.22 and 2.58 ± 0.22 in the 4-bin image, and 1.83 ± 0.12 and 2.54 ± 0.18 in the 8 bin images (Figure 5a) (Table 2).

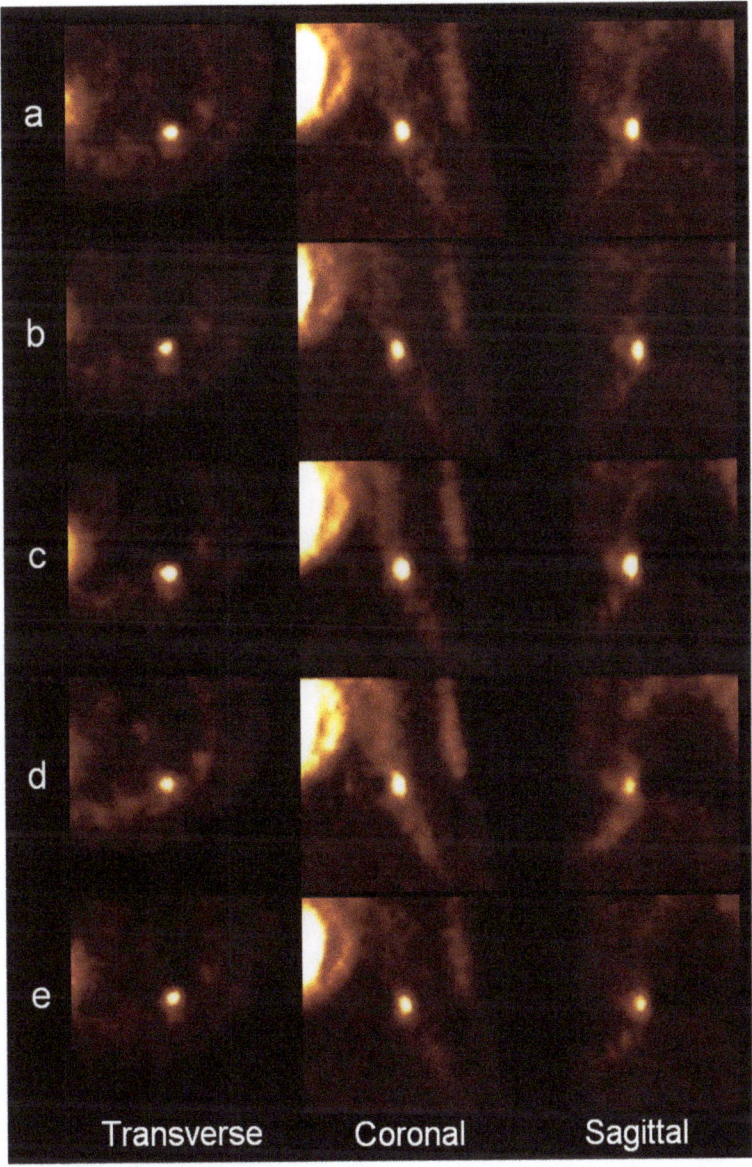

Figure 3. PET images of the molecular sieve in the lung region; (**a**) a static PET image, (**b**) a PET image corrected using a fiducial marker, (**c**) an image corrected using 3D VIBE MRI, (**d**) an image corrected using 2D FLASH MRI, (**e**) an image corrected using a 2D tagged MRI.

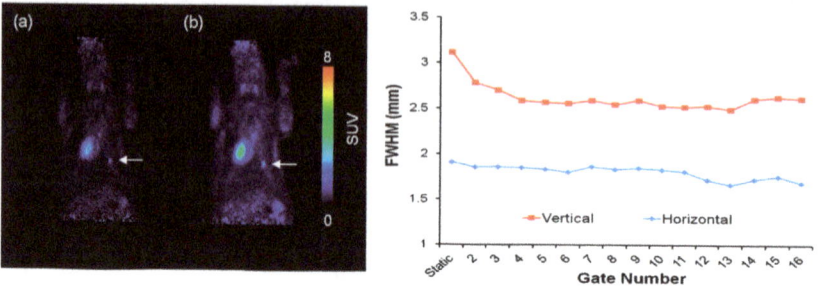

Figure 4. Motion correction PET image and result of FWHM in vertical and horizontal directions in the lung. (**a**) No motion correction PET image, (**b**) motion corrected PET image.

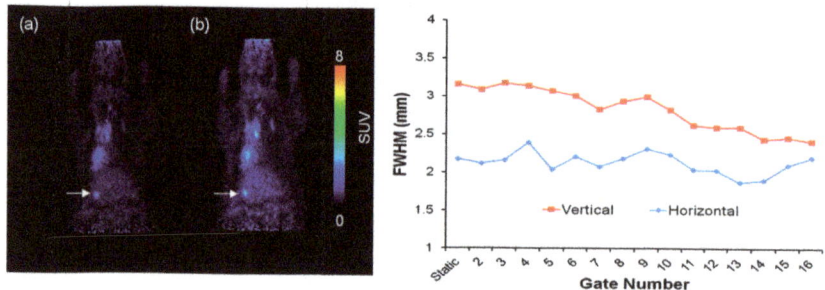

Figure 5. Motion correction PET image and result of FWHM in vertical and horizontal direction of liver. (**a**) No motion correction PET image, (**b**) motion corrected PET image.

Table 1. Estimated count (counts/s) and estimated SNR in lung.

Estimated count (counts/s) in lung	
High-activity group	low-activity group
9.31 ± 0.36	3.49 ± 0.32
8.12 ± 0.06	3.57 ± 0.45
7.72 ± 0.09	3.27 ± 0.52
Evaluated SNR in lung	
High-activity group	low-activity group
108.07 ± 11.01	32.57 ± 1.44
51.69 ± 2.90	11.01 ± 2.87
28.79 ± 0.61	8.96 ± 3.75

Table 2. Horizontal and vertical FWHM in lung.

Static Image	4 Bin Images	8 Bin Images
1.91 ± 0.17	1.85 ± 0.22	1.83 ± 0.12
3.11 ± 0.01	2.58 ± 0.22	2.54 ± 0.18

The result for the liver region exhibited a sharp decline in SNR and improvement in FWHM with the increase in gate number, as with the preceding result of the lung region. Estimated counts (counts/s) in the liver target of the high-activity group were 4.17 ± 0.07, 4.29 ± 0.26 and 4.18 ± 0.18, and in the low-activity group were 2.18 ± 0.06, 2.08 ± 0.08 and 2.13 ± 0.12 for static, 4 bin and 8 bin images, respectively. Evaluated SNR in the liver target of the high-activity group was 40.89 ± 4.89, 18.83 ± 0.50 and 13.52 ± 0.86, and in the low-activity group was 23.52 ± 4.40, 11.49 ± 1.02 and 7.96 ± 0.58 for static, 4 bin and 8 bin images, respectively (Table 3). Horizontal and vertical FWHMs were 2.18 ± 0.06 and 3.16 ± 0.13 in the static images, 2.39 ± 0.13 and 3.14 ± 0.00 in the 4 bin images, and

2.18 ± 0.07 and 2.94 ± 0.19 in the 8 bin images (Figure 5b). The liver region showed a higher slope of fitting line in the vertical FWHM graph (0.0553) when compared to the lung region (0.0177) (Table 4).

Table 3. Estimated count (counts/s) and estimated SNR.

Estimated count (counts/s) in liver	
High-activity group	low-activity group
4.17 ± 0.07	2.18 ± 0.06
4.29 ± 0.26	2.08 ± 0.08
4.18 ± 0.18	2.13 ± 0.12
Evaluated SNR in liver	
High-activity group	low-activity group
40.89 ± 4.89	23.52 ± 4.40
18.83 ± 0.50	11.49 ± 1.02
13.52 ± 0.86	7.96 ± 0.58

Table 4. Horizontal and vertical FWHM.

Static Image	4 Bin Images	8 Bin Images
2.18 ± 0.06	2.39 ± 0.13	2.18 ± 0.07
3.16 ± 0.13	3.14 ± 0.00	2.94 ± 0.19

3.6. Motion Corrected PET Image

Motion correction of small animal PET images was realized by affine transformation. Figure 6 presents images of an artificial tumor in lung region both before and after motion correction. Horizontal and vertical FWHMs were evaluated from each image for comparison, as shown in Table 5. In the lung region, horizontal and vertical FWHMs showed values of 2.04 and 2.63 before correction, and 1.89 and 2.11 after correction. Figure 7 also presents the image of an artificial tumor in the liver region both before and after motion correction. In the liver region, the previously mentioned criteria showed the values of 2.87 and 3.21 before correction, and 2.35 and 2.89 after correction.

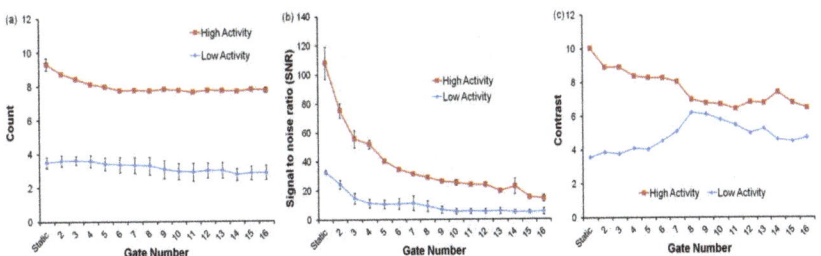

Figure 6. Gate number effects on the (**a**) count, (**b**) SNR, (**c**) contrast in high- and low-activity PET data.

Table 5. Horizontal and vertical FWHM values of an ^{18}F-FDG PET image in the lung region.

FWHM	Uncorrected	PET Motion Correction (Fiducial)	Using 3D MRI Motion Correction (VIBE)	Using 2D MRI Motion Correction (FLASH)	Using 2D MRI Motion Correction (Tagging)
Horizontal	3.39 ± 0.08	3.31 ± 0.22	3.65 ± 0.05	2.99 ± 0.04	2.77 ± 0.06
Vertical	5.03 ± 0.11	4.54 ± 0.26	4.59 ± 0.06	4.51 ± 0.05	4.05 ± 0.08

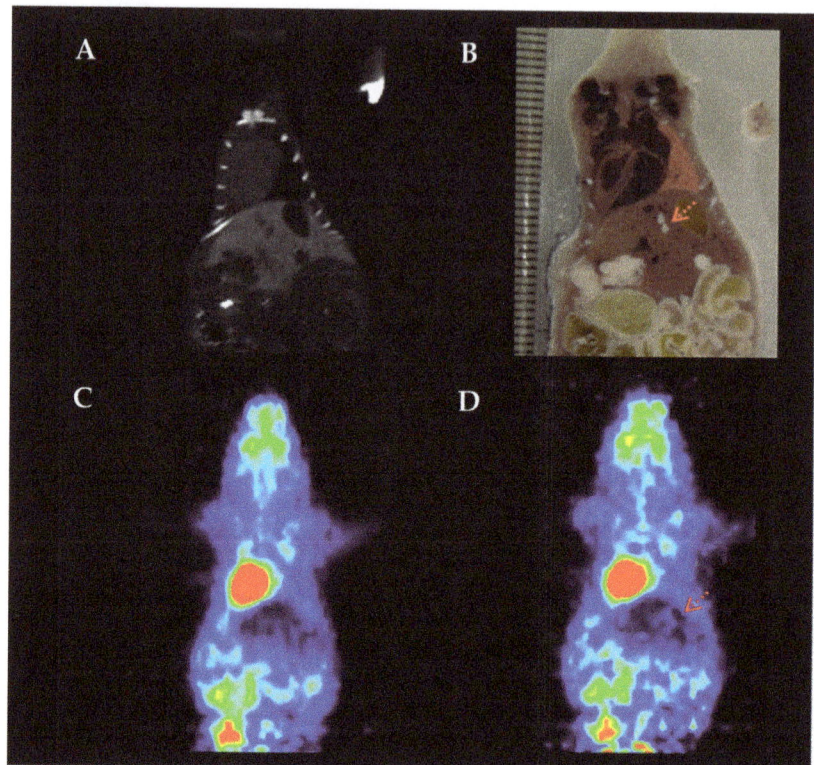

Figure 7. Detection of specific areas in liver. (**A**) Acquired CT data before PET scan, (**B**) Slice section of small animal, (**C**) high-activity PET image, (**D**) low-activity PET image.

4. Discussion

In the present work, we describe region-adaptive tumor evaluation by internal motion estimation for quantitative improvement of PET image [25]. It is hard to estimate real internal motion with conventional methods using external markers or external monitoring devices. Often, a surgical approach is necessary to determine tumor activity and internal motion during PET imaging [15]. Even though the fiducial mark is set by reference value, actual activity is difficult to measure due to the partial volume effect, the scatter effect or the attenuation effect [26]. Therefore, we tried quantitative estimation by surgical planting of artificial tumors of predetermined activity. The internal organ motion of small animals was measured from artificial lesions imitated by molecular sieves in the body. Surgery to insert artificial lesions containing radiopharmaceuticals in the lung and liver regions was performed after anterior thoracotomy. Suture, which followed the insertion, was appropriately performed, and we confirmed the absence of abnormal vital signs similar to preoperative conditions. The ^{18}F adsorbed well into artificial tumors because of the immersion of the molecular sieves in ethanol before the initiation of study, for better enhancement of adsorptive power [27]. The Pluronic F-127 hydrogel that was used as coating material aided the artificial lesion to maintain activity while minimizing variation in the body. Therefore, the count of the target region was four times greater than the count of the organ region even after FDG was distributed completely over the entire body. The quantitative estimation was possible because this count ratio, which meant a high contrast, was indicated in the whole image.

The internal motion data were evaluated from inserted molecular sieves in the lung and liver region, respectively. Upon comparison of the obtained data with the monitoring data, the internal motion data were not identical to the monitoring data as presented in Figure 3. The inserted molecular sieves in the lung and liver regions showed different internal organ motion. Movement patterns of molecular sieves were different between each region. The internal motion in the lung region showed higher variation than the liver region. Monitoring signals presenting only total motion would be a problem for tumor quantification, because each region showed different motion according to the nearest organ.

Gated PET images showed that there was no proportional improvement in the count, SNR and FWHM according to increased number of gates. In fact, a drastic reduction in SNR was observed with increased gate numbers because of the increase in noise due to loss of count. The obtained result exhibited overall improvement in horizontal and vertical FWHM with an increase in gate number.

Molecular sieves were classified into two groups (high and low) based on the amount of activity, which meant artificial tumor intensity. Although SNR was reduced in both groups according to increase gate number, contrast was increased in low-activity groups from 2 bin to 8 bin (Figure 4). The effect of an increase in gate number on the high-activity group was no stronger than the low-activity group; on the contrary, contrast deteriorated continuously in the high-activity group. This result indicates that high gate numbers are not necessary in imaging for terminal tumors or high-intensity tumors, but are essential for low-intensity tumor quantification. Moreover, gating of low-intensity tumors could aid in evaluation of new radiopharmaceuticals, because low-activity substances are mostly used in research and development.

We also recognized that vertical FWHM was more influenced by gate number than horizontal FWHM, because of the movement patterns of thoracic abdomen organs. The movement of lung and liver caused by respiration and heartbeat created a difference between FWHM and actual size of molecular sieve.

The internal motion of lung and liver showed different patterns and variance. Therefore, the gate number for motion correction should be differently set, depending on the organ motion. The vertical FWHM of the liver region showed higher slope when compared to the lung region, from which we concluded that the impact of gating in the liver region was greater than in the lung region. As can be seen in Figures 4 and 5, when the gate number is 4 bin, the result in the lung region shows that count and SNR were appropriately maintained, while improvement in FWHM was observed. However, there was no significant improvement in FWHM when gating more than 4 bin (4 bin: 17.09%, 8 bin: 18.39%). The result for the liver region in 8 bin shows that count and SNR were preserved, while FWHM was sufficiently improved. Gating with few gate numbers in the liver region revealed little change in FWHM improvement in contrast to the lung region (4 bin: 0.57%, 8 bin: 7.02%). This indicated that tumor imaging is needed for at least 8 bin gating in liver region.

Motion correction was executed by affine transformation, as shown in Figure 6. A significant difference was observed from the visible image, and we also confirmed improvement in images evaluated by FWHM. Table 5 presents the details of quantitative improvement in images of each region through motion correction. We ascertained that the motion correction using regional adaptive gate images resulted in better spatial resolution for all the regions. Our preclinical study proposed that in future, the internal motion estimation method could be applied to human clinical studies, which provide the possibility of motion-conjecture modeling without employing any external monitoring systems.

The limitation of this study is that it is difficult to directly observe the motion of internal organs, such as the liver. Molecular sieves were used for indirect observation of internal organs, but the molecular sieves did not settle well in internal organs and moved, making it difficult to observe the organ motion. It is necessary to develop a model that predicts the movement of other internal organs, as well as a breathing model, in order to overcome the limitations of motion correction. In this paper, we described regional adaptive PET image acquisition by internal motion estimation using artificial tumors. Our study demonstrated that a radioactive molecular sieve inserted into the body can be used as an artificial tumor for accurate estimation of internal organ motion. We confirmed the necessity of gating in low-intensity tumor quantification by carrying out a comparative analysis between high- and low-activity groups. Gating in low-intensity tumors could assist in the research of new radiopharmaceuticals. Estimated internal motion revealed differences in movement pattern and variation according to organ region in small animals. Based on this evidence, we could determine the optimal gate number and perform motion correction in accordance with the motion characteristics of each organ. The presented adaptive PET imaging technique based on tumor region allowed us to obtain the regional motion-corrected image, which resolved the disadvantage of gated PET. In consequence, we could quantitatively improve tumor evaluation by considering tumor region and tumor intensity.

In high-dose PET images, the targeted internal organs are clearly visible, but the background is also strongly visible. Because of this, it is difficult to analyze internal organ motion with a severe background, such as the liver. As shown in the results of this experiment, using low-dose PET showed that movement correction was possible not only in the lungs with a moderate background, but also in the liver with a severe background.

Author Contributions: Conceptualization, S.-K.W. and Y.J.L.; methodology, S.-K.W.; software, S.-K.W.; validation, S.-K.W., I.O.K. and Y.J.L.; formal analysis, S.-K.W.; investigation, S.-K.W.; resources, Y.J.L. and E.K.R.; data curation, S.-K.W.; writing—original draft preparation, S.-K.W.; writing—review and editing, B.-C.K.; visualization, I.O.K.; supervision, S.-K.W.; project administration, S.-K.W.; funding acquisition, S.-K.W. All authors have read and agreed to the published version of the manuscript.

Funding: This work was supported by the National Research Foundation of Korea (NRF) grant funded by the Korea government (Ministry of Science and ICT) (No. 2020M2D9A1094070, No. 2019M2D2A1A02057204).

Institutional Review Board Statement: All protocols of this study were approved by the Institutional Animal Care and Use Committee of the Korea Institute of Radiological and Medical Science (KIRAMS 2012-13).

Informed Consent Statement: Informed consent was obtained from all subjects involved in the study.

Data Availability Statement: Data sharing not applicable.

Conflicts of Interest: The authors declare no conflict of interest.

References

1. Lu, Y.; Fontaine, K.; Mulnix, T.; Onofrey, J.A.; Ren, S.; Panin, V.; Jones, J.; Casey, M.E.; Barnett, R.; Kench, P.; et al. Respiratory motion compensation for PET/CT with motion information derived from matched attenuation-corrected gated PET data. *J. Nucl. Med.* **2018**, *59*, 1480–1486. [CrossRef]
2. Holman, B.F.; Cuplov, V.; Millner, L.; Endozo, R.; Maher, T.M.; Groves, A.M.; Hutton, B.F.; Thielemans, K. Improved quantitation and reproducibility in multi-PET/CT lung studies by combining CT information. *EJNMMI Phys.* **2018**, *5*, 14. [CrossRef]
3. Mizuno, H.; Saito, O.; Tajiri, M.; Kimura, T.; Kuroiwa, D.; Shirai, T.; Inaniwa, T.; Fukahori, M.; Miki, K.; Fukuda, S. Commissioning of a respiratory gating system involving a pressure sensor in carbon-ion scanning radiotherapy. *J. Appl. Clin. Med. Phys.* **2019**, *20*, 37–42. [CrossRef]
4. LoPresti, P.G.; Finn, W.E. Fiber-optic sensor system for rapid positioning of a microelectrode array. *Appl. Opt.* **1998**, *37*, 3426–3431. [CrossRef] [PubMed]
5. Hurley, S.; Spangler-Bickell, M.; Deller, T.; Bradshaw, T.; Jansen, F.; McMillan, A. Data-driven rigid motion correction of PET brain images using list mode reconstruction. *J. Nucl. Med.* **2019**, *60* (Suppl. 1), 1358.
6. Guo, R.; Petibon, Y.; Ma, Y.; El Fakhri, G.; Ying, K.; Ouyang, J. MR-based motion correction for cardiac PET parametric imaging: A simulation study. *EJNMMI Phys.* **2018**, *5*, 3. [CrossRef]
7. Luengo Morato, Y.; Ovejero Paredes, K.; Lozano Chamizo, L.; Marciello, M.; Filice, M. Recent Advances in Multimodal Molecular Imaging of Cancer Mediated by Hybrid Magnetic Nanoparticles. *Polymers* **2021**, *13*, 2989. [CrossRef]
8. Meier, J.G.; Wu, C.C.; Cuellar, S.L.B.; Truong, M.T.; Erasmus, J.J.; Einstein, S.A.; Mawlawi, O.R. Evaluation of a novel elastic respiratory motion correction algorithm on quantification and image quality in abdominothoracic PET/CT. *J. Nucl. Med.* **2019**, *60*, 279–284. [CrossRef]

9. Lehtonen, E.; Teuho, J.; Koskinen, J.; Jafari Tadi, M.; Klén, R.; Siekkinen, R.; Rives Gambin, J.; Vasankari, T.; Saraste, A. A Respiratory Motion Estimation Method Based on Inertial Measurement Units for Gated Positron Emission Tomography. *Sensors* **2021**, *21*, 3983. [CrossRef] [PubMed]
10. Ippoliti, M.; Lukas, M.; Brenner, W.; Schatka, I.; Furth, C.; Schaeffter, T.; Makowski, M.R.; Kolbitsch, C. Respiratory motion correction for enhanced quantification of hepatic lesions in simultaneous PET and DCE-MR imaging. *Phys. Med. Biol.* **2021**, *66*, 095012. [CrossRef]
11. Zhong, Y.; Kalantari, F.; Zhang, Y.; Shao, Y.; Wang, J. Quantitative 4D-PET reconstruction for small animal using SMEIR-reconstructed 4D-CBCT. *IEEE Trans. Radiat. Plasma Med. Sci.* **2018**, *2*, 300–306. [CrossRef] [PubMed]
12. Munoz, C.; Kunze, K.P.; Neji, R.; Vitadello, T.; Rischpler, C.; Botnar, R.M.; Nekolla, S.G.; Prieto, C. Motion-corrected whole-heart PET-MR for the simultaneous visualisation of coronary artery integrity and myocardial viability: An initial clinical validation. *Eur. J. Nucl. Med. Mol. Imaging* **2018**, *45*, 1975–1986. [CrossRef]
13. Fuin, N.; Catalano, O.A.; Scipioni, M.; Canjels, L.P.; Izquierdo-Garcia, D.; Pedemonte, S.; Catana, C. Concurrent respiratory motion correction of abdominal PET and dynamic contrast-enhanced–MRI using a compressed sensing approach. *J. Nucl. Med.* **2018**, *59*, 1474–1479. [CrossRef] [PubMed]
14. Munoz, C.; Neji, R.; Kunze, K.P.; Nekolla, S.G.; Botnar, R.M.; Prieto, C. Respiratory-and cardiac motion-corrected simultaneous whole-heart PET and dual phase coronary MR angiography. *Magn. Reson. Med.* **2019**, *81*, 1671–1684. [CrossRef]
15. Kyme, A.Z.; Fulton, R.R. Motion estimation and correction in SPECT, PET and CT. *Phys. Med. Biol.* **2021**, *66*, 18TR02. [CrossRef]
16. Jaudet, C.; Filleron, T.; Weyts, K.; Didierlaurent, D.; Vallot, D.; Ouali, M.; Zerdoud, S.; Dierickx, O.L.; Caselles, O.; Courbon, F. Gated 18F-FDG PET/CT of the lung using a respiratory spirometric gating device: A feasibility study. *J. Nucl. Med. Technol.* **2019**, *47*, 227–232. [CrossRef] [PubMed]
17. Wang, S.; Shang, D.; Meng, X.; Sun, X.; Ma, Y.; Yu, J. Effects of respiratory motion on volumetric and positional difference of GTV in lung cancer based on 3DCT and 4DCT scanning. *Oncol. Lett.* **2019**, *17*, 2388–2392. [CrossRef]
18. Nuvoli, S.; Fiore, V.; Babudieri, S.; Galassi, S.; Bagella, P.; Solinas, P.; Spanu, A.; Madeddu, G. The additional role of 18F-FDG PET/CT in prosthetic valve endocarditis. *Eur. Rev. Med. Pharmacol. Sci.* **2018**, *22*, 1744–1751. [PubMed]
19. Avella, D.M.; Manjunath, Y.; Singh, A.; Deroche, C.B.; Kimchi, E.T.; Staveley-O'Carroll, K.F.; Mitchem, J.B.; Kwon, E.; Li, G.; Kaifi, J.T. 18F-FDG PET/CT total lesion glycolysis is associated with circulating tumor cell counts in patients with stage I to IIIA non-small cell lung cancer. *Transl. Lung Cancer Res.* **2020**, *9*, 515. [CrossRef] [PubMed]
20. Mirus, M.; Tokalov, S.V.; Abramyuk, A.; Heinold, J.; Prochnow, V.; Zöphel, K.; Kotzerke, J.; Abolmaali, N. Noninvasive assessment and quantification of tumor vascularization using [18F] FDG-PET/CT and CE-CT in a tumor model with modifiable angiogenesis—An animal experimental prospective cohort study. *EJNMMI Res.* **2019**, *9*, 55. [CrossRef]
21. Nie, S.; Hsiao, W.W.; Pan, W.; Yang, Z. Thermoreversible Pluronic® F127-based hydrogel containing liposomes for the controlled delivery of paclitaxel: In vitro drug release, cell cytotoxicity, and uptake studies. *Int. J. Nanomed.* **2011**, *6*, 151.
22. Robin, P.; Bourhis, D.; Bernard, B.; Abgral, R.; Querellou, S.; Duc-Pennec, L.; Le Roux, P.-Y.; Salaün, P.-Y. Feasibility of Systematic Respiratory-Gated Acquisition in Unselected Patients Referred for 18F-Fluorodeoxyglucose Positron Emission Tomography/Computed Tomography. *Front. Med.* **2018**, *5*, 36. [CrossRef] [PubMed]
23. Manber, R.; Thielemans, K.; Hutton, B.F.; Wan, S.; Fraioli, F.; Barnes, A.; Ourselin, S.; Arridge, S.; Atkinson, D. Clinical impact of respiratory motion correction in simultaneous PET/MR, using a joint PET/MR predictive motion model. *J. Nucl. Med.* **2018**, *59*, 1467–1473. [CrossRef] [PubMed]
24. Petibon, Y.; Sun, T.; Han, P.; Ma, C.; El Fakhri, G.; Ouyang, J. MR-based cardiac and respiratory motion correction of PET: Application to static and dynamic cardiac 18F-FDG imaging. *Phys. Med. Biol.* **2019**, *64*, 195009. [CrossRef]
25. Yu, J.W.; Woo, S.-K.; Lee, Y.J.; Kim, J.S.; Lee, K.C.; Kim, M.H.; Ji, Y.H.; Kang, J.H.; Kim, B.I.; Choi, C.W. Region adaptive PET gating using internal motion estimation. In Proceedings of the 2011 IEEE Nuclear Science Symposium Conference Record, Valencia, Spain, 23–29 October 2011; pp. 2948–2951.
26. Cherry, S.R.; Sorenson, J.A.; Phelps, M.E. *Physics in Nuclear Medicine*, 4th ed.; Elsevier Health Sciences, 2012. Available online: https://www.sciencedirect.com/book/9781416051985/physics-in-nuclear-medicine#book-info (accessed on 14 November 2021).
27. Wagener, K.; Worm, M.; Pektor, S.; Schinnerer, M.; Thiermann, R.; Miederer, M.; Frey, H.; Rösch, F. Comparison of linear and hyperbranched polyether lipids for liposome shielding by 18F-radiolabeling and positron emission tomography. *Biomacromolecules* **2018**, *19*, 2506–2516. [CrossRef]

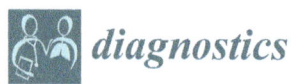

Article

Automated Motion Analysis of Bony Joint Structures from Dynamic Computer Tomography Images: A Multi-Atlas Approach

Benyameen Keelson [1,2,3,*], Luca Buzzatti [4], Jakub Ceranka [2,3], Adrián Gutiérrez [1], Simone Battista [5], Thierry Scheerlinck [6], Gert Van Gompel [1], Johan De Mey [1], Erik Cattrysse [4], Nico Buls [1] and Jef Vandemeulebroucke [1,2,3]

[1] Department of Radiology, Vrije Universiteit Brussel (VUB), Universitair Ziekenhuis Brussel (UZ Brussel), 1090 Brussels, Belgium; Adrian.Gutierrez@uzbrussel.be (A.G.); Gert.VanGompel@uzbrussel.be (G.V.G.); johan.demey@uzbrussel.be (J.D.M.); Nico.Buls@uzbrussel.be (N.B.); jefvdmb@etrovub.be (J.V.)
[2] Department of Electronics and Informatics (ETRO), Vrije Universiteit Brussel (VUB), 1050 Brussels, Belgium; jceranka@etrovub.be
[3] IMEC, Kapeldreef 75, B-3002 Leuven, Belgium
[4] Department of Physiotherapy, Human Physiology and Anatomy (KIMA), Vrije Universiteit Brussel (VUB), Vrije Universiteit, 1090 Brussel, Belgium; luca.buzzatti@vub.be (L.B.); Erik.Cattrysse@vub.be (E.C.)
[5] Department of Neurosciences, Rehabilitation, Ophthalmology, Genetics, Maternal and Child Health, Campus of Savona, University of Genova, 17100 Savona, Italy; simone.battista@edu.unige.it
[6] Department of Orthopaedic Surgery and Traumatology, Vrije Universiteit Brussel (VUB), Universitair Ziekenhuis Brussel (UZ Brussel), 1090 Brussels, Belgium; Thierry.Scheerlinck@uzbrussel.be
* Correspondence: bkeelson@etrovub.be

Citation: Keelson, B.; Buzzatti, L.; Ceranka, J.; Gutiérrez, A.; Battista, S.; Scheerlinck, T.; Van Gompel, G.; De Mey, J.; Cattrysse, E.; Buls, N.; et al. Automated Motion Analysis of Bony Joint Structures from Dynamic Computer Tomography Images: A Multi-Atlas Approach. *Diagnostics* **2021**, *11*, 2062. https://doi.org/10.3390/diagnostics11112062

Academic Editor: Carlo Ricciardi

Received: 18 August 2021
Accepted: 2 November 2021
Published: 7 November 2021

Publisher's Note: MDPI stays neutral with regard to jurisdictional claims in published maps and institutional affiliations.

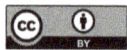

Copyright: © 2021 by the authors. Licensee MDPI, Basel, Switzerland. This article is an open access article distributed under the terms and conditions of the Creative Commons Attribution (CC BY) license (https://creativecommons.org/licenses/by/4.0/).

Abstract: Dynamic computer tomography (CT) is an emerging modality to analyze in-vivo joint kinematics at the bone level, but it requires manual bone segmentation and, in some instances, landmark identification. The objective of this study is to present an automated workflow for the assessment of three-dimensional in vivo joint kinematics from dynamic musculoskeletal CT images. The proposed method relies on a multi-atlas, multi-label segmentation and landmark propagation framework to extract bony structures and detect anatomical landmarks on the CT dataset. The segmented structures serve as regions of interest for the subsequent motion estimation across the dynamic sequence. The landmarks are propagated across the dynamic sequence for the construction of bone embedded reference frames from which kinematic parameters are estimated. We applied our workflow on dynamic CT images obtained from 15 healthy subjects on two different joints: thumb base ($n = 5$) and knee ($n = 10$). The proposed method resulted in segmentation accuracies of 0.90 ± 0.01 for the thumb dataset and 0.94 ± 0.02 for the knee as measured by the Dice score coefficient. In terms of motion estimation, mean differences in cardan angles between the automated algorithm and manual segmentation, and landmark identification performed by an expert were below 1°. Intraclass correlation (ICC) between cardan angles from the algorithm and results from expert manual landmarks ranged from 0.72 to 0.99 for all joints across all axes. The proposed automated method resulted in reproducible and reliable measurements, enabling the assessment of joint kinematics using 4DCT in clinical routine.

Keywords: dynamic CT; motion analysis; musculoskeletal imaging; registration; segmentation; multi-atlas segmentation

1. Introduction

Musculoskeletal (MSK) conditions are a leading cause of disability in four of the six World Health Organization regions [1] and a major contributor to years lived with disability (YLD) [2]. MSK diseases affect more than one out of every two persons in the United States age 18 and older and nearly three out of four age 65 and older [3]. For instance, patellar instability, which is a disease where the patella bone dislocates out from the patellofemoral joint, accounts for 3% of all knee injuries [4]. Patients with this condition can have debilitating pain, which can limit basic function, and develop long term arthritis overtime. Understanding the complexity of such conditions and improving the results of therapeutic interventions remains a challenge. Combining kinematic information of joints with detailed analysis of joint anatomy can provide useful insight and help therapeutic decision making. X-ray imaging techniques and their quantitative analysis are helpful to better understand and manage some MSK conditions, but the 2D nature of the images make detailed kinematic analysis challenging [5]. Dynamic computer tomography (4D-CT) enables acquisition of a series of high temporal-resolution 3D CT datasets of moving structures. Various phantom studies [6–9] demonstrated the validity and feasibility of dynamic CT for evaluating MSK diseases. Several patient studies have been conducted investigating different joint disorders of the wrist, knee, hip, shoulder and foot [10–12]. However, the accurate and reproducible detection of joint motion or subtle changes over time in clinical routine requires image analysis procedures such as image registration. This refers to the estimation of a spatial transformation which aligns a reference image and a corresponding target image.

Currently, few computer-aided diagnostic tools are available for dynamic MSK image data analysis, thus limiting the clinical applicability of quantitative motion analysis from these images. Reasons for this include the complexity and heterogeneity of the musculoskeletal system and the associated challenges in motion estimation of these structures. MSK structures can move with respect to each other, and motion can therefore not be assessed using a global rigid registration. Moreover, in most applications of dynamic MSK imaging, the piece-wise rigid motion of the individual bones is of primary interest for extracting kinematic parameters. The principal challenges for non-rigid registration are the magnitude and complexity of osteoarticular motion, often also including sliding structures, leading to poor accuracies or implausible deformation [13]. Block matching techniques have been proposed to improve robustness [14,15]. Several authors have proposed methods to account for sliding motion [16,17], but most rely on prior segmentations of bones of interest. Motion estimation of MSK structures is therefore commonly performed using prior manual segmentations of the bony structures, limiting registration to a region of interest and obtaining individual bone motion to facilitate estimation of kinematics [6,8]. However, manual bone segmentation is labor intensive and hinders application in clinical routine.

D'Agostino et al. [18] made use of image registration in estimating kinematics of the thumb to study the Screw-home mechanism. They investigated extreme positions (i.e., maximal Ex–Fl and maximal Ab–Ad) by means of an iterative closest-point algorithm. Their approach required manual segmentations of each bone for each position to generate 3D surface models. Such an approach can be labor intensive when analyzing dynamic sequences of multiple time frames or bone positions. Furthermore, the quantitative description of joint kinematics requires the reconstruction of the bone positions and orientation relative to a laboratory reference frame [19]. Skeletal anatomic landmarks help to provide what is known as bone-embedded reference frames. This determines the estimated motion of the joints in relation to anatomical axes defined on the bones. The manual identification of these anatomical landmarks on the CT images can also be a labor-intensive step. A few algorithms for automatic localization of skeletal landmarks have been proposed in literature [20–22]. Techniques based on machine learning algorithms which learn distinctive image features on annotated data have also been presented [22]. These techniques usually require a significant amount of annotated data to yield good results. In general, most of these approaches detect geometrical features that match the shape properties of these landmarks [20,23]. However, none of these approaches have been applied for the computation of kinematics from dynamic images.

In this work, we propose an automated framework for motion estimation of bony structures obtained from dynamic CT acquisitions. Changes in joint functionality are of diagnostic importance, the proposed automated workflow can help in quantitatively monitoring joint health as well as the impact of therapeutic interventions.

2. Materials and Methods

2.1. Subject Recruitment

After approval from our institution's Medical Ethics Committee (B.U.N 143201733617) and written informed consent, 15 healthy volunteers (7 females, 8 males) were recruited to participate in this dynamic CT study. Ages of participants ranged from (22 to 36). Five subjects (3 females, 2 males) had a CT scan of the thumb, and 10 subjects (4 females, 6 males) had a CT scan of one of the knees. To be eligible for the study, participants should not have reported joint pain in the previous 6 months prior to the study.

2.2. CT Acquisitions

All images were acquired with a clinical 256-slice Revolution CT (GE Healthcare, Waukesha, WI, USA). The dynamic acquisition protocol consisted of low-dose images (effective dose < 0.02 mSv) obtained in cine mode. Volunteers were instructed to perform cyclic joint movements: opposition-reposition movement of the thumb ($n = 5$) and flexion-extension of the knee ($n = 10$). Static scans were also acquired of each joint without motion (Figure 1). Thumb base images were acquired with the patient sitting with a 90-degree flexed elbow, with the thumb directed upwards and the forearm in a neutral rotation. Images of the knee were acquired in full extension. The dynamic scans were acquired with a tube rotation time of 0.28 s and a total dynamic acquisition time of 6 s. This generated 15 timeframes, each composed of a 3D CT dataset. Videos of the dynamic images are available as Supplementary Data (Video S1 and S2). Details of the scan parameters are shown in Table 1. In each dynamic dataset, an image with the joint in a position similar to the static scans was selected as reference image. The selected reference image served as the input to the multi-atlas segmentation step.

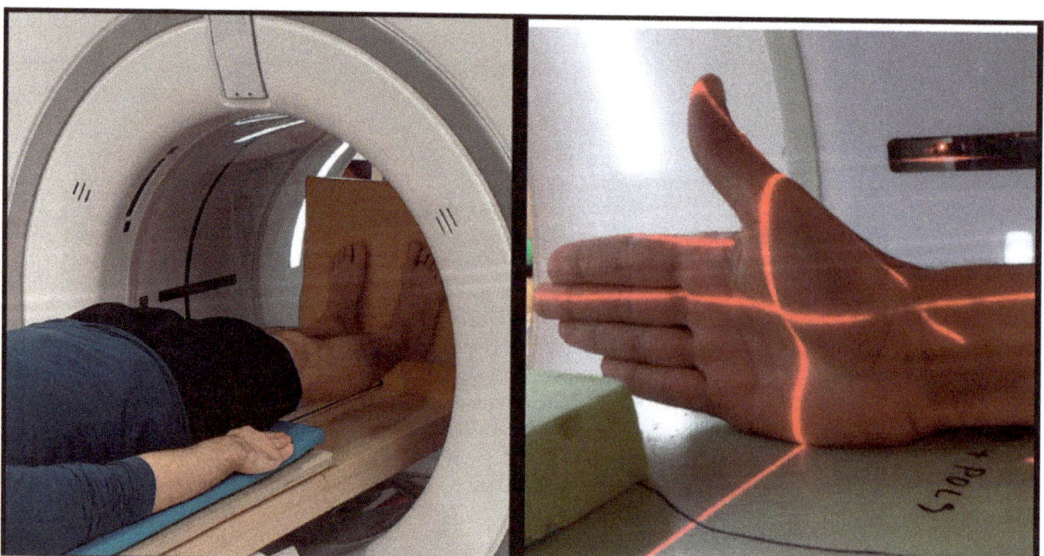

Figure 1. The figure shows the positioning in the gantry of the CT.

Table 1. Overview of scan parameters for the dynamic and static acquisitions.

	Dynamic Acquisition	Static Acquisitions
Knee		
Tube Voltage	80 kV	120 kV
Tube current	50 mA	80 mA
Tube rotation time	0.28 s	0.28 s
Reconstructed slice thickness	2.5 mm	2.5 mm
Field of View	500 mm	500 mm
Collimation	256 × 0.625 mm	256 × 0.625 mm
Dose length product	107.91 mGycm	23.06 mGycm
* CTDI	6.74 mGy	1.44 mGy
Thumb		
Tube Voltage	80 kV	120 kV
Tube current	50 mA	80 mA
Tube rotation time	0.28 s	0.28 s
Reconstructed slice thickness	1.25 mm	1.25 mm
Field of View	300 mm	300 mm
Collimation	192 × 0.625 mm	192 × 0.625 mm
Dose length product	156.45 mGycm	19.58 mGycm
CTDI	13 mGy	1.63 mGy

* Computed tomography dose index.

2.3. Atlas Dataset

Atlases of the thumb base and knee were created based on the static CT scan datasets. Manual bone segmentations were performed in collaboration with an expert in bone anatomy using ITKSnap's [24] active contour mode, followed by morphological operations and manual refinement. The patella, femur and tibia were segmented for the knee images. First, metacarpal bone and the trapezium were segmented for the thumb base. For each joint we created two separate left and right atlases. As the knee datasets were obtained with both legs in the gantry, we used an automated post-processing step for axis of symmetry detection and splitting, to separate the left from the right sides. For each dataset, a total of 9 anatomical landmarks were manually identified on the bones of interest by three expert readers. The expert readers had varying levels of expertise and training. "Reader 1" was a physiotherapist and musculoskeletal radiology research fellow with 6 years of experience, "reader 2" was an orthopedic surgeon with 30 years of experience and "reader 3" was an orthopedic surgeon specialized in hand, wrist and upper limb pathology with 4 years of experience. The mean of landmarks identified by all readers were used in the creation of the atlas anatomical landmarks for the automated algorithm.

2.4. Multi-Atlas Segmentation

The multi-atlas segmentation (MAS) consisted of a three-step process: (1) a pairwise registration of the image to be segmented (reference image) to the set of atlases to find optimal transformations that align each atlas to the reference image, (2) the propagation of the atlas labels onto the reference image using the corresponding transformations from step 1, and (3) a fusion step which combines all labels into a single final segmentation.

The pairwise registration step can be mathematically represented by the optimization problem below

$$\hat{\mu} = \operatorname*{argmin}_{\mu} C\big(f(x), g_n\big((T_\mu(x))\big)\big) \tag{1}$$

where f represents the reference image to be segmented, g_n is the individual atlas images and x is the spatial coordinate over the image. T is the sought spatial transformation with parameters μ which aligns the two images. The cost function C is composed of a similarity metric and (in the case of deformable registration) a regularization penalty.

We implemented a three-stage registration process employing a rigid, affine and a deformable transform based on free-form deformations using cubic B-Splines [25]. Each stage was initialized from the previous solution. We also investigated different similarity metrics for the pairwise registration (normalized cross correlation (NCC), mean squared difference (MSD) and mutual information (MI)) [26] and evaluated their impact on the accuracy of the segmentation results. The parameters used in the pairwise multi-atlas registration are summarized in Table 2. All registrations were implemented using the open source Elastix registration software package [27]. The labels associated to each atlas were propagated to the reference image using the spatial transformation obtained from the final registration stage. We also evaluated the influence on the segmentation accuracy of three label fusion techniques (majority voting [28] (MV), global normalized cross correlation (GNCC) [29] and local normalized cross correlation (LNCC)) [30] as implemented in NiftySeg [31]. For the latter two fusion techniques, the impact of the hyperparameters k (kernel size) and r (number of highest ranked atlases used) was assessed.

Table 2. Registration parameters used for the multi-atlas registration.

Parameter	First Stage	Second Stage	Final Stage
Similarity Metric	(MSD/MI/NCC) *	(MSD/MI/NCC) *	(MSD/MI/NCC) *
Regulariser	/	/	Bending energy
Transform	Rigid	Affine	B-Spline
Multi Resolution levels	4	4	4
Number of histogram bins used for MI	32	32	32
Sampler	Random	Random	Random
Max iterations	2000	1000	1000
Number of samples	2000	2000	2000
Optimizer	Stochastic Gradient Descent	Stochastic Gradient Descent	Stochastic Gradient Descent

* All three metrics were investigated.

2.5. Dynamic Registration Framework

Motion estimation in the dynamic sequence was achieved through rigid registration in which computation of the similarity was limited to the bone of interest and its immediate vicinity. The multi-atlas segmentation approach was applied to the static reference 3DCT dataset using atlas images priorly obtained and corresponding to different subjects. The segmented reference images served as regions of interest for the rigid registration of each bone to its equivalent in the dynamic sequence. The segmented bones were dilated with a kernel radius of 3 voxels to ensure neighboring regions would be considered during the registration process. MSD was chosen as the similarity metric for this intrasubject monomodal registration because it yielded accurate results and was the least computationally demanding. We implemented a sequential intensity-based registration whereby subsequent registrations were initialized with the results of the previous registration (Figure 2II). A series of rigid transformation matrices ($T_{bone,t}$) were obtained for each bone of interest and for each time point (t). These transformation matrices aligned each bone in the reference image to its corresponding position in the dynamic sequence. The general workflow of our proposed approach is depicted in Figure 2.

2.6. Landmark Propagation and Kinematic Parameters Estimation

Anatomical landmarks from the atlases were propagated onto each of the bones of interest in the reference images, using the spatial transformation obtained from the final registration stage of the MAS step. A majority voting was done to decide the winning landmark, where each landmark votes based on the local-normalized cross-correlation (LNCC) of the registered atlas to the given target at that location. Propagation of the anatomical landmarks to subsequent time frames was then performed using the estimated transformation matrices of the dynamic registration step. With these landmarks expressed in the global coordinate system (GCS) of the CT, we computed three-unit vectors, $\vec{i}, \vec{j}, \vec{k}$, to define bone embedded reference frames for each time frame. Orientation of the axis of the reference frames followed ISB recommendations [32,33].

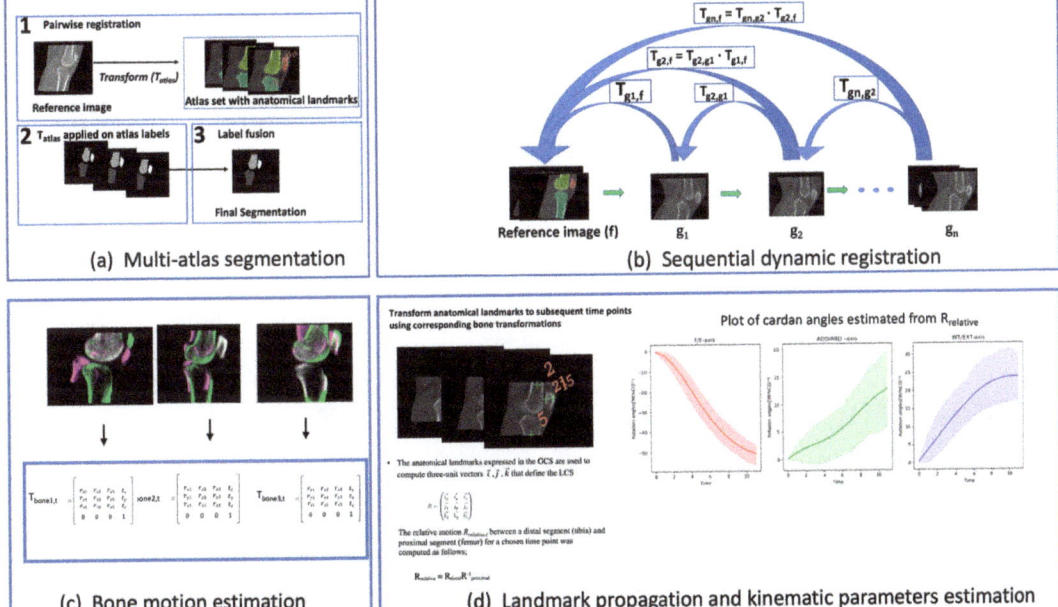

Figure 2. A general overview of the workflow for obtaining in vivo kinematics of bony structures. (**a**) shows the 3-step multi-atlas segmentation stage for obtaining segmentations of the reference image and propagation of anatomical landmarks. (**b**) shows the sequential dynamic registration workflow, each bone in the first time point of the dynamic sequence (g1) was aligned to the corresponding bone in the reference image (f) by the transformation ($T_{g1,f}$) via a rigid registration. The registration between the second time point (g2) and the reference image was initialized with the previous transformation to obtain the transformation $T_{g2,f}$. Subsequent time point registrations followed the same procedure. (**c**) shows an overlay of the registered bones along with transformation matrices ($T_{bone,t}$) from which motions are estimated for each bony structure. (**d**) shows the propagation of the anatomical landmarks from the reference image to other time points using the corresponding bone transformations. Local coordinate systems (bone embedded reference frames) are defined using these landmarks. Cardan angles are estimated from unit vectors constructed using the local coordinate system to generate kinematic plots.

The relative motion $R_{relative,t}$ between a distal segment (tibia or trapezium) and proximal segment (femur or 1st metacarpus) for a chosen time point was computed as follows;

$$R_{realative,t} = R_{distal,t}\, R_{proximal,t}^{-1} \qquad (2)$$

where R is a 3×3 rotation matrix constructed from the three-unit vectors as in Equation (3)

$$R = \begin{bmatrix} i_x & i_y & i_z \\ j_x & j_y & j_z \\ k_x & k_y & k_y \end{bmatrix} \qquad (3)$$

Cardan angles were then subsequently extracted from results of (2) using a ZXY sequence for the thumb base and ZYX for the knee joint.

2.7. Validation

The MAS pipeline was validated by a leave-one-out cross-validation (LOOCV) experiment for each joint, in which data from one subject was taken as target, while the remaining were used as atlases. Success of the segmentation was evaluated using overlap and distance measures. Overlap measures consisted of false positive error (FP) and false negative error (FN) volume fractions as well as Dice coefficients (DC) [34],

$$DC(A,B) = \frac{2|A \cap B|}{|A| + |B|} \quad (4)$$

$$FP(A,B) = \frac{|B \setminus A|}{|B|} \quad (5)$$

$$FN(A,B) = \frac{|A \setminus B|}{|A|} \quad (6)$$

where A, represents the ground truth (manual) binary segmentation and B represented the segmentation obtained by MAS. In addition, Euclidean distance maps of the ground truth manual segmentations and the surface of the corresponding segmentation obtained from the atlas-based method, were used to compute the Hausdorff distance [34]. Equation (7) shows the definition of the Hausdorff distance.

$$h(A,B) = max\{dist(A,B), dist(B,A)\}, \quad (7)$$

where

$$dist(A,B) = \max_{x \in A} \min_{y \in B} ||x - y|| \quad (8)$$

We quantified the impact of introducing MAS in the dynamic registration workflow. We used the 3D Scale Invariant Feature Transform (SIFT) [35] to automatically detect a set of corresponding landmarks between the reference image and the moving image. The landmarks were checked manually to ensure an accurate and even distribution of points across all bones of interest. The Target Registration Error (TRE) was then computed as the distance between the landmarks detected on the moving image and the landmarks of the reference image transformed using results of the registration. We compared the TREs of our proposed approach to those obtained using expert manual segmentations as well as a direct B-Spline deformable registration of the whole image, initialized from a rigid + affine registration without segmentation.

Kinematic parameters obtained via our automated anatomic landmark detection were compared to those estimated using manually defined landmarks (obtained from the 3 different readers). Bland-Altman plots were created to show differences in kinematic parameters estimated with our proposed approach to that obtained using the mean of all readers as an approximation of the ground truth. We computed absolute agreement intraclass correlation coefficients (ICCs) under a two-way mixed effects model [ICC(2,k)] [36] to compare kinematic parameters obtained by the automated algorithm and those obtained using manually identified landmarks by the three human readers.

2.8. Statistical Analysis

Statistical analysis was performed using Statistical Package for Social Sciences (SPSS v23, IBM Corp, Armonk, NY, USA). We analyzed the influence of the choice of metric (NCC, MI, MSD) for the MAS registration as well as the impact of the different label fusion techniques (LNCC, GNCC, MV). Data distribution was checked using a Shapiro-Wilk test for normality [37]. Non-parametric tests were chosen since not all variables were normally distributed. To compare the fusion techniques, we used a non-parametric Friedman test for repeated measures. When the Friedman test was statistically significant, a post-hoc Wilcoxon signed-rank analysis was performed. Furthermore, the Wilcoxon signed rank test [38] was used to check for statistical significance between the mean TRE obtained by the proposed approach and the baseline method ($p = 0.05$). The distribution of the landmark identification error in the leave-one-out experiments was analyzed using descriptive statistics (median and maximal error) and box plots.

3. Results
3.1. Multi-Atlas Segmentation

Figure 3 summarizes the results of the segmentations using overlap measures. We successfully segmented the bones of interest for both the knee and thumb dataset resulting in mean Dice coefficients above 0.90. No significant differences were observed between the three investigated similarity metrics ($X2 = 4.7$, $p = 0.09$). We therefore chose MSD in subsequent experiments because of the low computational complexity.

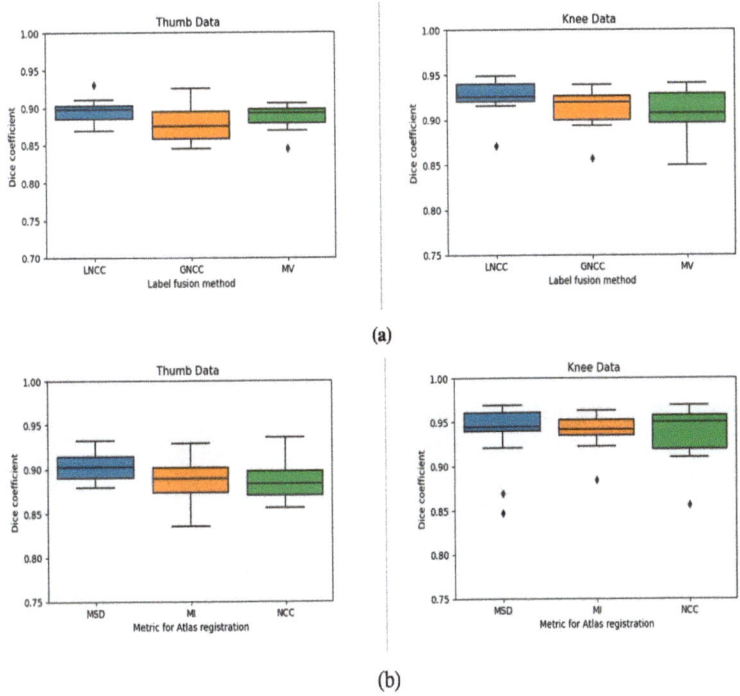

Figure 3. (a) Box plots of label fusion techniques against Dice coefficient for the two joints. These results are generated using MI as the similarity metric for the pairwise registrations. Parameters for LNCC were k = 5, r = 3 and for GNCC r = 3. (b) Plots of similarity metrics (used in the pairwise registration between atlases and images to be segmented) against Dice coefficient for the two joints.

Concerning the label fusion, the Friedman test showed significant differences between the label fusion techniques. Post-hoc Wilcoxon signed rank tests revealed that LNCC was significantly better than GNCC for all joints ($p < 0.001$).

The hyperparameters, kernel size (k) and the number of highest ranked atlases (r), had a marginal impact on the Dice score (Figure 4). Consequently, we selected LNCC with k = 5 and r = 3 to obtain the final automatic segmentations. Table 3 summarizes the quantitative results of these experiments. An example of the volume rendered segmentation for the two joints using LNCC (k = 5, r = 3) is shown in Figure 5.

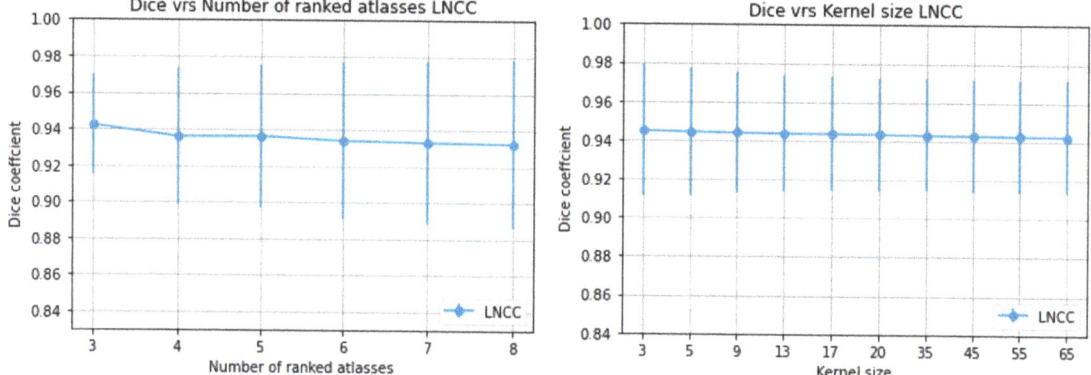

Figure 4. (**a**) Plot of Dice coefficient against number of highest ranked atlases (r) for a fixed kernel size = 5 voxels and (**b**) dice coefficient against kernel size (k) for a fixed r = 3 for the knee.

Table 3. Segmentation evaluation criteria results (Mean ± SD) over the leave-one-out cross-validation for the 2 joints using LNCC (k = 5, r = 3).

Joint	Dice Score	FP	FN	Mean Surface Distance (mm)	Max Surface Distance (mm)	SD Surface Distance (mm)
Thumb	0.90 ± 0.01	0.08 ± 0.02	0.14 ± 0.03	0.53 ± 0.05	4.89 ± 1.25	0.68 ± 0.05
Knee	0.94 ± 0.02	0.05 ± 0.02	0.06 ± 0.02	0.42 ± 0.16	4.91 ± 1.13	0.66 ± 0.18

FP = false positive error fraction, FN = false negative error fraction.

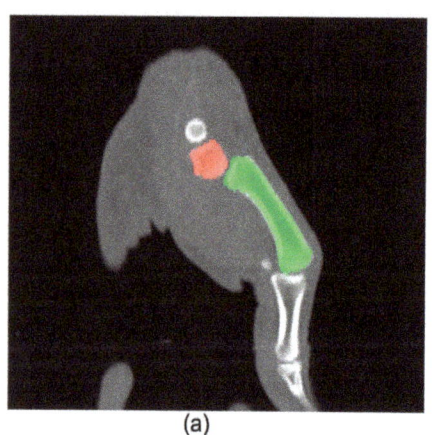
(**a**)

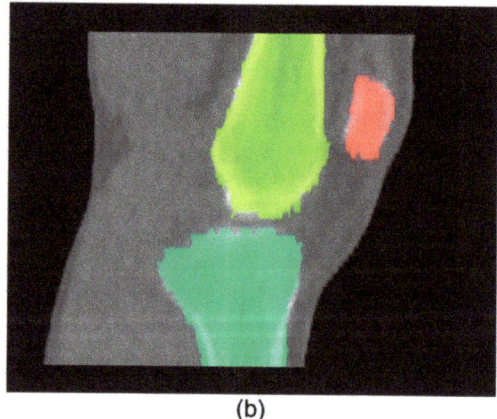
(**b**)

Figure 5. Segmentation result of our multi-atlas multi-label segmentation for (**a**) thumb base and (**b**) knee joint.

3.2. Dynamic Registration

The box plots in Figure 6a show the TRE results of the dynamic registration step. Introducing our MAS approach in the dynamic registration framework successfully registered the dynamic sequences and performed on par (Wilcoxon 2-tailed ranked test; $p = 0.51$) with a manual segmentation-guided approach. As a comparison, we also evaluated the TRE of a direct deformable registration, without prior segmentation of the bones. The large values for the TRE obtained indicate the registration often failed, resulting in poor overlap and confirming the challenging nature of the problem.

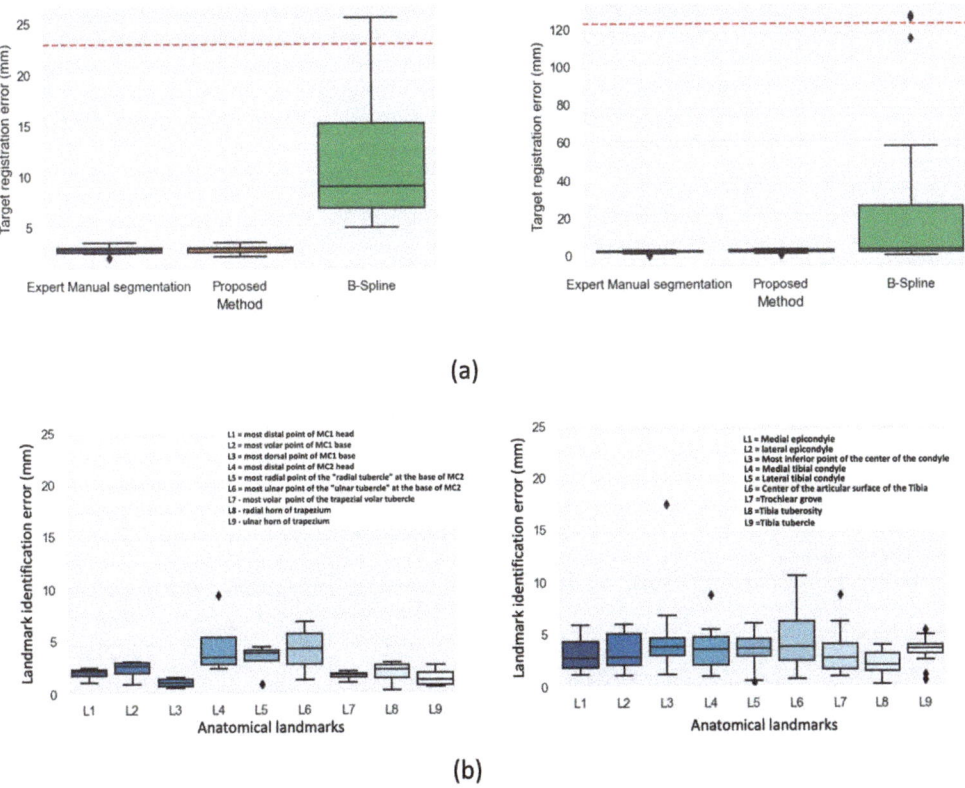

Figure 6. (**a**) Box plots showing TRE results of the piecewise rigid dynamic registration step for thumb base (top-left, $n = 5$) and the knee joint (top-right, $n = 10$). Results are shown for the expert manual segmentation approach, our multi-atlas guided approach (MAS) and a deformable registration (B-Spline). Dashed red lines indicate TRE for unregistered images (**b**) landmark identification error of the automatic anatomic landmark identification approach compared to the mean of all readers across 9 landmarks for thumb base (bottom-left) and the knee joint (bottom-right). The names of the anatomical landmarks are shown as inserts on the graphs.

3.3. Landmark Propagation

Concerning the landmark identification accuracy, Figure 6b summarizes the landmark identification error of the automatic algorithm to the mean of all readers taken as ground-truth. The femur center diaphysis and tibia center diaphysis landmarks used for estimating the femoral and tibial axes were omitted in the landmark identification error plots of Figure 6b. These points were eliminated because the images had to be cropped at those areas due to image artifacts. Consequently, the deformable registration employed in the final stage of the MAS mapped these landmarks outside the image regions for some subjects. While this had no impact on the computation of the bone-embedded reference frames, it resulted in high landmark identification errors. We therefore replaced these two landmarks with the most inferior point at the center of the condyle and center of the articular surface of the tibia. Each graph shows the distribution of distance errors of the landmarks for the leave-one-out test images, with median errors below 5 mm for all landmarks on both the thumb base and knee joint. The highest values of the median error for the knee are found for the most inferior point of the center of the condyle (L3) and center of the articular surface of the tibia (L6) with median errors of 4.8 mm and 4.3 mm respectively. For the thumb base, median errors of 4.7 mm and 4.2 mm were observed for the most distal point of the second metacarpal (L4) and the most ulnar point of the ulnar tubercle at the base of the second metacarpal (L6).

3.4. Kinematic Parameters

Performance of the proposed algorithm in estimating kinematic parameters is summarized in Figure 7a for the thumb base and Figure 7b for the knee joint. Results of cardan angles using our proposed approach are plotted together with results from manually identified landmarks of the 3 readers on the same graph. Shaded regions represent 95% Confidence Interval from the leave-one-out experiments.

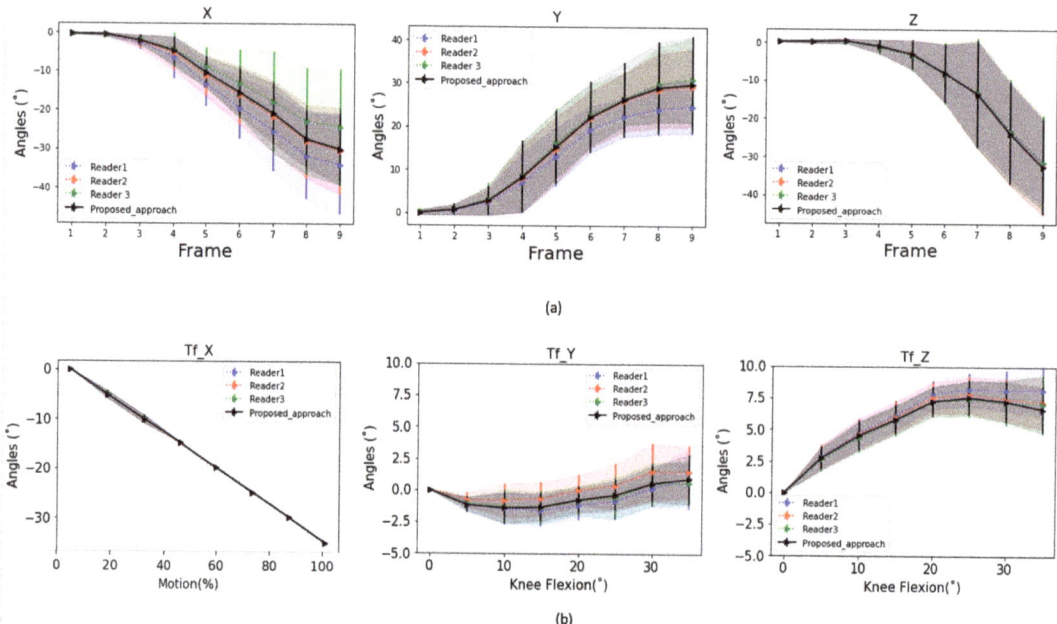

Figure 7. (**a**) 1st Metacarpal bone motion (cardan angles) showing an opposition movement of the thumb from neutral to full opposition. The plots show results using the proposed approach compared to using manual landmarks identified by three readers. X represents the Flexion (−)/Extension (+) axis, Y is the Adduction (−)/Abduction (+) and Z represents the Internal (+)/External (−) rotation axis; (**b**) Tibiofemoral (Tf) joint motion (cardan angles) obtained in leave-one-out validation on 10 subjects for the first 30° of knee flexion. The plots show results using the proposed approach compared to using manual landmarks identified by the three readers. Shaded regions represent 95% Confidence Interval over all subjects. (**a**) Tf_X represents the Flexion (−)/Extension (+) axis, Tf_Y represents Adduction (−)/Abduction (+) axis and TF_Z represents Internal (+)/External (−) rotation axis.

The Bland-Altman plots in Figure 8 also show the limits of agreement between our proposed approach and the manual approach for both the thumb base and knee joint. As in Figure 6b, results shown in Figure 8 are computed against the mean of all 3 readers. Our proposed approach produces kinematic parameters which fall within the limits of agreement of all three readers as is evident in Figure 8. Intraclass correlation (ICC) between cardan angles from the algorithm and results from expert manual landmarks ranged from 0.72 to 0.99 for all joints across all axes as detailed in Table 4.

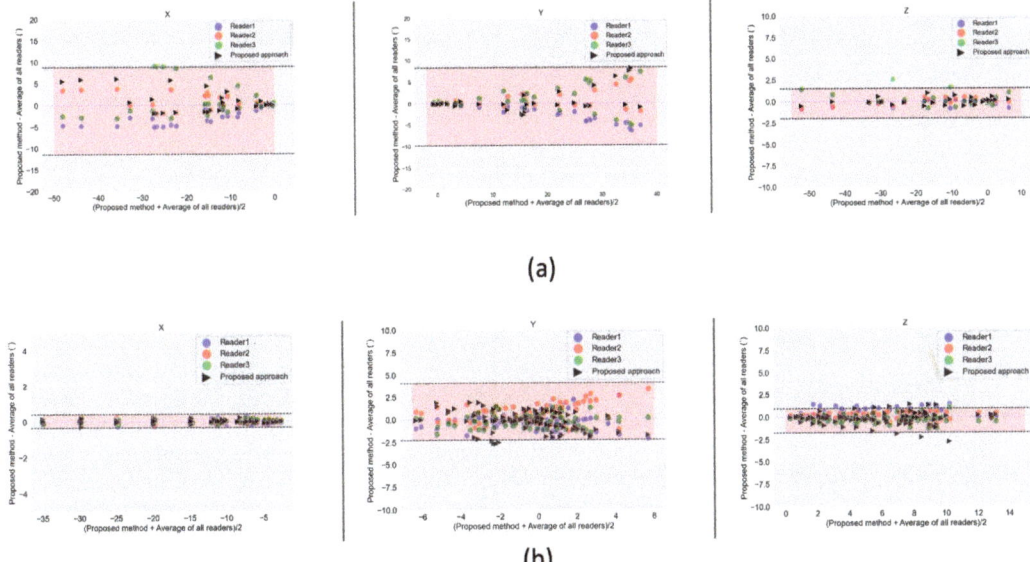

Figure 8. Bland Altman plots showing the limits of agreement between our proposed approach for kinematic parameter estimation (cardan angles) and a manual landmark identification (by three readers) approach for (**a**) thumb base; (**b**) knee. The mean of landmarks identified by the three readers is compared to our multi-atlas segmentation and landmark propagation approach. Shaded regions represent the limits of agreement of the three readers combined.

Table 4. ICCs of cardan angles obtained by expert readers and by the proposed automated workflow (Auto) for the three axes for the thumb and knee.

Thumb	* AUTO		
	X	Y	Z
Reader 1	0.99	0.99	0.99
Reader 2	0.95	0.94	0.99
Reader 3	0.92	0.94	0.99
Reader AVG	0.95	0.97	0.99
Knee	X	Y	Z
Reader 1	0.99	0.72	0.96
Reader 2	0.99	0.76	0.95
Reader 3	0.99	0.83	0.94
* Reader AVG	0.99	0.82	0.96

* Auto: the proposed automated workflow, * Reader AVG: the average of all three reader.

3.5. Discussion

We proposed an automated method for kinematic assessment of bony joint structures, based on multi-atlas segmentation of bony structures and landmark propagation. We evaluated this on a dataset of dynamic CT acquisitions of the thumb base and knee joint. Experiments were conducted to investigate the influence of the similarity metric in the MAS registration step, and we observed no significant differences in the choice of metric, allowing us to use MSD for our study. In case the dynamic sequence is from a different modality as the atlas (CBCT, MRI), alternative metrics such as NCC and MI will need to be tested.

The choice of the label fusion technique had an influence on the accuracy of the final segmentation, with LNCC performing better than the other fusion techniques. This can be attributed to the fact that LNCC computes a local normalized cross-correlation similarity using a 3D kernel and selects the best matching atlases based on this to be used in a majority vote. This captured the spatially varying nature of the registration accuracy and (locally) ignore poorly registered atlases that might misguide the final segmentation result. Our findings are in line with the work of Ceranka et al. [26] and Arabi et al. [39], both showing a better performance of the LNCC label fusion technique. The impact of both r and k on LNCC was marginal.

The impact of the number of atlases was not investigated in this study. Ceranka et al. [24] performed an analysis on the influence of the number of atlases on the quality of the segmentation of skeletal structures in whole-body MRIs and only found a marginal improvement above six atlases. The number of atlases used in this current study ($n = 4$ for thumb, $n = 9$ for knee) yielded Dice coefficients of 0.90 ± 0.01 for the thumb and 0.94 ± 0.02 for the knee. We believe that increasing the number of atlases for the thumb may increase segmentation accuracy further.

Our MAS approach with the best label fusion technique (LNCC, $k = 5$, $r = 3$) facilitated the segmentation of reference images, which were introduced in the dynamic registration framework. Accuracy of the dynamic registration workflow was evaluated using TRE. We compared the TRE results of our approach with results obtained using manually segmented images and observed no significant difference with our proposed approach ($p = 0.51$). Conversely, direct deformable registration of the joint images, without prior segmentation, led to mean errors around 10 mm and failed registrations (outliers).

The use of anatomical landmark propagation to define local bone-embedded reference frames further justifies the need for a multi-atlas segmentation approach for the segmentation of bones of interest. The spatial transformation obtained from the MAS automates the detection of anatomical landmarks in reference images. These landmarks can be propagated across the entire dynamic sequence automatically using transformations obtained from the dynamic registration step. Moreover, metrics based on changes of bone landmarks distance over time such as tibial-tuberosity trochlear groove [40] (used for subject with patella instability) can be extracted using the same approach. This can facilitate orthopedic diagnosis and surgical planning. Our automated landmark approach for estimating kinematics performed on par to the manual identification of landmarks by three independent readers, as shown by the Bland-Altman plots with mean differences falling within the limits of agreement of the readers across all axes for both joints. Beside cardan angles, other parameters such as bone surface contacts can be calculated from the obtained transformation matrices [41,42]. Our proposed approach uses a set of annotated datasets (atlases) but requires a reduced number ($n = 5$, $n = 10$ for thumb and knee) as it belongs to the group of methods that make use of image registration. This contrasts with machine learning algorithms, [22], which rely on a significant amount of annotated data in training to yield good results.

Similar algorithms to the proposed method both in terms of multi-atlas methodology and anatomical landmarks identified are presented in [43,44]. Our current study however demonstrated the generalizability of the proposed approach to other joints by applying it on dynamic CT of the knee and thumb. In [44], the authors proposed an algorithm for automatic anatomical measurements in the knee based on landmarks on CBCT images. A comparison between our approach and [44] can only be made on the knee data. Taking into consideration corresponding anatomical landmarks, L7 in our work corresponds to FT1 in [44], L8 corresponds to TT1, L5 to TP8 and L4 to TP9. Other potential corresponding points were excluded in the error analysis of [44] because they were not associated with any specific anatomical features. The average LDE of available points for comparison is 3.75 mm for [44] against 4.27 mm in our work. In general, our approach reaches comparable accuracy to previously reported algorithms for musculoskeletal applications [45,46] which reported median errors from ~2.5 to ~6 mm. Furthermore, results obtained from the kinematic analysis are within the limit of agreements of the three independent readers.

A potential limitation of the proposed approach is the computationally expensive pairwise registrations needed in the MAS step. Segmentation of a single subject using

$n = 10$ atlases was completed in 40 min on a 2.6 GHz Intel Core i7 16 GB ram computer. To speed up this step, approaches which involve selecting relevant atlases as opposed to a registration with all available atlases can be considered [47–49]. The use of the capabilities of GPU processors have also been proposed to help accelerate the registration step [50].

Another potential limitation of this study is the definition of ground-truth anatomical landmarks on the atlas dataset. The mean of the three readers and error analysis was also done with respect to the mean of all the readers. There is however the potential of introducing errors if one of the readers' landmarks are poorly defined. A potential solution is to propose a consensus framework like that proposed in [51], for combining segmentations.

Furthermore, this study only involved 15 healthy subjects which limits making detailed inferences from the obtained kinematic parameters. The homogenous nature of the study population (in terms of age and health status) also means the atlases were constructed with bones that do not exhibit unique or pathological morphology. Processing a new subject with such morphological variants may limit the success of the MAS step as well as the anatomic landmark propagation. Nonetheless, the deformable registration stage introduced in the workflow could compensate for some of the variations in morphology. It is also likely that manual landmark identification would be equally challenging in such situations.

3.6. Conclusions

Quantitative imaging modalities are becoming increasingly useful in understanding and evaluating MSK conditions, with dynamic CT being a promising tool [52]. The 4D MSK images generated from this technique are however not intuitive and in general require automated image analysis procedures to extract quantitative estimates of joint kinematics. We proposed a multi-atlas multi-label bone segmentation and landmark propagation approach and used it as an input for the kinematic analysis of dynamic CT images of two joints. Our method performed on par with commonly used approaches requiring manual segmentation and landmark identification. As such, it contributes to the build-up of an automated workflow for the post-processing of dynamic CT MSK images. Such quantitative assessment could increase the clinical value of radiologic examinations as it adds a functional dimension to morphological data.

Future studies will include reducing the time for the computationally expensive pairwise registrations of the MAS and the dynamic registration step by means of GPU implementation. The introduction of deep learning and conventional machine learning methods will also be considered using results of this study as annotated data.

Supplementary Materials: The following are available online at https://www.mdpi.com/article/10.3390/diagnostics11112062/s1, Video S1: dynamic CT volume render thumb, Video S2: dynamic CT of Knee.

Author Contributions: Conceptualization, B.K., L.B., A.G.; methodology, B.K., J.C.; software, B.K., J.C., A.G.; validation, B.K., L.B. and A.G.; formal analysis, B.K., L.B., S.B.; investigation, B.K., L.B., A.G.; resources, N.B., J.V., J.D.M.; data curation, S.B.; writing—original draft preparation, B.K.; writing—review and editing, B.K., L.B., N.B., J.V., E.C., T.S., G.V.G.; visualization, B.K.; supervision, N.B., J.V.; project administration, J.D.M.; funding acquisition, T.S., N.B., J.V., E.C., J.D.M., G.V.G. All authors have read and agreed to the published version of the manuscript.

Funding: This research was funded by an Interdisciplinary Research Project grant from Vrije Universiteit Brussel IRP10 (1 July 2016–30 June 2021).

Institutional Review Board Statement: The study was conducted according to the guidelines of the Declaration of Helsinki and approved by the Institutional Review Board (or Ethics Committee) of UZ Brussel Medical Ethics Committee (B.U.N 143201733617, 23 August 2019).

Informed Consent Statement: Informed consent was obtained from all subjects involved in the study.

Data Availability Statement: Data supporting this study can be obtained by contacting the corresponding author.

Acknowledgments: Special thanks to Mattias Nicolas Bossa, Kjell Van Royen and Tjeerd Jager for proofreading this manuscript.

Conflicts of Interest: The authors declare no conflict of interest.

References

1. Vos, T.; Allen, C.; Arora, M.; Barber, R.M.; Bhutta, Z.A.; Brown, A.; Carter, A.; Casey, D.C.; Charlson, F.J.; Chen, A.Z.; et al. Global, regional, and national incidence, prevalence, and years lived with disability for 354 diseases and injuries for 195 countries and territories, 1990–2017: A systematic analysis for the Global Burden of Disease Study 2017. *Lancet* **2018**, *392*, 1789–1858. [CrossRef]
2. Vos, T.; Flaxman, A.D.; Naghavi, M.; Lozano, R.; Michaud, C.; Ezzati, M.; Shibuya, K.; A Salomon, J.A.; Abdalla, S.; Aboyans, V.; et al. Years lived with disability (YLDs) for 1160 sequelae of 289 diseases and injuries 1990–2010: A systematic analysis for the Global Burden of Disease Study 2010. *Lancet* **2012**, *380*, 2163–2196. [CrossRef]
3. Musculoskeletal Conditions | BMUS: The Burden of Musculoskeletal Diseases in the United States, (n.d.). Available online: https://www.boneandjointburden.org/fourth-edition/ib2/musculoskeletal-conditions (accessed on 21 October 2021).
4. Fithian, D.C.; Paxton, E.W.; Stone, M.L.; Silva, P.; Davis, D.K.; Elias, D.A.; White, L. Epidemiology and Natural History of Acute Patellar Dislocation. *Am. J. Sports Med.* **2004**, *32*, 1114–1121. [CrossRef]
5. Buckler, A.J.; Bresolin, L.; Dunnick, N.R.; Sullivan, D.C. For the Group A Collaborative Enterprise for Multi-Stakeholder Participation in the Advancement of Quantitative Imaging. *Radiology* **2011**, *258*, 906–914. [CrossRef]
6. Buzzatti, L.; Keelson, B.; Apperloo, J.; Scheerlinck, T.; Baeyens, J.-P.; Van Gompel, G.; Vandemeulebroucke, J.; De Maeseneer, M.; De Mey, J.; Buls, N.; et al. Four-dimensional CT as a valid approach to detect and quantify kinematic changes after selective ankle ligament sectioning. *Sci. Rep.* **2019**, *9*, 1291. [CrossRef] [PubMed]
7. Gervaise, A.; Louis, M.; Raymond, A.; Formery, A.-S.; Lecocq, S.; Blum, A.; Teixeira, P.A.G. Musculoskeletal Wide-Detector CT Kinematic Evaluation: From Motion to Image. *Semin. Musculoskelet. Radiol.* **2015**, *19*, 456–462. [CrossRef]
8. Kerkhof, F.; Brugman, E.; D'Agostino, P.; Dourthe, B.; van Lenthe, H.G.; Stockmans, F.; Jonkers, I.; Vereecke, E. Quantifying thumb opposition kinematics using dynamic computed tomography. *J. Biomech.* **2016**, *49*, 1994–1999. [CrossRef] [PubMed]
9. Tay, S.-C.; Primak, A.N.; Fletcher, J.G.; Schmidt, B.; Amrami, K.K.; Berger, R.A.; McCollough, C.H. Four-dimensional computed tomographic imaging in the wrist: Proof of feasibility in a cadaveric model. *Skelet. Radiol.* **2007**, *36*, 1163–1169. [CrossRef] [PubMed]
10. Demehri, S.; Thawait, G.K.; Williams, A.A.; Kompel, A.; Elias, J.J.; Carrino, J.A.; Cosgarea, A.J. Imaging Characteristics of Contralateral Asymptomatic Patellofemoral Joints in Patients with Unilateral Instability. *Radiology* **2014**, *273*, 821–830. [CrossRef]
11. Forsberg, D.; Lindblom, M.; Quick, P.; Gauffin, H. Quantitative analysis of the patellofemoral motion pattern using semi-automatic processing of 4D CT data. *Int. J. Comput. Assist. Radiol. Surg.* **2016**, *11*, 1731–1741. [CrossRef]
12. Rauch, A.; Arab, W.A.; Dap, F.; Dautel, G.; Blum, A.; Teixeira, P.A.G. Four-dimensional CT Analysis of Wrist Kinematics during Radioulnar Deviation. *Radiology* **2018**, *289*, 750–758. [CrossRef]
13. Risser, L.; Vialard, F.-X.; Baluwala, H.Y.; Schnabel, J.A. Piecewise-diffeomorphic image registration: Application to the motion estimation between 3D CT lung images with sliding conditions. *Med. Image Anal.* **2013**, *17*, 182–193. [CrossRef] [PubMed]
14. Jain, J.; Jain, A. Displacement Measurement and Its Application in Interframe Image Coding. *IEEE Trans. Commun.* **1981**, *29*, 1799–1808. [CrossRef]
15. Ourselin, S.; Roche, A.; Prima, S.; Ayache, N. Block Matching: A General Framework to Improve Robustness of Rigid Registration of Medical Images. In *Logic-Based Program Synthesis and Transformation*; Springer: Berlin/Heidelberg, Germany, 2000; pp. 557–566.
16. Commowick, O.; Arsigny, V.; Isambert, A.; Costa, J.; Dhermain, F.; Bidault, F.; Bondiau, P.; Ayache, N.; Malandain, G. An efficient locally affine framework for the smooth registration of anatomical structures. *Med. Image Anal.* **2008**, *12*, 478–481. [CrossRef]
17. Makki, K.; Borotikar, B.; Garetier, M.; Brochard, S.; BEN Salem, D.; Rousseau, F. In vivo ankle joint kinematics from dynamic magnetic resonance imaging using a registration-based framework. *J. Biomech.* **2019**, *86*, 193–203. [CrossRef] [PubMed]
18. D'Agostino, P.; Dourthe, B.; Kerkhof, F.; Stockmans, F.; Vereecke, E.E. In vivo kinematics of the thumb during flexion and adduction motion: Evidence for a screw-home mechanism. *J. Orthop. Res.* **2016**, *35*, 1556–1564. [CrossRef] [PubMed]
19. Donati, M.; Camomilla, V.; Vannozzi, G.; Cappozzo, A. Anatomical frame identification and reconstruction for repeatable lower limb joint kinematics estimates. *J. Biomech.* **2008**, *41*, 2219–2226. [CrossRef]
20. Subburaj, K.; Ravi, B.; Agarwal, M. Automated identification of anatomical landmarks on 3D bone models reconstructed from CT scan images. *Comput. Med. Imaging Graph.* **2009**, *33*, 359–368. [CrossRef]
21. Bier, B.; Aschoff, K.; Syben, C.; Unberath, M.; Levenston, M.; Gold, G.; Fahrig, R.; Maier, A. Detecting Anatomical Landmarks for Motion Estimation in Weight-Bearing Imaging of Knees. *Tools Algorithms Constr. Anal. Syst.* **2018**, *11074 LNCS*, 83–90. [CrossRef]
22. Ebner, T.; Stern, D.; Donner, R.; Bischof, H.; Urschler, M. Towards Automatic Bone Age Estimation from MRI: Localization of 3D Anatomical Landmarks. In *Implementation of Functional Languages*; Springer: Berlin/Heidelberg, Germany, 2014; Volume 17, pp. 421–428.
23. Amerinatanzi, A.; Summers, R.K.; Ahmadi, K.; Goel, V.K.; Hewett, T.E.; Nyman, J.E. Automated Measurement of Patient-Specific Tibial Slopes from MRI. *Bioengineering* **2017**, *4*, 69. [CrossRef]
24. Yushkevich, P.A.; Piven, J.; Hazlett, H.C.; Smith, R.G.; Ho, S.; Gee, J.C.; Gerig, G. User-guided 3D active contour segmentation of anatomical structures: Significantly improved efficiency and reliability. *NeuroImage* **2006**, *31*, 1116–1128. [CrossRef] [PubMed]

25. Rueckert, D.; Sonoda, L.; Hayes, C.; Hill, D.; Leach, M.; Hawkes, D. Nonrigid registration using free-form deformations: Application to breast MR images. *IEEE Trans. Med. Imaging* **1999**, *18*, 712–721. [CrossRef] [PubMed]
26. Ceranka, J.; Verga, S.; Kvasnytsia, M.; Lecouvet, F.; Michoux, N.; De Mey, J.; Raeymaekers, H.; Metens, T.; Absil, J.; Vandemeulebroucke, J. Multi-atlas segmentation of the skeleton from whole-body MRI—Impact of iterative background masking. *Magn. Reson. Med.* **2020**, *83*, 1851–1862. [CrossRef] [PubMed]
27. Klein, S.; Staring, M.; Murphy, K.; Viergever, M.A.; Pluim, J.P.W. elastix: A Toolbox for Intensity-Based Medical Image Registration. *IEEE Trans. Med. Imaging* **2009**, *29*, 196–205. [CrossRef]
28. Xu, L.; Krzyzak, A.; Suen, C. Methods of combining multiple classifiers and their applications to handwriting recognition. *IEEE Trans. Syst. Man Cybern.* **1992**, *22*, 418–435. [CrossRef]
29. Aljabar, P.; Heckemann, R.; Hammers, A.; Hajnal, J.; Rueckert, D. Multi-atlas based segmentation of brain images: Atlas selection and its effect on accuracy. *NeuroImage* **2009**, *46*, 726–738. [CrossRef]
30. Artaechevarria, X.; Munoz-Barrutia, A.; de Solórzano, C.O. Combination Strategies in Multi-Atlas Image Segmentation: Application to Brain MR Data. *IEEE Trans. Med. Imaging* **2009**, *28*, 1266–1277. [CrossRef]
31. GitHub—KCL-BMEIS/NiftySeg, (n.d.). Available online: https://github.com/KCL-BMEIS/NiftySeg (accessed on 25 May 2021).
32. Wu, G.; Van Der Helm, F.C.; Veeger, H.E.J.; Makhsous, M.; Van Roy, P.; Anglin, C.; Nagels, J.; Karduna, A.R.; McQuade, K.; Wang, X.; et al. ISB recommendation on definitions of joint coordinate systems of various joints for the reporting of human joint motion—Part II: Shoulder, elbow, wrist and hand. *J. Biomech.* **2005**, *38*, 981–992. [CrossRef]
33. Wu, G.; Siegler, S.; Allard, P.; Kirtley, C.; Leardini, A.; Rosenbaum, D.; Whittle, M.; D'Lima, D.D.; Cristofolini, L.; Witte, H.; et al. ISB recommendation on definitions of joint coordinate system of various joints for the reporting of human joint motion—Part I: Ankle, hip, and spine. *J. Biomech.* **2002**, *35*, 543–548. [CrossRef]
34. Insight Journal (ISSN 2327-770X)—Introducing Dice, Jaccard, and Other Label Overlap Measures To ITK, (n.d.). Available online: https://www.insight-journal.org/browse/publication/707 (accessed on 25 May 2021).
35. Cheung, W.; Hamarneh, G. N-SIFT: N-Dimensional Scale Invariant Feature Transform for Matching Medical Images. In Proceedings of the 2007 4th IEEE International Symposium on Biomedical Imaging: From Nano to Macro, Arlington, VA, USA, 12–15 May 2007; Institute of Electrical and Electronics Engineers (IEEE): Manhattan, NY, USA, 2007; pp. 720–723.
36. Koo, T.K.; Li, M.Y. A Guideline of Selecting and Reporting Intraclass Correlation Coefficients for Reliability Research. *J. Chiropr. Med.* **2016**, *15*, 155–163. [CrossRef]
37. Shapiro, S.S.; Wilk, M.B. An Analysis of Variance Test for Normality (Complete Samples). *Biometrika* **1965**, *52*, 591. [CrossRef]
38. Williams, W.A. Statistical Methods (8th ed.). *J. Am. Stat. Assoc.* **1991**, *86*, 834–835. Available online: https://go.gale.com/ps/i.do?p=AONE&sw=w&issn=01621459&v=2.1&it=r&id=GALE%7CA257786252&sid=googleScholar&linkaccess=fulltext (accessed on 25 May 2021). [CrossRef]
39. Arabi, H.; Zaidi, H. Comparison of atlas-based techniques for whole-body bone segmentation. *Med. Image Anal.* **2017**, *36*, 98–112. [CrossRef]
40. Williams, A.A.; Elias, J.J.; Tanaka, M.J.; Thawait, G.K.; Demehri, S.; Carrino, J.A.; Cosgarea, A.J. The relationship between tibial tuberosity-trochlear groove distance and abnormal patellar tracking in patients with unilateral patellar instability. Imaging Characteristics of Contralateral Asymptomatic Patellofemoral Joints in Patients with Unilateral Instability. *Arthroscopy* **2016**, *32*, 55–61. [PubMed]
41. Yang, Z.; Fripp, J.; Chandra, S.S.; Neubert, A.; Xia, Y.; Strudwick, M.; Paproki, A.; Engstrom, C.; Crozier, S. Automatic bone segmentation and bone-cartilage interface extraction for the shoulder joint from magnetic resonance images. *Phys. Med. Biol.* **2015**, *60*, 1441–1459. [CrossRef]
42. Wang, K.K.; Zhang, X.; McCombe, D.; Ackland, D.C.; Ek, E.T.; Tham, S.K. Quantitative analysis of in-vivo thumb carpometacarpal joint kinematics using four-dimensional computed tomography. *J. Hand Surg. Eur. Vol.* **2018**, *43*, 1088–1097. [CrossRef] [PubMed]
43. Jacinto, H.; Valette, S.; Prost, R. Multi-atlas automatic positioning of anatomical landmarks. *J. Vis. Commun. Image Represent.* **2018**, *50*, 167–177. [CrossRef]
44. Brehler, M.; Thawait, G.; Kaplan, J.; Ramsay, J.; Tanaka, M.J.; Demehri, S.; Siewerdsen, J.H.; Zbijewski, W. Atlas-based algorithm for automatic anatomical measurements in the knee. *J. Med. Imaging* **2019**, *6*, 026002. [CrossRef]
45. Baek, S.; Wang, J.-H.; Song, I.; Lee, K.; Lee, J.; Koo, S. Automated bone landmarks prediction on the femur using anatomical deformation technique. *Comput. Des.* **2012**, *45*, 505–510. [CrossRef]
46. Phan, C.-B.; Koo, S. Predicting anatomical landmarks and bone morphology of the femur using local region matching. *Int. J. Comput. Assist. Radiol. Surg.* **2015**, *10*, 1711–1719. [CrossRef]
47. Langerak, T.R.; Berendsen, F.F.; Van Der Heide, U.A.; Kotte, A.N.T.J.; Pluim, J.P.W. Multiatlas-based segmentation with preregistration atlas selection. *Med. Phys.* **2013**, *40*, 091701. [CrossRef] [PubMed]
48. Van Rikxoort, E.M.; Isgum, I.; Arzhaeva, Y.; Staring, M.; Klein, S.; Viergever, M.A.; Pluim, J.P.; Van Ginneken, B.B. Adaptive local multi-atlas segmentation: Application to the heart and the caudate nucleus. *Med. Image Anal.* **2010**, *14*, 39–49. [CrossRef] [PubMed]
49. Duc, A.K.H.; Modat, M.; Leung, K.K.; Cardoso, M.J.; Barnes, J.; Kadir, T.; Ourselin, S. Using Manifold Learning for Atlas Selection in Multi-Atlas Segmentation. *PLoS ONE* **2013**, *8*, e70059. [CrossRef]

50. Han, X.; Hibbard, L.S.; Willcut, V. GPU-accelerated, gradient-free MI deformable registration for atlas-based MR brain image segmentation. In Proceedings of the 2009 IEEE Computer Society Conference on Computer Vision and Pattern Recognition Workshops, Miami, FL, USA, 20–25 June 2009; Institute of Electrical and Electronics Engineers (IEEE): Manhattan, NY, USA, 2009; pp. 141–148.
51. Warfield, S.K.; Zou, K.H.; Wells, W.M. Simultaneous Truth and Performance Level Estimation (STAPLE): An Algorithm for the Validation of Image Segmentation. *IEEE Trans. Med. Imaging* **2004**, *23*, 903–921. [CrossRef] [PubMed]
52. Cuadra, M.B.; Favre, J.; Omoumi, P. Quantification in Musculoskeletal Imaging Using Computational Analysis and Machine Learning: Segmentation and Radiomics. *Semin. Musculoskelet. Radiol.* **2020**, *24*, 50–64. [CrossRef]

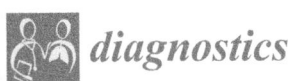

Article

Remote Gait Type Classification System Using Markerless 2D Video

Pedro Albuquerque [1], João Pedro Machado [2], Tanmay Tulsidas Verlekar [3,*], Paulo Lobato Correia [1] and Luís Ducla Soares [2]

[1] Instituto de Telecomunicações, Instituto Superior Técnico, Universidade de Lisboa, Av. Rovisco Pais 1, 1049-001 Lisboa, Portugal; pedro.flores.albuquerque@tecnico.ulisboa.pt (P.A.); plc@lx.it.pt (P.L.C.)
[2] Instituto de Telecomunicações, Instituto Universitário de Lisboa (ISCTE-IUL), Av. das Forças Armadas, 1649-026 Lisboa, Portugal; jpsmo11@iscte-iul.pt (J.P.M.); lds@lx.it.pt (L.D.S.)
[3] Department of CSIS and APPCAIR, BITS Pilani, K K Birla, Goa Campus, Goa 403726, India
* Correspondence: tanmayv@goa.bits-pilani.ac.in

Abstract: Several pathologies can alter the way people walk, i.e., their gait. Gait analysis can be used to detect such alterations and, therefore, help diagnose certain pathologies or assess people's health and recovery. Simple vision-based systems have a considerable potential in this area, as they allow the capture of gait in unconstrained environments, such as at home or in a clinic, while the required computations can be done remotely. State-of-the-art vision-based systems for gait analysis use deep learning strategies, thus requiring a large amount of data for training. However, to the best of our knowledge, the largest publicly available pathological gait dataset contains only 10 subjects, simulating five types of gait. This paper presents a new dataset, GAIT-IT, captured from 21 subjects simulating five types of gait, at two severity levels. The dataset is recorded in a professional studio, making the sequences free of background camouflage, variations in illumination and other visual artifacts. The dataset is used to train a novel automatic gait analysis system. Compared to the state-of-the-art, the proposed system achieves a drastic reduction in the number of trainable parameters, memory requirements and execution times, while the classification accuracy is on par with the state-of-the-art. Recognizing the importance of remote healthcare, the proposed automatic gait analysis system is integrated with a prototype web application. This prototype is presently hosted in a private network, and after further tests and development it will allow people to upload a video of them walking and execute a web service that classifies their gait. The web application has a user-friendly interface usable by healthcare professionals or by laypersons. The application also makes an association between the identified type of gait and potential gait pathologies that exhibit the identified characteristics.

Keywords: assisted living; gait classification; pathology identification; remote diagnosis; web application

1. Introduction

Gait can be defined as the act of locomotion, involving periodic body movements, such as sequences of loading and unloading of the limbs [1]. The study and analysis of gait in a medical context can contribute to the diagnosis and monitoring of pathologies that affect people's gait [2]. For this reason, the automatic classification of the type of gait is gathering interest, with many approaches already available in the literature [3,4]. Of these approaches, vision-based solutions appear to be especially interesting since image sequences can be captured with relatively simple setups, e.g., with a single 2D camera [5]. This enables the capture of gait data in a clinical environment or even at home, with most of the processing required to analyze the observed gait done remotely. A prototype based on this idea is proposed in this paper to enable the remote classification of people's gait.

Most state-of-the-art vision-based systems for gait classification rely on deep learning strategies [6–8]. They involve the use of Convolutional Neural Networks (CNN), such as

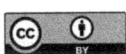

VGG-19 [9], pre-trained on the ImageNet [10], and fine-tuned using gait datasets. Fine-tuning requires relatively smaller datasets to adjust an existing CNN to perform better on a related problem. The quality of this adjustment and the expected results depend on the richness and suitability of the used datasets. However, most publicly available datasets containing different types of gait are captured from a limited number of healthy subjects simulating gait pathologies. Most datasets contain simulations because of the ethical and privacy concerns involved in sharing data from real patients. However, simulating pathologies with all its complexity is seldom correctly executed.

This paper presents a new gait dataset, GAIT-IT, containing 21 subjects and five types of gait, at two severity levels, simulated following instructions provided using an illustrative video, an oral explanation, and a short walking demonstration. The gait video sequences are captured in a professional studio with a chroma-keying background, resulting in a high contrast between the foreground and the background. These characteristics of the dataset are helpful for training a reliable gait type classification system.

The paper also presents a novel gait type classification system based on a CNN architecture. It drastically reduces the number of trainable parameters, compared to the state-of-the-art, thus having lower memory requirements and faster execution times. The proposed system is trained using the GAIT-IT dataset and tested using also a publicly available dataset containing simulations of the corresponding gait pathologies. The results suggest that the proposed system has significant generalization ability, as it can correctly associate available gait types with the corresponding pathologies. The results also highlight the effectiveness of the proposed system to operate in a relatively noisy acquisition setup of the GAIT-IST dataset, which was captured using a cell phone in an 'at home'-like setting, with a wall as background and without particular care taken with the illumination, which came from a side window and the ceiling fluorescent lamps. Additionally, the distance from the camera to the subjects is different in the GAIT-IT and GAIT-IST datasets.

A third contribution of this paper is a web application for gait assessment. It is the prototype of a remote healthcare system, performing diagnosis by analyzing video sequences captured and uploaded from a cellphone or a personal computer. The web service identifies the type of gait and associates it to a possible gait related pathology. All computations are performed on the server, and the results are returned in a user-friendly manner, with images highlighting the parts of the gait that contribute more to the diagnosis.

1.1. Related Work

A rich characterization of gait information can be obtained through the use of different types of sensors, including [3]:
1. floor-based sensors;
2. wearable sensors;
3. vision-based sensors.

Floor-based sensors are used to detect ground reaction force [11], or the pressure exerted on the area under the foot [3]. It typically provides limited information for gait classification and the equipment used is restricted to constrained spaces. Wearable sensors are portable, allowing data acquisition of three-dimensional information related to walking patterns over long periods of time [4,12]. However, their performance can be influenced by the sensor placement. If sensor placement is not completed carefully, walking can become uncomfortable, which can then affect the quality of gait data acquired. Additionally, if an 'at-home' scenario is envisaged, for self-monitoring, then it is not guaranteed that sensors will be correctly applied, and the captured data may not be the intended type. In summary, sensor placement should always be completed under the supervision of trained professionals.

Vision-based systems have the advantage of being unobtrusive and not requiring a complicated cooperation of the subject. Marker-based systems are considered as the gold standard approach for gait analysis [13], using special markers placed on key body parts to track them and obtain kinematic features from the observed motion. However, these often require specialized personnel to ensure correct setup and calibration. On the other hand, a markerless approach can be more suitable for application in less constrained environments [14].

Markerless vision-based systems for gait analysis typically follow a model-based or an appearance-based approach [15]. In the model-based approach, gait representations are created by fitting a model to the input sequence of images or silhouettes, using prior knowledge of the human body (structural model) or its motion (motion model) [16]. An example includes using two Kinect sensors with perpendicular viewing directions, acquiring both RGB and depth information to create a 3D model based on the movement of skeleton parts [17]. This model combines static features (e.g., distances between joints) and dynamic features (e.g., speed, stride length or the body's center of mass movement). In the appearance-based approach, gait is represented without assuming prior knowledge of human motion. A sequence of binary silhouettes is typically obtained using background subtraction, as illustrated in Figure 1a. As long as a well performing background subtraction method is used, the resulting silhouettes are mostly free from background clutter and the influence of illumination changes. The desired gait representation can then be derived using the sequence of binary silhouettes. A widely used representation called the Gait Energy Image (GEI) [18] is obtained by averaging the cropped, normalized in size and horizontally aligned binary silhouettes belonging to a gait cycle, according to Equation (1).

$$GEI(x,y) = \frac{1}{N} \sum_{i=1}^{N} B_i(x, y) \qquad (1)$$

In Equation (1), N represents the number of frames in one (or multiple) gait cycle(s). $B_i(x, y)$ is a binary silhouette image, with x and y being pixel coordinates. The resulting GEI is a grey-level image implicitly representing, in a single image, the subject's shape and motion along the gait cycle, as illustrated in Figure 1b,c. The GEI representation is robust against noise in individual frames.

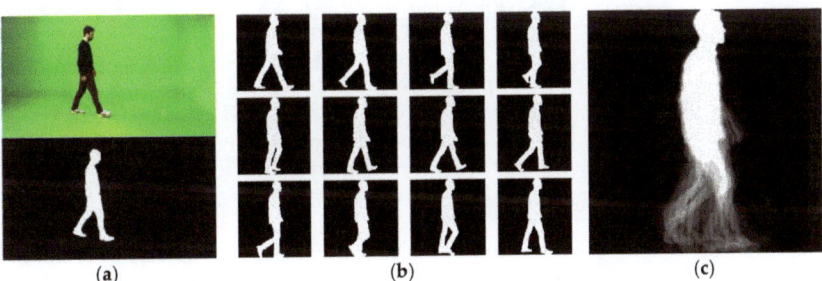

Figure 1. Example of (**a**) background subtraction, (**b**) binary silhouettes and (**c**) GEI.

A second representation considered for the presentation of results in this paper is the Skeleton Energy Image (SEI) [6], a hybrid between model- and appearance-based approaches—see Figure 2c. It starts by obtaining skeleton models for every available image of the walking person, using Open Pose [19]. Open Pose is a neural network trained to locate the positions of key joints of a human body on a 2D image, as illustrated in Figure 2a. With a skeleton image for each frame, the SEI can then be obtained with the same method used for GEI computation. The SEI was reported to achieve better pathological gait classification results than the GEI, as the SEI focuses on the dynamic movement characteristics and not on the physical constitution and clothing of a subject [6].

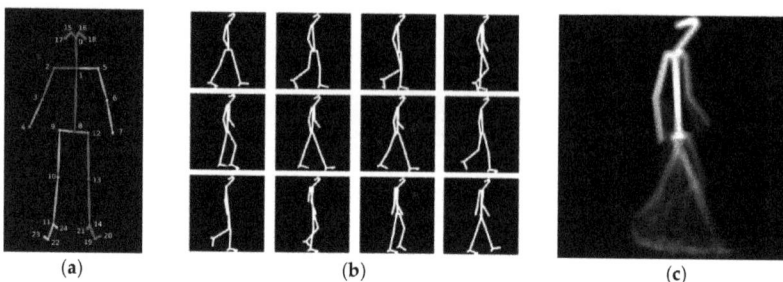

Figure 2. Example of (**a**) output of Open Pose [19], (**b**) skeleton images and (**c**) SEI.

1.1.1. Gait Classification Systems

Systems for the classification of gait types often use the gait representation directly, they compute a set of biomechanical features, or use a combination of both. For instance, the work reported in [20] describes two approaches, one using leg angles as features, and another one using the GEI. A set of normalized gait features is proposed in [21], including the step length, stance and swing phase durations, or the amount and broadness of limb movements, to quantify gait impairments. The last decade has witnessed the emergence of deep learning strategies for feature extraction in image recognition and classification with very good results, including gait analysis systems. The solution presented in [8] adopts the GEI for gait representation and uses the VGG-19 [9], pre-trained on a subset of ImageNet [10], for feature extraction. Transfer learning is used to repurpose the CNN for pathological gait classification, with the last layers of the VGG-19 network being trained using GEIs computed from the INIT dataset [21]. Linear Discriminant Analysis (LDA) was used for classification and the system's performance is tested using two other pathological gait datasets: DAI [22] and DAI2 [20]. Another deep learning approach, also based on the VGG-19, is adopted in [6] for pathological gait classification, using both GEI and SEI gait representations. In this case, the pre-trained CNN is fine-tuned with data from the GAIT-IST dataset [6]. Other deep learning approaches include the use of Recurrent Neural Networks (RNNs) that are able to learn correlations between inputs in a time series, such as the application of a bidirectional Long-Short Term Memory (LSTM) [23] network for pathological gait classification based on sequences of lower limb flexion angles [7]. Given the good performance reported in the literature, this paper also considers a deep learning solution to perform gait type classification.

1.1.2. Gait Datasets

Publicly available gait datasets are created either for biometric recognition, or for gait type classification. Datasets for recognition include subjects walking normally, possibly with some covariates such as different speeds, different types of shoes, different clothing or carrying different items. The purpose of gait type datasets is to capture sequences reflecting different kinds of impairments, notably to mimic the effects of some pathological conditions. Since sharing data from real patients raises ethical and data privacy issues, the publicly available impaired gait datasets are captured from healthy subjects simulating a selection of gait impairments. To the best of our knowledge, there are four gait impairment datasets publicly available, as listed below. All the sequences in these datasets are captured from a canonical viewpoint and recorded in controlled environments.

The DAI dataset [22] contains binary silhouettes of five subjects. It has 15 healthy gait sequences, and 15 sequences with random gait impairment simulations, for a total of 30 gait sequences. The subjects are captured walking over a distance of 3 m using both the RGB camera of a Kinect sensor and a smartphone.

The DAI2 dataset [20] also considers five subjects, but contains a total of 75 gait sequences. Each subject simulates four pathologies (Parkinson's, diplegia, hemiplegia and neuropathy), as well as normal walking gait. Each condition was recorded 3 times, while walking along a distance of 8 m.

The INIT dataset [21] contains binary silhouettes of 10 subjects (9 males, 1 female), for a total of 80 sequences. Every subject is recorded 2twodifferent times, at 30 fps, capturing multiple gait cycles and simulating seven different gait impairments (in addition to a healthy gait sequence): (i) right arm motionless; (ii) half motion of the right arm; (iii) left arm motionless; (iv) half motion of the left arm; (v) full body impairments; (vi) half motion of the right leg; and (vii) half motion of the left leg.

The GAIT-IST dataset [6] considers 10 subjects, with a total of 360 gait sequences. The dataset includes the same four pathologies considered in DAI2, with two severity levels for each, two directions of walking, and two repetitions per subject, except for the normal gait. It is the largest pathological gait dataset publicly available. Video sequences were captured using a smartphone camera, with a resolution of 1280×720 pixels, mounted on a tripod at about 1.5 m above the ground and at a distance of about 4 m from the target.

Of the above datasets, some include impairments that are very easy to simulate, but which may not be directly related to any specific gait pathology. Other datasets include simulations of the gait pathologies, which are harder for healthy people to simulate. The proposed GAIT-IT dataset simulates different gait types that can be associated with known pathologies. Healthy volunteers were instructed on how to perform the simulations by watching detailed explanation videos, as well as personal interaction to clarify questions and see a short demonstration of the main walking characteristics related to the pathologies to simulate. GAIT-IT also doubles the number of subjects relatively to the largest publicly available dataset.

2. Materials and Methods

This paper presents three novel contributions:
1. proposal of a new, larger, gait type dataset: GAIT-IT;
2. a gait type classification system;
3. a remote diagnosing web application.

2.1. GAIT-IT Dataset

The proposed GAIT-IT dataset (available at http://www.img.lx.it.pt/GAIT-IT/ accessed on 3 September 2021) captures a larger number of subjects, with significantly more variations than the existing publicly available datasets. The sequences are captured at a higher quality and with a better contrast between the subject and the background. GAIT-IT is recorded in the professional studio of FCT I FCCN, Lisbon, Portugal (https://www.fccn.pt/en/colaboracao/estudio/ accessed date 25 July 2021), on two different days. The studio includes controlled artificial lighting and a green background, ideal for chroma-keying segmentation, resulting in high-quality sequences, free from background camouflage and other artifacts. Two professional 4K video cameras are used to capture synchronized gait sequences, one with a side view, at approximately 3 m from the target, and the other with a front/rear view, at about half a meter from the walking start position. Both cameras stood on tripods at 1.75 m from the ground.

The GAIT-IT dataset contains simulations of five different types of gait. For each type, except normal, two levels of severity are captured. The subjects provide four gait sequences per severity level. This corresponds to a subject walking twice from left to right and from right to left, from the side view. The sequences are captured on two different days where 21 volunteers (19 males and 2 females) between the age range of 20 to 56 years participated, with a mean of 29.5 and a standard deviation of 11.6—see Figure 3. Thus, GAIT-IT dataset includes a total of 828 gait sequences. Having some subjects captured on different days, allows intra-subject variations in the simulations. Before capturing the sequences, the subjects are instructed on how to simulate the various gait types and severity levels, as summarized below [24].

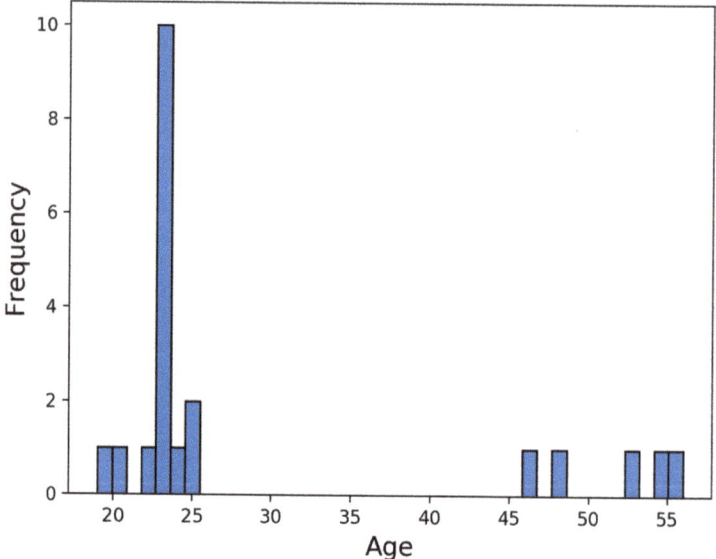

Figure 3. Subjects' age distribution.

The scissor gait commonly associated with diplegia affects both sides of the body. A subject adopts a forward leaning posture and walks by dragging both feet in a circular motion. For the second severity level the overall bending is accentuated, along with leg and arm movements.

The spastic gait commonly associated with hemiplegia affects only one side of the body. The leg is dragged in a circular motion, with a broader reach for the second severity, while the right arm remains still and held close to the waist, or flexed against the chest in the second severity level.

The steppage gait commonly associated with neuropathy leads to foot drop. Subjects tend to lift their knees higher than normal to avoid dragging their toes on the floor. In the second severity level, the lift of the leg and the forward swing are exaggerated.

The propulsive gait commonly associated with Parkinson's diseases is characterized by a stooped posture, with both arms held close to the chest and the lower limbs flexed and rigid. Subjects are asked to attempt simulating general and erratic body shaking while taking small and relatively fast steps. The second severity level involves an overall exaggeration of these symptoms.

The captured sequences are processed to produce four different representations:

1. sequence of binary silhouettes;
2. sequence of skeletal images;
3. GEIs;
4. SEIs.

GEI and SEI representations are obtained for each gait cycle, as well as for the complete set of gait cycles available per sequence. The spatial dimension of the produced gait representations is 224 × 224 pixels. The binary silhouettes are cropped and overlapped following Equation (1) to obtain the gait representations. All representations consider a framerate of 10 fps. The main steps for obtaining the gait representations are as follows.

The extraction of binary silhouettes relies on chroma-keying segmentation. A frame containing only the background is represented in the HSV color space and the histograms of the hue (H), saturation (S) and value (V) components are computed. Then, all pixels in gait sequences with HSV values outside the background range are classified as belonging to the walking subject. Finally, a morphological filtering operation is applied to remove noise. A sample result is presented in Figure 1a. Skeleton computation relies on locating key anatomical parts in the gait images, using the Open Pose [19] software, which uses a multi-stage CNN to automatically detect a total of 135 body, hand, facial and foot key points in each frame of a video, operating in real-time. In the current implementation, only 25 key points corresponding to the body are captured, as illustrated in Figure 2a. The GEIs and SEIs are computed following Equation (1). An example of the gait representations obtained from the GAIT-IT dataset is illustrated in Figure 1c (GEI) and Figure 2c (SEI).

2.2. Gait Type Classification System

The state-of-the-art vision-based systems for gait type classification rely on deep learning using pre-trained CNNs, which are then fine-tuned by transfer learning with task-specific datasets. This strategy is employed as most gait type datasets contain a limited amount of training data. Since the proposed GAIT-IT dataset provides a considerable increase in the amount of data available for training, rather than fine-tuning a complex network, this paper proposes a novel lightweight CNN, specifically trained to perform gait type classification. The architecture of the proposed CNN is illustrated in Figure 4.

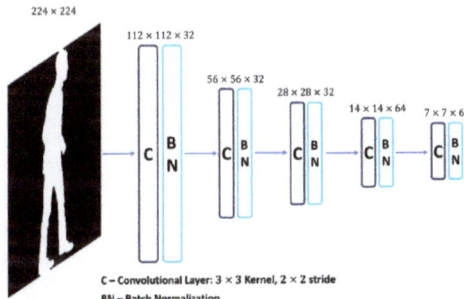

Figure 4. The proposed gait type classification CNN architecture.

The proposed system accepts a GEI or SEI as an input, which is processed using five convolutional layers. This option follows the type of architectures adopted in the Kaggle MNIST challenge [25,26], which also process binary images. As in the architectures of popular CNNs, such as VGG-16, the proposed system adopts a 3×3 filter size and a stride of 2 for the convolutional layers. A total of 32 feature maps, or filters, is considered in the first convolutional layer, being doubled for the last two layers. Each convolutional layer is followed by batch normalization, to adjust and scale the outputs to have a mean value close to 0 and a standard deviation close to 1. Bounding the values that pass between layers helps to stabilize and speedup the training process.

To perform classification, the features computed by the final convolutional layer are flattened and passed on to a fully connected neural network, consisting of two dense layers with a dropout [27] of 0.5 between them. The first dense layer has 512 units and the second layer has five units, corresponding to the five considered gait types, with a softmax activation function to output class probabilities. The proposed system is trained using categorical cross entropy and the Adam algorithm [28], with the Nesterov momentum variation [29]. The learning rate is set to 0.001.

2.3. A Remote Diagnostic Web Application Prototype

This paper also proposes the prototype of a system that allows remote gait diagnosis. It could assist healthcare professionals to identify patients requiring immediate attention and further examination, as well as monitor the evolution of existing gait pathologies, without the need of physical interaction with the patient. The usefulness of such a system is made more evident under the COVID-19 pandemic.

The proposed remote diagnostic web application runs the proposed gait type classification system on its server. It can be access by issuing HTTP requests to the web service. The web interface allows uploading a video sequence or a compact gait representation, notably a GEI or a SEI. It then executes the web service and returns the results to be presented in way that can be easily interpreted by the user.

The web application offers two different modes of operations:
1. basic mode;
2. advanced mode.

The basic mode is a simple interface to be used in a clinical environment or at home. It assumes a simple setup which involves filming a subject using a 2D camera, e.g., using a cellphone's camera. The user interface, illustrated in Figure 5a, allows the user to upload the video, and the web application generates a GEI (or SEI) representation. The gait representation is processed by the web service using the proposed gait type classification system, which checks if the identified features could be associated to a specific gait pathology. The user can then visualize the parts of the body that contributed to the diagnostic using a saliency representation [30] and class-activation maps (grad-CAM) [31]. Figure 6 illustrates results for two different types of gait, suggesting that spastic gait is identified by the characteristic movement of the feet, while propulsive gait is identified by the type of feet movement and the bending of the spine. The diagnostic can optionally be sent to a specified e-mail address. The interface is designed to remotely obtain a preliminary diagnostic, and to help visualize the body motions that deviate from a healthy gait.

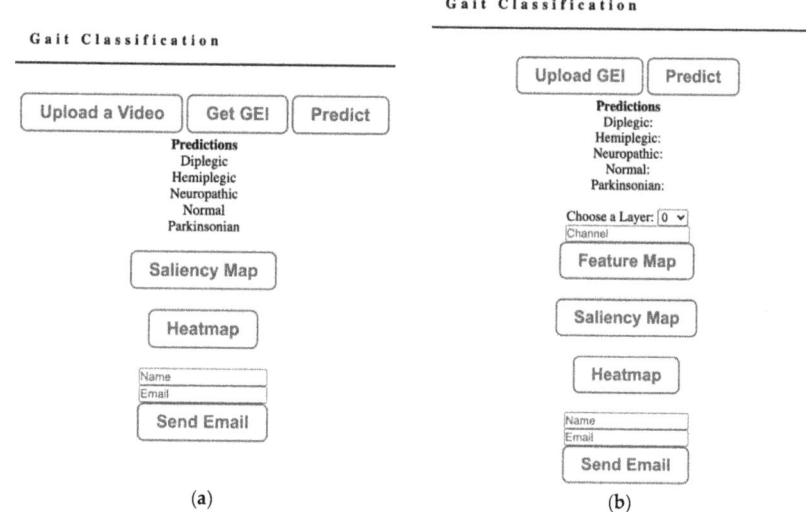

Figure 5. Web service user interface modes of operation: (**a**) basic, (**b**) advanced.

The advanced mode uses the interface illustrated in Figure 5b, providing additional details for those interested in analyzing the operation of the classification system. It allows users to visualize the feature maps generated by specified convolutional layers. The visualization of the feature maps can offer a low-level insight into the training process. It also allows users to directly upload GEIs or SEIs to the system.

The remote diagnostic web application prototype can be further improved to allow training the classification system with different gait representations. The visualization of detailed features supported by the advanced user interface mode can provide an important insight to understand the operation of the classification system.

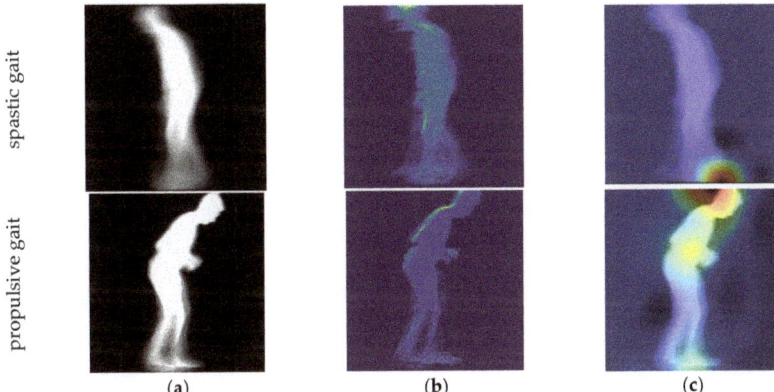

Figure 6. Output of the visualizer (**a**) GEI, (**b**) saliency feature map, (**c**) class activation map.

3. Results

The proposed gait type classification system is evaluated using a 10-fold cross-validation protocol on the GAIT-IT dataset. To emphasize the proposed system generalization capability, a second set of evaluation results considers the proposed system trained on the GAIT-IT dataset and tested on GAIT-IST. To compare the proposed system performance with the state-of-the-art, the systems presented in [6,8] are considered here for benchmarking. These systems use a solution based on VGG-19, pre-trained on Imagenet, and then fine-tuned using GEIs [6] and SEIs [8]. Those systems are re-implemented and fine-tuned using the GAIT-IT dataset, for fairness of the presented comparisons.

First, the proposed and the state-of-the-art systems [6,8] are evaluated using a 10-fold cross-validation protocol. The GAIT-IT dataset is split into training and test sets, where the subjects in each set are mutually exclusive. The test set for each fold is defined as $V_k = \{S_i, S_{i+1}, S_{i+2}\}$, where $i = 2 \times k - 1$, k is the fold iteration and S_i represents one of the 21 subjects. This arrangement ensures the use of every subject in the test set at least once, thus reducing training bias. The cross-validation results are presented in Table 1. Table 2 additionally compares the neural network model size and the execution times for the proposed and the state-of-the-art [6,8] systems, using a personal computer equipped with an AMD Ryzen 7 1700X processer, 32 GB RAM and a GTX 1070 GPU with 8 GB.

Table 1. Cross-validation results obtained using the GAIT-IT dataset.

Gait Classification System	Input	Accuracy (%)
Fine-Tuned VGG-19 [8]	GEI	94.0
Fine-Tuned VGG-19 [6]	SEI	93.6
Proposed system	GEI	93.4
Proposed system	SEI	92.6

Table 2. Number of parameters, storage space, training and execution time (milliseconds) required by the VGG-19 [6,8] and the proposed systems.

Gait Classification System	Parameters	Size (Mb)	Execution Time (ms)	
			Train	Test
Fine-Tuned VGG-19 [6,8]	139,330,565	558.4	15	6
Proposed system	1,684,421	6.8	1	1

Training and testing a classification system using the same dataset can raise the issue of overfitting. To address this issue, a cross-dataset evaluation is additionally performed using the GAIT-IST [6] and the proposed GAIT-IT datasets. This second set of evaluations are conducted by training the proposed and the state-of-the-art [6,8] systems using all available subjects from the GAIT-IT dataset, and then testing the gait type classification systems using all the available subjects from the GAIT-IST dataset. It should be noted that GAIT-IST dataset acquisition setup is significantly different from GAIT-IT, with acquisition performed using a cell phone camera, under a ceiling light. Table 3 reports the obtained classification accuracy results, while Table 4 reports the corresponding confusion matrix. Training with GAIT-IST or DAI2 was not considered as those datasets are significantly smaller and some of the available silhouettes contain segmentation errors. The other publicly available datasets discussed in Section 1.1.2 were not considered because they include simulations of limb movement impairments, rather than gait types, and their size is small.

Table 3. Cross-dataset results obtained using GAIT-IT for training and GAIT-IST for testing.

Gait Classification System	Input	Accuracy (%)
Fine-Tuned VGG-19 [8]	GEI	86.4
Fine-Tuned VGG-19 [6]	SEI	85.1
Proposed system	GEI	89.8
Proposed system	SEI	86.4

Table 4. Confusion matrix for the proposed gait type classification system representing an average score of GEI and SEI inputs (%).

		Predicted Class				
	Gait Type	Scissor (Diplegic)	Spastic (Hemiplegic)	Steppage (Neuropathic)	Normal (Healthy)	Propulsive (Parkinsonian)
True Class	Scissor	87	7	0	0	5
	Spastic	9	89	2	0	0
	Steppage	0	2	97	1	0
	Normal	0	0	0	99	0
	Propulsive	5	0	0	0	95

4. Discussion

The average classification accuracy obtained using 10-fold cross validation, reported in Table 1, suggests that the proposed system's performance, achieving a classification accuracy of 93.4% and 92.6% on GEI and SEI gait representations, respectively, is equivalent to the state-of-the-art [6,8]. However, it should be noted that the proposed system has a much lower computational complexity, due to the significantly smaller number of trainable parameters and the consequent reduction of static and dynamic memory needed to store and execute the system—see Table 2. The proposed system, represented in hdf5 [32] file format, is 83 times smaller than the state-of-the-art VGG-19 system. The proposed gait type classification system also executes significantly faster, which is of great importance for considering the deployment of a diagnostics web service to operate over the Internet. Table 2 also reports training and execution time for the proposed and the state-of-the-art [6,8] systems, showing that the proposed system operates 15 times faster during training and six times faster when processing a request.

The cross-dataset results reported in Table 3 suggest that the proposed system generalizes better than the state-of-the-art VGG-19 systems [6,8]. The proposed system improves the average classification accuracy by 3.4% and 1.3% using GEIs and SEIs, respectively. A possible explanation for this increase may be that the deeper CNN architecture requires significantly more data for fine-tuning, and to avoid overfitting to the seen training data. Thus, the shallower CNN model of the proposed gait type classification system appears to be more suitable for operation with datasets with limited training data.

Table 4 reports results of classification across five different types of gait when testing with the GAIT-IST dataset [6]. This test assumes an association between the gait types simulated in the novel GAIT-IT dataset (scissor, spastic, steppage, propulsive and normal), and the gait pathologies simulated in the GAIT-IST dataset (diplegic, hemiplegic, neuropathic, Parkinsonian, healthy), with the results obtained confirmed to be a reasonable assumption.

To further analyze the proposed system's performance, the confusion matrix presented in Table 4 highlights the prediction errors made by the proposed system. From these results it can be inferred that normal gait is the easiest to classify, with a classification accuracy of 99%., while the scissor gait is the most difficult to classify, with a classification accuracy of 87%. This can be due to the scissor gait GEIs' showing a similar appearance to spastic and propulsive GEIs, as these three types of gait involve a limited leg movement. The spastic gait performs slightly better with an average classification accuracy of 89%. The distinct walking pattern of steppage gait allows the system to achieve an average classification accuracy of 97%. Propulsive gait achieved the next best classification accuracy of 95% as it involves a stooped posture along with the restricted leg movements. Finally, it can be concluded that the proposed gait type classification system can be used to successfully identify gait impairments from 2D video sequences, which may be captured using the pervasive smartphone devices (as considered in the GAIT-IST dataset).

5. Conclusions

This paper presents the prototype of a web application for remote gait diagnostic system. The application, to be used over the Internet, implements a web service that executes a gait type classification system on the server, returning results to be reported using a user-friendly graphical interface. The novel gait type classification system is based on a shallow CNN architecture, whose performance is equivalent to the state-of-the-art classification systems [6,8], while showing two distinct advantages:

1. The proposed deep learning model is 83 times smaller than the one considered by state-of-the-art solutions [6,8]. This reduces the memory requirements and improves the execution time, which is significant when operating over the Internet;
2. The shallower network model achieves a better fit using the GAIT-IT dataset, which contains data from only 21 subjects, as confirmed by the cross-database test results. This is significant as the proposed web application accepts video sequences captured under different conditions and environments.

The paper also presents GAIT-IT dataset, containing 828 gait sequences, captured from 21 subjects simulating five different types of gait. The sequences were captured using two synchronized cameras, capturing both the sagittal and frontal views. The dataset contains silhouettes, skeletons, GEIs and SEIs.

Since this work focuses on the sagittal view, future work can consider the integration of frontal view analysis. The combination of orthogonal viewpoints can result in more discriminative features, leading to an improved classification system. Furthermore, different deep network architectures can be considered to explore the temporal nature of gait. The web application prototype is presently hosted as a web service in a private network, and after further development, e.g., to allow training the system with additional types of gaits and other gait representations, it might be made publicly available. The model is also be released in GitHub (https://github.com/jpsmachado/Gait-WebApp.git accessed date 23 July 2021).

Another possible future direction can include extending the GAIT-IT dataset to incorporate sequences from real patients. Since all the existing publicly available datasets, including GAIT-IT dataset, are composed of simulations, testing the proposed system with real patients will allow further validation of its performance in classifying gait pathologies.

Author Contributions: P.A., J.P.M., T.T.V., P.L.C. and L.D.S. participated in the design of the proposed system. J.P.M. and P.A. led the software implementation. P.A., J.P.M., T.T.V., P.L.C. and L.D.S. participated in the preparation and review of the manuscript. All authors have read and agreed to the published version of the manuscript.

Funding: This work was partly funded by FCT/MCTES under the project UIDB/50008/2020.

Institutional Review Board Statement: Not applicable.

Informed Consent Statement: Not applicable as the dataset consists of silhouettes and skeletal coordinates.

Data Availability Statement: The GAIT-IT dataset is available at http://www.img.lx.it.pt/GAIT-IT/ (accessed on 3 September 2021).

Conflicts of Interest: The authors declare no conflict of interest. The funders had no role in the design of the study; in the collection, analyses, or interpretation of data; in the writing of the manuscript, or in the decision to publish the results.

References

1. Kirtley, C. *Clinical Gait Analysis: Theory and Practice*; Elsevier Health Sciences: New York, NY, USA, 2006.
2. Boyd, J.E.; Little, J.J. Biometric gait recognition. In *Advanced Studies in Biometrics*; Springer: Berlin/Heidelberg, Germany, 2005; pp. 19–42.
3. Muro-De-La-Herran, A.; Garcia-Zapirain, B.; Mendez-Zorrilla, A. Gait analysis methods: An overview of wearable and non-wearable systems, highlighting clinical applications. *Sensors* **2014**, *14*, 3362–3394. [CrossRef] [PubMed]
4. Ailisto, H.J.; Lindholm, M.; Mantyjarvi, J.; Vildjiounaite, E.; Makela, S.-M. Identifying people from gait pattern with accelerometers. *Biom. Technol. Hum. Identif. Int. Soc. Opt. Photonics* **2005**, *5779*, 7–14.
5. Verlekar, T.T.; Soares, L.D.; Correia, P.L. Automatic classification of gait impairments using a marker-less 2D video-based system. *Sensors* **2018**, *18*, 2743. [CrossRef] [PubMed]
6. Loureiro, J.; Correia, P.L. Using a skeleton gait energy image for pathological gait classification. In Proceedings of the 15th IEEE International Conference on Automatic Face and Gesture Recognition, Buenos Aires, Argentina, 16–20 May 2020; pp. 410–414.
7. Khokhlova, M.; Migniot, C.; Morozov, A.; Sushkova, O.; Dipanda, A. Normal and pathological gait classification LSTM model. *Artif. Intell. Med.* **2019**, *94*, 54–66. [CrossRef] [PubMed]
8. Verlekar, T.T.; Soares, L.D.; Correia, P.L. Using transfer learning for classification of gait pathologies. In Proceedings of the IEEE International Conference on Bioinformatics and Biomedicine (BIBM), Madrid, Spain, 3–6 December 2018; pp. 2376–2381.
9. Simonyan, K.; Zisserman, A. Very deep convolutional networks for large-scale image recognition. *arXiv* **2014**, arXiv:1409.1556, preprint.
10. Deng, J.; Dong, W.; Socher, R.; Li, L.-J.; Li, K.; Li, F.-F. Imagenet: A large-scale hierarchical image database. In Proceedings of the IEEE Conference on Computer Vision and Pattern Recognition, Miami, FL, USA, 20–25 June 2009; pp. 248–255.
11. Slijepcevic, D.; Zeppelzauer, M.; Gorgas, A.M.; Schwab, C.; Schüller, M.; Baca, A.; Breiteneder, C.; Horsak, B. Automatic classification of functional gait disorders. *IEEE J. Biomed. Health Inform.* **2018**, *22*, 1653–1661. [CrossRef] [PubMed]
12. Mannini, A.; Trojaniello, D.; Cereatti, A.; Sabatini, A. A Machine Learning Framework for Gait Classification Using Inertial Sensors: Application to Elderly, Post-Stroke and Huntington's Disease Patients. *Sensors* **2016**, *16*, 134. [CrossRef] [PubMed]
13. Vanrenterghem, J.; Gormley, D.; Robinson, M.; Lees, A. Solutions for representing the whole-body centre of mass inside cutting manoeuvres based on data that is typically available for lower limb kinematics. *Gait Posture* **2010**, *31*, 517–521. [CrossRef] [PubMed]
14. Verlekar, T.; Vroey, H.; Claeys, K.; Hallez, H.; Soares, L.; Correia, P. Estimation and validation of temporal gait features using a markerless 2D video system. *Comput. Methods Programs Biomed.* **2019**, *175*, 45–51. [CrossRef] [PubMed]
15. Wang, J.; She, M.; Nahavandi, S.; Kouzani, A. A review of vision-based gait recognition methods for human identification. In Proceedings of the International Conference on Digital Image Computing: Techniques and Applications, Sydney, Australia, 1–3 December 2010; pp. 320–327.
16. Verlekar, T.; Correia, P.; Soares, L. Gait recognition using normalized shadows. In Proceedings of the 25th European Signal Processing Conference (EUSIPCO), Kos Island, Greece, 28 August–2 September 2017; pp. 936–940.
17. Wang, Y.; Sun, J.; Li, J.; Zhao, D. Gait recognition based on 3D skeleton joints captured by kinect. In Proceedings of the IEEE International Conference on Image Processing (ICIP), Phoenix, AZ, USA, 25–28 September 2016; pp. 3151–3155.
18. Han, J.; Bhanu, B. Individual recognition using gait energy image. *IEEE Trans. Pattern Anal. Mach. Intell.* **2005**, *28*, 316–322. [CrossRef] [PubMed]
19. Cao, Z.; Hidalgo, G.; Simon, T.; Wei, S.; Sheikh, Y. Open pose: Realtime multi-person 2D pose estimation using part affinity fields. *arXiv* **2018**, arXiv:1812.08008.
20. Nieto-Hidalgo, M.; García-Chamizo, J. Classification of pathologies using a vision based feature extraction. In Proceedings of the International Conference on Ubiquitous Computing and Ambient Intelligence, Philadelphia, PA, USA, 7–10 November 2017; pp. 265–274.
21. Ortells, J.; Herrero-Ezquerro, M.; Mollineda, R. Vision-based gait impairment analysis for aided diagnosis. *Med Biol. Eng. Comput.* **2018**, *56*, 1553–1564. [CrossRef] [PubMed]
22. Nieto-Hidalgo, M.; Ferrández-Pastor, F.; Valdivieso-Sarabia, R.; Mora-Pascual, J.; García-Chamizo, J. Vision based extraction of dynamic gait features focused on feet movement using RGB camera. In *Ambient Intelligence for Health*; Springer: Cham, Switzerland, 2015; pp. 155–166.

23. Hochreiter, S.; Schmidhuber, J. Long Short-Term Memory. *Neural Comput.* **1997**, *9*, 1735–1780. [CrossRef] [PubMed]
24. Stanford School of Medicine. Gait Abnormalities. Available online: https://stanfordmedicine25.stanford.edu/the25/gait.html (accessed on 3 September 2021).
25. Digit Recognizer. Available online: https://www.kaggle.com/c/digit-recognizer/overview (accessed on 3 September 2021).
26. Deotte, C. How to Choose CNN Architecture MNIST. Available online: https://www.kaggle.com/cdeotte/how-to-choose-cnn-architecture-mnist (accessed on 3 September 2021).
27. Srivastava, N.; Hinton, G.; Krizhevsky, A.; Sutskever, I.; Salakhutdi-nov, R. Dropout: A simple way to prevent neural networks from overfitting. *J. Mach. Learn. Res.* **2014**, *15*, 1929–1958.
28. Kingma, D.; Ba, J. Adam: A method for stochastic optimization. In Proceedings of the 3rd International Conference on Learning Representations, ICLR, San Diego, CA, USA, 7–9 May 2015; pp. 1–15.
29. Nesterov, Y. A method for solving the convex programming problem with convergence rate $O(1/k^2)$. *Dokl. Akad. Nauk Sssr.* **1983**, *269*, 543–547.
30. Simonyan, K.; Vedaldi, A.; Zisserman, A. Deep inside convolutional networks: Visualizing image classification models and saliency maps. *arXiv* **2013**, arXiv:1312.6034.
31. Selvaraju, R.; Cogswell, M.; Das, A.; Vedantam, R.; Parikh, D.; Batra, D. Grad-cam: Visual explanations from deep networks via gradient-based localization. In Proceedings of the IEEE international conference on computer vision, Venice, Italy, 22–29 October 2017; pp. 618–626.
32. Folk, M.; Heber, G.; Koziol, Q.; Pourmal, E.; Robinson, D. An overview of the HDF5 technology suite and its applications. In Proceedings of the EDBT/ICDT 2011 Workshop on Array Databases, Uppsala, Sweden, 25 March 2011; pp. 36–47.

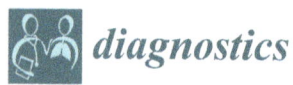

Review

Robot-Aided Motion Analysis in Neurorehabilitation: Benefits and Challenges

Mirjam Bonanno * and Rocco Salvatore Calabrò

IRCCS Centro Neurolesi Bonino Pulejo, Cda Casazza, S.S. 113, 98124 Messina, Italy; roccos.calabro@irccsme.it
* Correspondence: mirjam.bonanno@irccsme.it

Abstract: In the neurorehabilitation field, robot-aided motion analysis (R-AMA) could be helpful for two main reasons: (1) it allows the registration and monitoring of patients' motion parameters in a more accurate way than clinical scales (clinical purpose), and (2) the multitude of data produced using R-AMA can be used to build machine learning algorithms, detecting prognostic and predictive factors for better motor outcomes (research purpose). Despite their potential in clinical settings, robotic assessment tools have not gained widespread clinical acceptance. Some barriers remain to their clinical adoption, such as their reliability and validity compared to the existing standardized scales. In this narrative review, we sought to investigate the usefulness of R-AMA systems in patients affected by neurological disorders. We found that the most used R-AMA tools are the Lokomat (an exoskeleton device used for gait and balance rehabilitation) and the Armeo (both Power and Spring, used for the rehabilitation of upper limb impairment). The motion analysis provided by these robotic devices was used to tailor rehabilitation sessions based on the objective quantification of patients' functional abilities. Spinal cord injury and stroke patients were the most investigated individuals with these common exoskeletons. Research on the use of robotics as an assessment tool should be fostered, taking into account the biomechanical parameters able to predict the accuracy of movements.

Keywords: robot-aided motion analysis; objective motor assessment; biomechanics; neurorehabilitation

1. Introduction

In the field of neurorehabilitation, innovative technologies, such as robotic devices, have been widely used to treat and evaluate patients affected by motor impairment due to different neurological disorders (e.g., stroke, multiple sclerosis (MS), and spinal cord injury (SCI)) [1]. Compared with conventional rehabilitation approaches, robotic-assisted therapy (RAT) may have some advantages, including (i) guaranteeing repetitive, intensive, and task-oriented rehabilitation; (ii) reducing the physical burden on clinical therapists, giving them the possibility to treat more patients simultaneously; and (iii) quantitatively and objectively assessing patients' motor performance over time [2,3]. In particular, objective assessment of motor performance is a fundamental issue in neurorehabilitation [4]. In fact, clinical scales are still widely used in hospital settings, despite their validity and reliability being under debate. Robot-aided motion analysis (R-AMA) could be helpful for two main reasons: (i) it allows the registration and monitoring of patients' motion parameters in a more accurate way than clinical scales (clinical purpose), and (ii) the multitude of data produced using R-AMA can be used to build machine learning algorithms, detecting prognostic and predictive factors for better motor outcomes (research purpose). Specifically, motion analysis refers to the recording of three-dimensional movements of human body segments and the subsequent computation of meaningful parameters that describe human movement from raw kinematic parameters [5,6]. Motion analysis is commonly carried out through wearable and non-wearable sensors that are able to detect biomechanical parameters of movements [7]. Similarly, robotic devices, both end effectors and exoskeletons, through

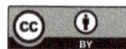

specific sensors, could allow the detection of passive or active range of motion, movement accuracy, and planning [8]. For example, Maggioni et al. [9] examined the possibilities of assessing lower extremity function using robots, with parameters such as range of motion (RoM), muscle strength, and proprioception. In fact, the Lokomat (which is a tethered exoskeleton) was used to assess joint position sense (i.e., proprioception) in patients with incomplete spinal cord injury. Despite their potential in clinical settings, robotic assessment tools have not gained widespread clinical acceptance. Some barriers to and doubts about their clinical adoption remain, such as their reliability and validity compared to the existing standardized scales and motion analysis.

In this narrative review, we aimed to investigate the usefulness of R-AMA systems in patients affected by neurological disorders.

2. Methods

Given the narrative nature of the paper, we only described the most relevant papers on the issue by searching for them on PubMed, IEEE Xplore, and Scopus, considering the period from 2010 to 2023. We chose this period because this past decade has witnessed the implementation of robotic devices in the neurorehabilitation field. To select evidence, we used the following keywords: "robotic device" OR "exoskeleton" AND "motor assessment" OR "biomechanical assessment" OR "biomechanical parameters" OR "lower limb assessment" OR "upper limb assessment" OR "motion analysis." Since this is a narrative review, we included the most relevant pilot studies, observational studies, randomized controlled trials, case–control studies, and systematic reviews, considering also the references of the selected articles, including only English papers. Each article was evaluated through the title, abstract, text, and scientific validity [10].

3. Motion Analysis and Its Biomechanical Contribution to Accuracy Prediction

Motion analysis involves registering the three-dimensional movements of human body segments and then calculating biomechanical parameters that describe human movement [11]. The modeling of human motion can be studied from different perspectives. For this purpose, various approaches are used to derive mathematical expressions that describe human motion. Newton's equations of motion are the fundamental tools for understanding the cause–effect relationship between the forces acting on a system and the resulting motion [12]. However, applying them to complex systems, such as human locomotion, which involve a large number of degrees of freedom, requires formulating and solving multiple equations, leading to high computational costs. The Euler–Lagrange method is used in multibody systems because it analyzes the entire system without studying the reaction and contact forces between the elements that comprise the system. This equation allows for the study of human motion by focusing solely on the mechanical energy of the system. The knowledge of motion equations allows researchers to identify problems and design mechanisms that seek to recognize or recover human movements [13]. Nowadays, motion analysis has evolved substantially in parallel with technological advancements, encompassing various applications, such as clinical gait analysis and 3D biomechanical modeling [14]. Biomechanical motion analysis is generally based on two types of models: the multibody model and the finite element model. The first type consists of a set of rigid or flexible bodies connected by joints, while the second type of motion analysis reconstructs internal strain, stress, or deformation in flexible bodies based on continuum mechanics theories [15,16].

Within a rehabilitation setting, quantitative analysis of human body kinematics is a powerful tool that has been used to understand the different biomechanical patterns of both healthy and pathological individuals [17]. Recently, biomechanical tools have also been developed, ranging from simple manual annotation of images to marker-based optical trackers and inertial sensor-based systems. Nowadays, motion analysis can be performed using marker-less systems that use sophisticated human body models, computer vision, and machine learning algorithms [17]. Biomechanical parameters that are considered during motion analysis include kinematic and kinetic parameters [18,19]. In particular, kinematic parameters [20] include the spatial and temporal aspects of movement. These parameters describe (a) the "static" direction during point-to-point movements; (b) the continuous change of position, speed, and acceleration, which can be further subdivided into its amplitude and direction components; or (c) combinations of these, such as movement trajectories.

4. Robotic Devices for Upper Limb Measurement

Kinematic (e.g., position, velocity, and acceleration) and kinetic (e.g., force, joint torque, and muscle activity) data are acquired from sensors affixed to robotic and passive mechanical devices to measure biomechanical aspects of upper extremities [21–28] (see more in Table 1).

Table 1. Studies about upper limb robotic-aided motion analysis performed in neurological disorders.

Reference No.	Robotic Device	Description	Usefulness of Robot-Aided Motion Analysis
[29]	Armeo®Power (Hocoma AG, Switzerland)	The Armeo®Power is a 6-degrees-of-freedom exoskeleton for upper limb rehabilitation.	Useful tool for the objective evaluation of upper limbs in post-stroke patients. The kinetic parameters of the motion analysis included kinetic parameters of the shoulder (flexion–extension, abduction and adduction, internal and external rotation), of the elbow (flexion–extension, prone–supination), of the wrist (flexion–extension), and of the hand (opening and closing). The values deriving from the valuation of the articular range were expressed in degrees; the values deriving from the evaluation of the force were expressed in Newton meters (Nm).
[30]	Armeo®Spring (Hocoma AG, Switzerland)	The Armeo®Spring device is an exoskeleton for upper limb rehabilitation. It is equipped with 7 goniometers and 1 pressure sensor, which permits free 3D arm movement. At the end of the robotic arm, there is a handle, which contains a pressure sensor, measuring the grip force.	The authors used the Armeo®Spring device to conduct a quantitative assessment of the precision, speed, and smoothness of upper limb motion. Among the several measures, the hand path ratio is the ratio between the actual path in the horizontal plane and the shortest-possible path, which reflects movement efficiency. The mean velocity and the number of peaks in the velocity profile were also assessed. Additionally, the normalized jerk (Norm Jerk), a measure of trajectory smoothness, was analyzed.
[31]	Armeo®Spring (Hocoma AG, Switzerland)	As described before	The Armeo®Spring was used to assess movement accuracy by measuring the hand path ratio, the mean velocity, and the number of peaks in the velocity profile. The authors concluded that the device should be integrated into the clinical evaluation of upper limb functions in post-stroke patients.
[32]	InMotion 2.0 (Bionik Laboratories, Watertown, MA, USA)	The InMotion 2.0 device is an end effector in which the subject moves their arm from a central target to 8 peripheral targets.	The authors assessed kinematic parameters of the upper limb, including elbow extension and shoulder flexion, abduction and external rotation of the shoulder, elbow flexion and shoulder extension, and adduction and internal rotation of the shoulder. These parameters, calculated at baseline, can assist clinicians in defining a rehabilitation program for post-stroke patients.
[33]	Gloreha Sinfonia (Idrogenet, Lumezzane BS, Italy –)	Gloreha Sinfonia is a robotic glove for hand rehabilitation to maintain range of motion (i.e., the flexion angle excursion of the finger metacarpophalangeal joints) of the patient's hand.	The authors objectively evaluated hand movements using the Gloreha Sinfonia glove in order to customize rehabilitation sessions according to patients' motor abilities. The angular values of the joints were assessed using bending sensors embedded in the glove.

These kinds of measures are commonly registered in post-stroke patients, who may present unilateral hemiplegic involvement. However, the percentage of studies dealing with R-AMA for upper limbs is still poor. It seems that the Armeo®Spring was the most used for this issue, followed by the Armeo®Power, InMotion 2.0, and Gloreha Sinfonia, as reported in Figure 1.

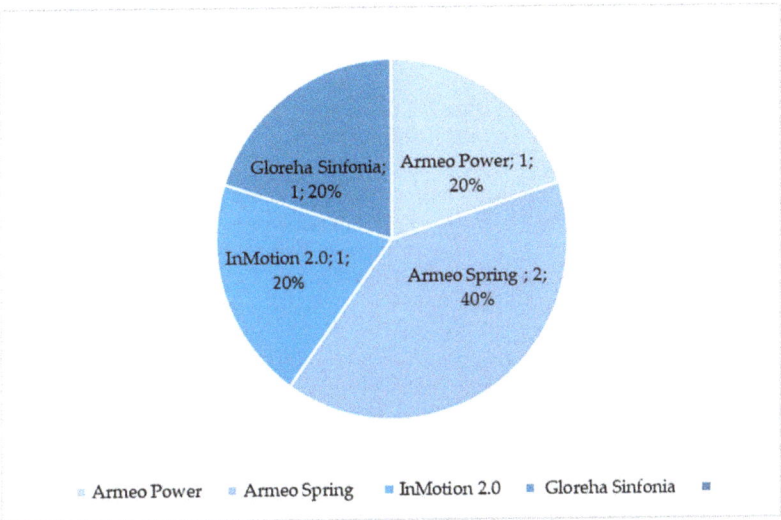

Figure 1. Percentage of selected articles reported in Table 1 dealing with upper limb robotic-aided motion analysis.

For example, one of the most used robotic devices in post-stroke neurorehabilitation is the Armeo®Power, an exoskeleton for upper limb training. Its efficacy in improving functional outcomes is already demonstrated in the literature [34,35]; however, few authors have investigated its role in assessing upper limb functions.

Specifically, this robotic device can evaluate specific kinematic parameters [36], as reported in Table 1. In addition, the Armeo®Power evaluates the range of joint movement, which is expressed in degrees, and the force of muscles, which is expressed in Newton meters (Nm). According to Galeoto et al. [29], the Armeo®Power can be considered an objective robotic tool compared to the Fugl–Meyer for upper limb (FM-UL) clinical scale items. The FM-UL clinical scale is the most used and reliable scale to assess motor functions, joint range of motion, joint pain, dysmetria, and tremor in post-stroke patients [37]. The authors found strong correlations between flexion synergy (forearm supination and elbow flexion) and results measured with the Armeo®Power. This suggests that the Armeo®Power is more accurate than the FM-UL clinical scale in evaluating upper limb movements [29].

Other researchers have also evaluated the motor function of stroke patients using robotic devices and measuring upper limb biomechanical features, such as movement velocity, accuracy, and smoothness in active training [30,31]. Merlo et al. [30] used the Armeo®Spring to conduct these measurements. To obtain objective data on upper limb functions, the Armeo®Spring calculates a set of numerical indices based on the 3D endpoint trajectory during the "vertical capture" task. The patient receives visual feedback of their hand position through a display, which is used to facilitate rehabilitation exercises. Indeed, the derived indices (movement velocity, accuracy, and smoothness) are easy to share with clinicians because they describe the motor impairment of the upper limb [28].

For example, the loss of movement accuracy can be related to a reduction in sensibility, whereas the decrease in velocity refers to paresis/paralysis, and the loss of smoothness refers to an abnormal muscle tone (spasticity) [38]. However, before implementing them in clinical practice, these indices must be validated by comparing them with other clinical scales. In their study, Longhi et al. [31] analyzed three aspects of upper limb (UL) evaluation. First, they examined the ability of the Armeo®Spring to distinguish between stroke patients and healthy subjects. Second, they assessed the validity of the indices used to measure movement. Lastly, they investigated the concurrent validity of these indices by comparing them with the Wolf Motor Function test, a clinically validated scale for assessing UL motor function. The authors' results confirmed the construct validity of the three indices, which is consistent with the findings of Merlo et al. [30]. This suggests that the Armeo®Spring can be a promising tool for objectively assessing UL motor skills. In addition, Goffredo et al. [32] performed a kinematic evaluation of the upper limb in post-stroke patients using the end effector InMotion 2.0.

The kinematic parameters were calculated from the trajectories recorded by the robot, starting from the central target and extending to the peripheral targets in various directions. The kinematic parameters described by the authors [32] refer to the functional abilities of the UL. However, the Armeo®Power and the Armeo®Spring cannot perform hand motion analysis due to their biomechanical architecture. To this aim, Cordella et al. [33] conducted a quantitative and objective assessment of hand movement in post-stroke patients using the Gloreha Sinfonia. The Gloreha Sinfonia is a robotic glove used to train hand motor functions, focusing on the recovery of range of motion [33]. Once calibrated, this glove allows an objective assessment of motor performance. In particular, the results of the authors [33] demonstrated that the Gloreha Sinfonia can measure angular values from bending sensors embedded in the glove.

Another concern that should be considered in clinical practice is the objective evaluation of spasticity. The Modified Ashworth Scale (MAS) is, in fact, the most commonly used clinical tool for assessing spasticity. However, it does have several limitations [39]. Indeed, de-la-Torre et al. [38] in their systematic review found that R-AMA based on data capture is effective for evaluating spasticity. However, it should be noted that cutting-edge algorithms provide a more predictive and analytical measure than the only variation between the original and the final status obtained from clinical scales [38]. Moreover, some authors [40] have evaluated muscle synergies in post-stroke patients using a robotic device. Muscle synergy specifically refers to the coordinated activation of both joints and muscles in order to execute purposeful movements [41,42]. Post-stroke patients tend to activate abnormal muscle synergies due to brain lesions in the corticospinal tract, which are further enhanced by hyperreflexia. This aspect is fundamental in establishing the most effective treatment for patients in the clinical rehabilitation setting. In this vein, Kung et al. [40] found that robotic devices, such as end effectors, can be used for long-term evaluation of muscle synergies.

They registered kinematic, kinetic, and electromyographic (EMG) signals during the tracking movement in order to develop biomechanical indices for evaluating muscle synergies. In fact, their results revealed that abnormal synergies can be assessed through two tracking directions: D2 (contra-proximal to ipsi-lateral) and D4 (left–right) [40]. Lastly, robotic devices can also measure muscle strength, as suggested by Toigo et al. [43]. In particular, the term "muscle strength" refers to force, moment, or power [43]. Robotic devices, including exoskeletons and end effectors, are equipped with force sensors for quantifying the interaction forces between the device and the patient [44]. These devices record raw sensor data on force during functional movements, enabling the extraction of valuable data detecting abnormal muscle synergies [43]. However, misalignments with the device and variations in the rotational axis of a joint can distort the results. Moreover, all kinematic and kinetic movement parameters are represented to some extent in the sensorimotor cortex. Distal movements of the hand, including movement direction and trajectories, can be discriminated in the sensorimotor cortex. This ability has potential applications in brain–computer interface technology [21].

5. Robotic Device for Lower Limb Assessment

Walking recovery in neurological patients is one of the most important goals planned by therapists [45]. In order to maximize the recovery of the walking function, it is important to define a personalized rehabilitation treatment, in addition to an accurate assessment to monitor patients' progress. In fact, both clinical and instrumental tools already exist to perform an accurate analysis of motion [45]. However, if the assessment protocol takes too much time to perform, clinicians and therapists may be reluctant to adopt them. A possible solution could involve the use of robotic devices in which the patient would undergo both training and assessment. In this study, Imoto et al. [46] used a novel gait training robot known as WelWalk WW-2000. This robot enables the adjustment of various gait parameters (such as time and mechanical assistance load) during the training session. The robot is equipped with sensors and a markerless motion capture system to detect altered gait patterns in stroke patients. This system can evaluate individuals' gait patterns and provide tailored rehabilitation gait training [46]. Generally, the objective assessment of the lower limb should consider the simultaneous measurement of joint angles, spatial and temporal parameters of gait, muscle strength, proprioception, and spasticity and/or muscle stiffness [47] (see Table 2).

Table 2. Studies about lower limb robotic-aided motion analysis performed on neurological patients.

Reference No.	Robotic Device	Description	Usefulness of Robot-Aided Motion Analysis
[46]	WelWalk (WW-2000, Toyota Motor Corporation, Aichi, Japan)	Knee-ankle-foot robot, low floor treadmill, safety suspension device for body weight support, monitor for patient use, 3D sensor, and control panel	Three-dimensional joint positions, lower limb tilt, and knee joint angle were recorded during a task using a 3D sensor, an inertial sensor, and a knee angle sensor. Two-dimensional joint positions collected using skeletal tracking software (VisionPose®, NEXT-SYSTEM Co., Ltd., Fukuoka, Japan) and depth data from the 3D sensor were used to estimate the three-dimensional coordinates of the joint positions. Bilateral hip, knee, ankle, and shoulder joints, as well as the midpoints of the shoulder and hip joints, were the predicted locations of the 3D joints. This objective gait analysis can be useful for individuals with hemiparetic stroke, as it provides individually tailored gait training based on these assessments.
[48]	Ekso (Ekso Bionics, San Rafael, CA 94901, USA)	Ekso a wearable unthethered exoskeleton. Motors power the hip and knee joints and all motion are started either through specific patient actions or the use of an external controller.	The authors conducted a comprehensive assessment by utilizing both kinematic and kinetic parameters, as well as EEG registrations, in patients with Parkinson's disease. In this way, clinicians can personalize the rehabilitation treatment with a device that could increase the treatment intensity and dose without burdening therapists.
[49]	Ekso (Ekso Bionics, San Rafael, CA 94901, USA)	As described before	Muscle synergies and activation profiles were extracted using non-negative matrix factorization. The authors' findings provided insights into the potential underlying mechanism for improving gait functions through exoskeleton-assisted locomotor training.
[50]	Lokomat (Hocoma AG, Switzerland)	The Lokomat is a robotic tethered exoskeleton with active hip–knee actuation and passive ankle control during the swing phase, in addition to a variable level of assistance.	The Lokomat was used to assess proprioception, which provides information about static position and movement sense, using custom software to measure joint position sense in the hip and knee. The authors demonstrated the usefulness of the Lokomat in measuring proprioception in SCI patients.

Table 2. *Cont.*

Reference No.	Robotic Device	Description	Usefulness of Robot-Aided Motion Analysis
[51]	Lokomat (Hocoma AG, Switzerland)	As described before	The authors proved the Lokomat's usefulness in objectively assessing proprioception at the hip and knee in people with SCI.
[52]	Lokomat (Hocoma AG, Switzerland)	As described before	Since lower limb kinesthesia deficits are common in SCI patients, the authors demonstrated that the Lokomat can serve as a valid and reliable robotic device for monitoring sensory function. Kinesthesia was evaluated using angular encoders of the hip and knee. During the analysis, a score was generated based on the difference between the initial angle and the final angle.

The Lokomat, which is a tethered exoskeleton, is one of most used robotic devices for gait training and for motion analysis in neurological disorders. In fact, 57% of the selected papers reported the use of the Lokomat in performing R-AMA, followed by Ekso and the WelWalk, as reported in Figure 2.

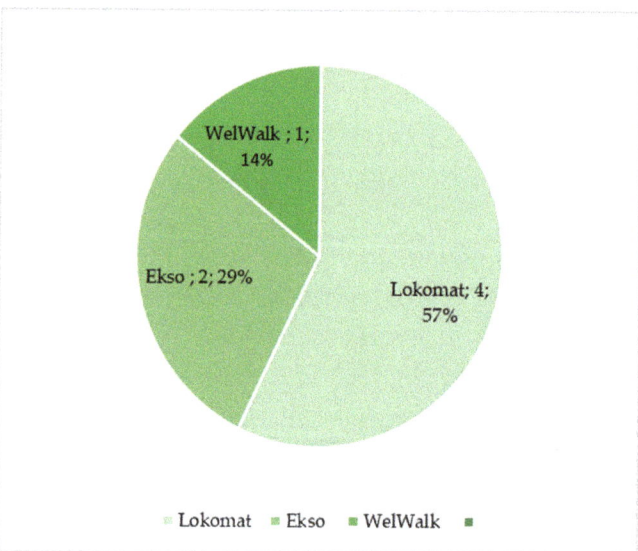

Figure 2. Percentage of selected articles reported in Table 2 dealing with lower limb robotic-aided motion analysis.

According to a systematic review [53], the Lokomat seems to be most suitable for the motion analysis of lower limbs. Maggioni et al. [54] used the Lokomat to perform a type of gait analysis, also adding force sensors and potentiometers. The authors successfully developed and tested a novel specific algorithm to assess walking through the Lokomat. Indeed, the Lokomat was used to calculate joint angles, assuming that those measured by the exoskeleton also corresponded to the human angles [54]. Mercado et al. [55] calculated joint angles in healthy subjects using the Denavit–Hartenberg notation and the Euler–Lagrange approach to process video recordings of movement. Another study [48] investigates the use of Ekso-GT, an overground exoskeleton, to assess gait parameters, such as stride time, stride length, gait speed, and gait events. Although Ekso does not provide a comprehensive report of gait parameters, these parameters and measurements can be derived from other calculations made by the exoskeleton. This allows for an accurate assessment of gait during training using mathematical models. In addition, exoskeletons, like Ekso, can be integrated with surface electromyography (sEMG) signals to monitor muscle synergies and muscular patterns during walking. According to a systematic review [56], the rectus femoris and vastus lateralis are the most frequently recorded muscles during gait. Indeed, the posterior calf muscles, which play a role in ankle and foot movement, have been less studied during gait training, despite their importance in the gait cycle. Similarly, Afzal et al. [49] investigated muscle synergies in patients with MS who were wearing an exoskeleton. EMG signals were recorded from seven muscles, including the vastus medialis, rectus femoris, biceps femoris, semitendinosus, soleus, medial gastrocnemius, and tibialis anterior muscles. The authors demonstrated that exoskeleton assistance does not alter the existing muscle synergies but it can induce a modification in neural commands [49].

Another point to consider is the evaluation of proprioception provided by robotic devices. Three studies [50–52] in spinal cord patients have addressed the evaluation of proprioception or kinesthesia using the Lokomat. In fact, the Lokomat is equipped with position sensors that are able to determine joint angles. For proprioception, the authors considered the difference between the target position and the achieved position for evaluation purposes [50,51]. Another author [52] evaluated kinesthesia by passively moving the lower limb in a specific direction while patients were wearing the exoskeleton.

6. Discussion

In this narrative review, we found that robotic devices may be used to assess motor behavior in patients with neurological disorders. Indeed, according to the few available studies, two main exoskeletons, namely the Lokomat and the Armeo®Spring, R-AMA may provide clinicians and researchers with reliable and more objective data regarding motion analysis of the lower and upper limbs, respectively [30,31,50–54]. In addition, upper limb R-AMA was tested only in post-stroke patients [29–31,33,36,37], while other neurological disorders were excluded. This issue could be related to the fact that the motor symptoms of other neurological pathologies, specifically those related to MS, are often complicated by ataxia or extrapyramidal signs. These complications have a negative impact on motion analysis [45]. Indeed, post-stroke patients manifest moderate-to-severe upper limb sequalae (mainly weakness with hypotonia in the acute phase) due to damage in the cortico-spinal tract [57]. Similarly, lower limb R-AMA was mostly performed on patients with SCI [50–52], who are characterized by severe lower limb motor impairments, mostly due to the traumatic interruption of central nervous pathways. Given that R-AMA was performed only in patients with moderate-to-severe motor impairment, future studies should take into account other levels of severity, as well as consider other pathologies. (e.g., MS, PD, and traumatic brain injury).

6.1. Benefits of Robotic-Aided Motion Analysis

Compared with conventional assessment methods, such as clinical scales or tests administered by physiotherapists and/or physicians, R-AMA offers several advantages. It can provide tri-axial measurements, analyze the patient's limb trajectory, accurately register spatial-temporal parameters of movement, and collect a large amount of data. Altogether, these elements allow for personalization of the rehabilitation path according to patients' needs. This personalized approach can be used to create a tailored patient profile, which includes a precise physiotherapy program. This program considers both traditional and cutting-edge devices for treatment. In recent years, the concept of personalized treatment has gained significant traction in various medical fields [58], including neurology and rehabilitation.

In this vein, the so-called "rehabilomics" sheds some light on the role of biomarkers in the clinical and rehabilitation setting [59]. This approach has primarily focused on the biological field, including proteomics, genomics, metabolomics, and other related areas. However, the kinematics and electrophysiological indicators can be considered biomarkers, as suggested by Garro et al. [60]. Indeed, the development of biomarkers based on the models of motor control mechanisms may be useful in a clinical context to understand healthy functions, disability, and rehabilitation progress. In this way, R-AMA can conduct a neuromechanical assessment, which examines the connection between neurological pathology and biomechanical issues [61] (Figure 3).

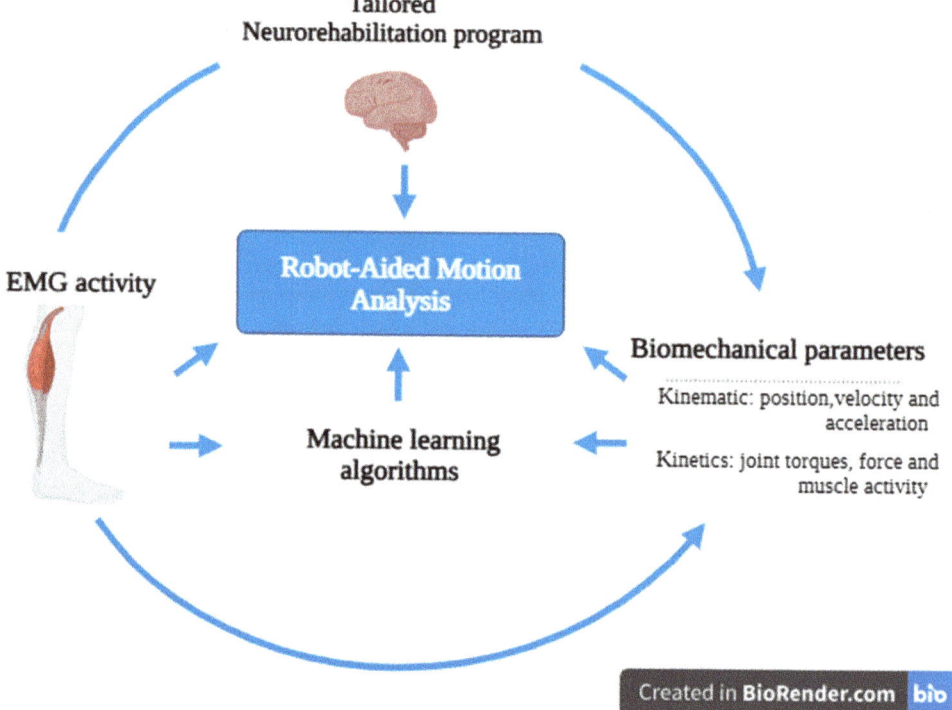

Figure 3. Graphic illustration showing the theoretical usefulness of robot-aided motion analysis in the field of neurorehabilitation. The figure was created with Biorender.com.

Legend: R-AMA could be useful to personalize neurorehabilitation programs, thanks to both biomarkers provided by EMG biosignals (on the left) and biomechanical parameters (on the right), including kinematic and kinetics. In the end, the great quantity of data obtained through R-AMA could be further used for MLA for individuating motor biomarkers involved in recovery prediction.

6.2. Challenges of Robotic-Aided Motion Analysis

To date, research on robotic devices has primarily focused on neuromotor training and recovery in patients with neurological disorders, without considering the potential role of these devices in objectively evaluating movement. However, physicians frequently criticize these technical solutions, claiming that the outcome measures offered by robotic devices are too abstract, do not translate into practical function, and lack ecological validity.

An important point that should be addressed is that robotic devices may require a lengthy setup time and the support of technical staff to operate. In the clinical setting, the physiotherapist has 30–60 min of rehabilitation treatment for each patient, and this could further discourage the use of robotic devices in clinical practice. Additionally, robotic devices, especially exoskeletons, must be perfectly aligned with the user to avoid undesired interaction forces [62]. These forces can result in an uncomfortable and unsafe human–robot interaction in the case of high forces or torques. Solutions to address misalignment of the joint's axes can include soft exoskeletons, which are constructed from soft textiles or elastomers. These exoskeletons offer greater user compliance compared to rigid robotic orthoses [63]. However, robotic devices are not available in all rehabilitation centers due to their costs, maintenance requirements, and the need for additional staff [64]. These may be some reasons why robot-based assessments have not yet been integrated into clinical practice on a large scale.

However, recent technological developments in the field of wearable devices, such as accelerometers and inertial sensors, have the advantage of providing objective motion analysis as low-cost and easy-to-use tools, as opposed to robotic devices [17,45]. In this sense, professional engineers should be encouraged to develop assessment technologies that are not constrained by practical limitations and administrative burdens. In our opinion, we must identify and overcome the barriers that prevent the translation of robotic evaluations to clinical application.

6.3. Future Perspectives: Combined Approaches and Beyond

The selection of motion biomarkers predicting recovery remains an open and under-debate question. According to Amrani El Yaakoubi et al. [56], EMG and biomechanical parameters together, including both kinetic and kinematic factors, are the most used predictors for lower limb movement. EMG is, in fact, sensitive to neuromuscular changes, particularly in post-stroke patients. The most common surface EMG analyses are time-domain and frequency-domain analyses. Specifically, among frequency-domain analyses, the mean frequency and median frequency are the most effective to assess muscle fatigue in post-stroke patients [65]. Hussain et al. [66] found that a machine learning neural network model based on EMG frequency domains has a high level of accuracy. However, the muscles that contribute the most to kinetic and kinematic prediction cannot currently be defined due to the heterogeneity of the results from the studies. In contrast, the kinematic assessment of the upper limb mainly includes the smoothness of the trajectory, as suggested by various authors [66,67]. Scano et al. [68] identified that post-stroke patients exhibit lower smoothness of trajectory, indicating difficulty in controlling the upper limb during multi-joint movements. Also, the authors found that elbow and shoulder joints showed a limited ROM, likely due to altered postural accommodation. In this view, analyzing EMG signals during upper limb functional activities with or without exoskeletons could be a future objective to achieve. Moreover, other biosignals, like EEG, can be used to control robotic devices through the brain–computer interface (BCI). An EEG-based brain-controlled robot is a robotic device that uses an EEG-based BCI to receive control commands from its user [69]. In the field of neurorehabilitation, EEG-based brain-controlled assistive robots are divided into manipulators and mobiles. Brain-controlled manipulators operate under direct BCI control, with user commands being sent to the robots. This is done without the need for additional assistance from robot intelligence elements [70]. In contrast, brain-controlled mobiles operate under shared BCI control, which involves combining a BCI system with an intelligent controller. Robots of this type are safer, less tiring for their users, and more accurate in interpreting and executing their commands [71,72]. Therefore, future developments in rehabilitation robotics should enable physicians to choose the most appropriate biomechanical parameters according to an individual patient's specific requirements. Future technological advancements in the assessment of motor performance should consider kinematic, EMG, and EEG signals. This aspect could be crucial in understanding how the brain's sensorimotor cortex encodes movements to achieve optimal neural control of motor performance. It also enables the differentiation between healthy and pathological characteristics. Hence, in order to guide the development of future robotic-based assessment tools, it is essential to foster multidisciplinary collaboration between clinical professionals (such as neurologists, physiatrists, and physiotherapists) and biomedical engineers.

7. Conclusions

In conclusion, the utility of R-AMA for both clinical and research purposes is still a subject of debate, although some promising findings have been reported regarding the effectiveness of the Lokomat and the Armeo. The motion analysis provided by these robotic devices is used to customize rehabilitation sessions, relying on the objective quantification of patients' functional abilities. It should be considered that clinical scales and tests used to monitor motor recovery in neurological patients are less accurate than motion analysis conducted by robotic devices. Next, research on the use of robotics and assessment tools should be encouraged. Future studies should be oriented toward two different frontiers: (1) understanding the most useful biomechanical parameters that can predict the accuracy of movements and (2) validating robotic device assessments for clinical purposes.

Author Contributions: Conceptualization, M.B. and R.S.C.; methodology, M.B.; validation, M.B. and R.S.C.; investigation, M.B. and R.S.C.; resources, R.S.C.; data curation, M.B.; writing—original draft preparation, M.B.; writing—review and editing, R.S.C.; visualization, M.B. and R.S.C.; supervision, R.S.C.; funding acquisition, R.S.C. All authors have read and agreed to the published version of the manuscript.

Funding: This study was supported by Current Research funds 2023, Ministry of Health, Italy.

Institutional Review Board Statement: Not applicable.

Informed Consent Statement: Not applicable.

Data Availability Statement: Not applicable.

Acknowledgments: The authors wish to thank Alex Donato for English editing.

Conflicts of Interest: The authors declare no conflict of interest.

References

1. Iandolo, R.; Marini, F.; Semprini, M.; Laffranchi, M.; Mugnosso, M.; Cherif, A.; De Michieli, L.; Chiappalone, M.; Zenzeri, J. Perspectives and Challenges in Robotic Neurorehabilitation. *Appl. Sci.* **2019**, *9*, 3183. [CrossRef]
2. Meng, W.; Liu, Q.; Zhou, Z.; Ai, Q.; Sheng, B.; Xie, S. Recent development of mechanisms and control strategies for robot-assisted lower limb rehabilitation. *Mechatronics* **2015**, *31*, 132–145. [CrossRef]
3. Rehmat, N.; Zuo, J.; Meng, W.; Liu, Q.; Xie, S.Q.; Liang, H. Upper limb rehabilitation using robotic exoskeleton systems: A systematic review. *Int. J. Intell. Robot. Appl.* **2018**, *2*, 283–295. [CrossRef]
4. Shishov, N.; Melzer, I.; Bar-Haim, S. Parameters and Measures in Assessment of Motor Learning in Neurorehabilitation; A Systematic Review of the Literature. *Front. Hum. Neurosci.* **2017**, *11*, 82. [CrossRef]
5. Roggio, F.; Ravalli, S.; Maugeri, G.; Bianco, A.; Palma, A.; Di Rosa, M.; Musumeci, G. Technological advancements in the analysis of human motion and posture management through digital devices. *World J. Orthop.* **2021**, *12*, 467–484. [CrossRef]
6. Crenna, F.; Rossi, G.B.; Berardengo, M. Filtering Biomechanical Signals in Movement Analysis. *Sensors* **2021**, *21*, 4580. [CrossRef] [PubMed]
7. Muro-de-la-Herran, A.; Garcia-Zapirain, B.; Mendez-Zorrilla, A. Gait analysis methods: An overview of wearable and non-wearable systems, highlighting clinical applications. *Sensors* **2014**, *14*, 3362–3394. [CrossRef]
8. Laut, J.; Porfiri, M.; Raghavan, P. The Present and Future of Robotic Technology in Rehabilitation. *Curr. Phys. Med. Rehabil. Rep.* **2016**, *4*, 312–319. [CrossRef]
9. Maggioni, S.; Melendez-Calderon, A.; van Asseldonk, E.; Klamroth-Marganska, V.; Lünenburger, L.; Riener, R.; van der Kooij, H. Robot-aided assessment of lower extremity functions: A review. *J. Neuroeng. Rehabil.* **2016**, *13*, 72. [CrossRef]
10. Green, B.N.; Johnson, C.D.; Adams, A. Writing narrative literature reviews for peer-reviewed journals: Secrets of the trade. *J. Chiropr. Med.* **2006**, *5*, 101–117. [CrossRef]
11. Ma, C.Z.-H.; Li, Z.; He, C. Advances in Biomechanics-Based Motion Analysis. *Bioengineering* **2023**, *10*, 677. [CrossRef] [PubMed]
12. Grimmer, M.; Zeiss, J.; Weigand, F.; Zhao, G.; Lamm, S.; Steil, M.; Heller, A. Lower limb joint biomechanics-based identification of gait transitions in between level walking and stair ambulation. *PLoS ONE* **2020**, *15*, e0239148. [CrossRef] [PubMed]
13. Sugihara, T.; Fujimoto, Y. Dynamics Analysis: Equations of Motion. In *Humanoid Robotics: A Reference*; Goswami, A., Vadakkepat, P., Eds.; Springer: Dordrecht, The Netherlands, 2017. [CrossRef]
14. Yeadon, M.; Pain, M. Fifty years of performance-related sports biomechanics research. *J. Biomech.* **2023**, *155*, 111666. [CrossRef] [PubMed]
15. Lerchl, T.; Nispel, K.; Baum, T.; Bodden, J.; Senner, V.; Kirschke, J.S. Multibody Models of the Thoracolumbar Spine: A Review on Applications, Limitations, and Challenges. *Bioengineering* **2023**, *10*, 202. [CrossRef] [PubMed]

16. Parashar, S.K.; Sharma, J.K. A review on application of finite element modelling in bone biomechanics. *Perspect. Sci.* **2016**, *8*, 696–698. [CrossRef]
17. Colyer, S.L.; Evans, M.; Cosker, D.P.; Salo, A.I.T. A Review of the Evolution of Vision-Based Motion Analysis and the Integration of Advanced Computer Vision Methods towards Developing a Markerless System. *Sports Med.-Open* **2018**, *4*, 24. [CrossRef]
18. Kwon, C.-W.; Yun, S.-H.; Koo, D.-K.; Kwon, J.-W. Kinetic and Kinematic Analysis of Gait Termination: A Comparison between Planned and Unplanned Conditions. *Appl. Sci.* **2023**, *13*, 7323. [CrossRef]
19. Aprile, I.; Rabuffetti, M.; Padua, L.; Di Sipio, E.; Simbolotti, C.; Ferrarin, M. Kinematic Analysis of the Upper Limb Motor Strategies in Stroke Patients as a Tool towards Advanced Neurorehabilitation Strategies: A Preliminary Study. *BioMed Res. Int.* **2014**, *2014*, 636123. [CrossRef]
20. Brihmat, N.; Loubinoux, I.; Castel-Lacanal, E.; Marque, P.; Gasq, D. Kinematic parameters obtained with the ArmeoSpring for upper-limb assessment after stroke: A reliability and learning effect study for guiding parameter use. *J. Neuroeng. Rehabil.* **2020**, *17*, 130. [CrossRef]
21. Branco, M.P.; de Boer, L.M.; Ramsey, N.F.; Vansteensel, M.J. Encoding of kinetic and kinematic movement parameters in the sensorimotor cortex: A Brain-Computer Interface perspective. *Eur. J. Neurosci.* **2019**, *50*, 2755–2772. [CrossRef]
22. Al-Mulla, M.R.; Sepulveda, F.; Colley, M. A Review of Non-Invasive Techniques to Detect and Predict Localised Muscle Fatigue. *Sensors* **2011**, *11*, 3545–3594. [CrossRef] [PubMed]
23. Schaefer, L.V.; Bittmann, F.N. Are there two forms of isometric muscle action? Results of the experimental study support a distinction between a holding and a pushing isometric muscle function. *BMC Sports Sci. Med. Rehabil.* **2017**, *9*, 11. [CrossRef] [PubMed]
24. Halilaj, E.; Rajagopal, A.; Fiterau, M.; Hicks, J.L.; Hastie, T.J.; Delp, S.L. Machine learning in human movement biomechanics: Best practices, common pitfalls, and new opportunities. *J. Biomech.* **2018**, *81*, 1–11. [CrossRef] [PubMed]
25. Giarmatzis, G.; Zacharaki, E.I.; Moustakas, K. Real-Time Prediction of Joint Forces by Motion Capture and Machine Learning. *Sensors* **2020**, *20*, 6933. [CrossRef] [PubMed]
26. Mundt, M.; Koeppe, A.; Bamer, F.; David, S.; Markert, B. Artificial Neural Networks in Motion Analysis—Applications of Unsupervised and Heuristic Feature Selection Techniques. *Sensors* **2020**, *20*, 4581. [CrossRef] [PubMed]
27. Ai, Q.; Liu, Z.; Meng, W.; Liu, Q.; Xie, S.Q. Machine Learning in Robot Assisted Upper Limb Rehabilitation: A Focused Review. *IEEE Trans. Cogn. Dev. Syst.* **2021**. [CrossRef]
28. Maura, R.M.; Parra, S.R.; Stevens, R.E.; Weeks, D.L.; Wolbrecht, E.T.; Perry, J.C. Literature review of stroke assessment for upper-extremity physical function via EEG, EMG, kinematic, and kinetic measurements and their reliability. *J. Neuroeng. Rehabil.* **2023**, *20*, 21. [CrossRef] [PubMed]
29. Galeoto, G.; Berardi, A.; Mangone, M.; Tufo, L.; Silvani, M.; González-Bernal, J.; Seco-Calvo, J. Assessment Capacity of the Armeo® Power: Cross-Sectional Study. *Technologies* **2023**, *11*, 125. [CrossRef]
30. Merlo, A.; Longhi, M.; Giannotti, E.; Prati, P.; Giacobbi, M.; Ruscelli, E.; Mancini, A.; Ottaviani, M.; Montanari, L.; Mazzoli, D. Upper limb evaluation with robotic exoskeleton. Normative values for indices of accuracy, speed and smoothness. *NeuroRehabilitation* **2013**, *33*, 523–530. [CrossRef]
31. Longhi, M.; Merlo, A.; Prati, P.; Giacobbi, M.; Mazzoli, D. Instrumental indices for upper limb function assessment in stroke patients: A validation study. *J. Neuroeng. Rehabil.* **2016**, *13*, 52. [CrossRef]
32. Goffredo, M.; Pournajaf, S.; Proietti, S.; Gison, A.; Posteraro, F.; Franceschini, M. Retrospective Robot-Measured Upper Limb Kinematic Data From Stroke Patients Are Novel Biomarkers. *Front. Neurol.* **2021**, *12*, 803901. [CrossRef] [PubMed]
33. Cordella, F.; Scotto, D.; Luzio, F.; Bravi, M.; Santacaterina, F.; Bressi, F.; Zollo, L. Hand motion analysis during robot-aided rehabilitation in chronic stroke. *J. Biol. Regul. Homeost. Agents* **2020**, *34* (Suppl. S3), 45–52. [PubMed]
34. Calabrò, R.S.; Russo, M.; Naro, A.; Milardi, D.; Balletta, T.; Leo, A.; Filoni, S.; Bramanti, P. Who May Benefit From Armeo Power Treatment? A Neurophysiological Approach to Predict Neurorehabilitation Outcomes. *PM&R* **2016**, *8*, 971–978. [CrossRef]
35. Calabrò, R.S.; Naro, A.; Russo, M.; Milardi, D.; Leo, A.; Filoni, S.; Trinchera, A.; Bramanti, P. Is two better than one? Muscle vibration plus robotic rehabilitation to improve upper limb spasticity and function: A pilot randomized controlled trial. *PLoS ONE* **2017**, *12*, e0185936. [CrossRef] [PubMed]
36. Palermo, E.; Hayes, D.R.; Russo, E.F.; Calabrò, R.S.; Pacilli, A.; Filoni, S. Translational effects of robot-mediated therapy in subacute stroke patients: An experimental evaluation of upper limb motor recovery. *PeerJ* **2018**, *6*, e5944. [CrossRef]
37. Santisteban, L.; Térémetz, M.; Bleton, J.-P.; Baron, J.-C.; Maier, M.A.; Lindberg, P.G. Upper Limb Outcome Measures Used in Stroke Rehabilitation Studies: A Systematic Literature Review. *PLoS ONE* **2016**, *11*, e0154792. [CrossRef]
38. De-La-Torre, R.; Oña, E.D.; Balaguer, C.; Jardón, A. Robot-Aided Systems for Improving the Assessment of Upper Limb Spasticity: A Systematic Review. *Sensors* **2020**, *20*, 5251. [CrossRef]
39. Bonanno, M.; De Luca, R.; Torregrossa, W.; Tonin, P.; Calabrò, R.S. Moving toward Appropriate Motor Assessment Tools in People Affected by Severe Acquired Brain Injury: A Scoping Review with Clinical Advices. *Healthcare* **2022**, *10*, 1115. [CrossRef]
40. Kung, P.-C.; Lin, C.-C.K.; Ju, M.-S. Neuro-rehabilitation robot-assisted assessments of synergy patterns of forearm, elbow and shoulder joints in chronic stroke patients. *Clin. Biomech.* **2010**, *25*, 647–654. [CrossRef]
41. Zhao, K.; Zhang, Z.; Wen, H.; Liu, B.; Li, J.; D'avella, A.; Scano, A. Muscle synergies for evaluating upper limb in clinical applications: A systematic review. *Heliyon* **2023**, *9*, e16202. [CrossRef]

42. Safavynia, S.A.; Torres-Oviedo, G.; Ting, L.H. Muscle Synergies: Implications for Clinical Evaluation and Rehabilitation of Movement. *Top. Spinal Cord Inj. Rehabil.* **2011**, *17*, 16–24. [CrossRef] [PubMed]
43. Toigo, M.; Flück, M.; Riener, R.; Klamroth-Marganska, V. Robot-assisted assessment of muscle strength. *J. Neuroeng. Rehabil.* **2017**, *14*, 103. [CrossRef] [PubMed]
44. Tiboni, M.; Borboni, A.; Vérité, F.; Bregoli, C.; Amici, C. Sensors and Actuation Technologies in Exoskeletons: A Review. *Sensors* **2022**, *22*, 884. [CrossRef]
45. Bonanno, M.; De Nunzio, A.M.; Quartarone, A.; Militi, A.; Petralito, F.; Calabrò, R.S. Gait Analysis in Neurorehabilitation: From Research to Clinical Practice. *Bioengineering* **2023**, *10*, 785. [CrossRef] [PubMed]
46. Imoto, D.; Hirano, S.; Mukaino, M.; Saitoh, E.; Otaka, Y. A novel gait analysis system for detecting abnormal hemiparetic gait patterns during robot-assisted gait training: A criterion validity study among healthy adults. *Front. Neurorobot.* **2022**, *16*, 1047376. [CrossRef] [PubMed]
47. Boudarham, J.; Hameau, S.; Zory, R.; Hardy, A.; Bensmail, D.; Roche, N. Coactivation of Lower Limb Muscles during Gait in Patients with Multiple Sclerosis. *PLoS ONE* **2016**, *11*, e0158267. [CrossRef]
48. Romanato, M.; Spolaor, F.; Beretta, C.; Fichera, F.; Bertoldo, A.; Volpe, D.; Sawacha, Z. Quantitative assessment of training effects using EksoGT®exoskeleton in Parkinson's disease patients: A randomized single blind clinical trial. *Contemp. Clin. Trials Commun.* **2022**, *28*, 100926. [CrossRef]
49. Afzal, T.; Zhu, F.; Tseng, S.-C.; Lincoln, J.A.; Francisco, G.E.; Su, H.; Chang, S.-H. Evaluation of Muscle Synergy During Exoskeleton-Assisted Walking in Persons With Multiple Sclerosis. *IEEE Trans. Biomed. Eng.* **2022**, *69*, 3265–3274. [CrossRef]
50. Domingo, A.; Marriott, E.; de Grave, R.B.; Lam, T. Quantifying lower limb joint position sense using a robotic exoskeleton: A pilot study. In Proceedings of the 2011 IEEE 12th International Conference on Rehabilitation Robotics: Reaching Users & the Community (ICORR 2011), Zurich, Switzerland, 29 June–1 July 2011; pp. 1–6.
51. Domingo, A.; Lam, T. Reliability and validity of using the Lokomat to assess lower limb joint position sense in people with incomplete spinal cord injury. *J. Neuroeng. Rehabil.* **2014**, *11*, 167. [CrossRef]
52. Chisholm, A.E.; Domingo, A.; Jeyasurya, J.; Lam, T. Quantification of Lower Extremity Kinesthesia Deficits Using a Robotic Exoskeleton in People With a Spinal Cord Injury. *Neurorehabilit. Neural Repair* **2016**, *30*, 199–208. [CrossRef]
53. Moeller, T.; Moehler, F.; Krell-Roesch, J.; Dežman, M.; Marquardt, C.; Asfour, T.; Stein, T.; Woll, A. Use of Lower Limb Exoskeletons as an Assessment Tool for Human Motor Performance: A Systematic Review. *Sensors* **2023**, *23*, 3032. [CrossRef] [PubMed]
54. Maggioni, S.; Lunenburger, L.; Riener, R.; Melendez-Calderon, A. Robot-aided assessment of walking function based on an adaptive algorithm. In Proceedings of the 2015 IEEE International Conference on Rehabilitation Robotics (ICORR 2015), Singapore, 11–14 August 2015; Yu, H., Ed.; IEEE: Piscataway, NJ, USA, 2015; pp. 804–809, ISBN 978-1-4799-1808-9.
55. Mercado, L.; Alvarado, L.; Quiroz-Compean, G.; Romo-Vazquez, R.; Vélez-Pérez, H.; Platas-Garza, M.; González-Garrido, A.A.; Gómez-Correa, J.; Morales, J.A.; Rodriguez-Liñan, A.; et al. Decoding the torque of lower limb joints from EEG recordings of pre-gait movements using a machine learning scheme. *Neurocomputing* **2021**, *446*, 118–129. [CrossRef]
56. El Yaakoubi, N.A.; McDonald, C.; Lennon, O. Prediction of Gait Kinematics and Kinetics: A Systematic Review of EMG and EEG Signal Use and Their Contribution to Prediction Accuracy. *Bioengineering* **2023**, *10*, 1162. [CrossRef] [PubMed]
57. Raghavan, P. Upper Limb Motor Impairment After Stroke. *Phys. Med. Rehabil. Clin. N. Am.* **2015**, *26*, 599–610. [CrossRef] [PubMed]
58. Spaulding, W.; Deogun, J. A Pathway to Personalization of Integrated Treatment: Informatics and Decision Science in Psychiatric Rehabilitation. *Schizophr. Bull.* **2011**, *37*, S129–S137. [CrossRef] [PubMed]
59. Cao, W.; Zhang, X.; Qiu, H. Rehabilomics: A state-of-the-art review of framework, application, and future considerations. *Front. Neurol.* **2023**, *14*, 1103349. [CrossRef] [PubMed]
60. Garro, F.; Chiappalone, M.; Buccelli, S.; De Michieli, L.; Semprini, M. Neuromechanical Biomarkers for Robotic Neurorehabilitation. *Front. Neurorobot.* **2021**, *15*, 742163. [CrossRef]
61. Úbeda, A.; Costa-Garcia, A.; Torricelli, D.; Vujaklija, I.; Del Vecchio, A. Editorial: Neuromechanical Biomarkers in Robot-Assisted Motor Rehabilitation. *Front. Neurorobot.* **2022**, *15*, 831113. [CrossRef]
62. Mallat, R.; Khalil, M.; Venture, G.; Bonnet, V.; Mohammed, S. Human-Exoskeleton Joint Misalignment: A Systematic Review. In Proceedings of the 2019 Fifth International Conference on Advances in Biomedical Engineering (ICABME), Tripoli, Lebanon, 17–19 October 2019; pp. 1–4.
63. Ramos, O.; Múnera, M.; Moazen, M.; Wurdemann, H.; Cifuentes, C.A. Assessment of Soft Actuators for Hand Exoskeletons: Pleated Textile Actuators and Fiber-Reinforced Silicone Actuators. *Front. Bioeng. Biotechnol.* **2022**, *10*, 924888. [CrossRef]
64. Calabrò, R.S.; Müller-Eising, C.; Diliberti, M.L.; Manuli, A.; Parrinello, F.; Rao, G.; Barone, V.; Civello, T. Who Will Pay for Robotic Rehabilitation? The Growing Need for a Cost-effectiveness Analysis. *Innov. Clin. Neurosci.* **2020**, *17*, 14–16.
65. McManus, L.; De Vito, G.; Lowery, M.M. Analysis and Biophysics of Surface EMG for Physiotherapists and Kinesiologists: Toward a Common Language With Rehabilitation Engineers. *Front. Neurol.* **2020**, *11*, 576729. [CrossRef] [PubMed]
66. Hussain, I.; Park, S.-J. Prediction of Myoelectric Biomarkers in Post-Stroke Gait. *Sensors* **2021**, *21*, 5334. [CrossRef] [PubMed]
67. Rohrer, B.; Fasoli, S.; Krebs, H.I.; Hughes, R.; Volpe, B.; Frontera, W.R.; Stein, J.; Hogan, N. Movement Smoothness Changes during Stroke Recovery. *J. Neurosci.* **2002**, *22*, 8297–8304. [CrossRef] [PubMed]

68. Schiefelbein, M.L.; Salazar, A.P.; Marchese, R.R.; Rech, K.D.; Schifino, G.P.; Figueiredo, C.S.; Cimolin, V.; Pagnussat, A.S. Upper-limb movement smoothness after stroke and its relationship with measures of body function/structure and activity—A cross-sectional study. *J. Neurol. Sci.* **2019**, *401*, 75–78. [CrossRef] [PubMed]
69. Korovesis, N.; Kandris, D.; Koulouras, G.; Alexandridis, A. Robot Motion Control via an EEG-Based Brain–Computer Interface by Using Neural Networks and Alpha Brainwaves. *Electronics* **2019**, *8*, 1387. [CrossRef]
70. Hekmatmanesh, A.; Nardelli, P.H.J.; Handroos, H. Review of the State-of-the-Art of Brain-Controlled Vehicles. *IEEE Access* **2021**, *9*, 110173–110193. [CrossRef]
71. Moioli, R.C.; Nardelli, P.H.J.; Barros, M.T.; Saad, W.; Hekmatmanesh, A.; Silva, P.E.G.; de Sena, A.S.; Dzaferagic, M.; Siljak, H.; Van Leekwijck, W.; et al. Neurosciences and Wireless Networks: The Potential of Brain-Type Communications and Their Applications. *IEEE Commun. Surv. Tutor.* **2021**, *23*, 1599–1621. [CrossRef]
72. Scano, A.; Guanziroli, E.; Mira, R.M.; Brambilla, C.; Tosatti, L.M.; Molteni, F. Biomechanical assessment of the ipsilesional upper limb in post-stroke patients during multi-joint reaching tasks: A quantitative study. *Front. Rehabil. Sci.* **2022**, *3*, 943397. [CrossRef]

Disclaimer/Publisher's Note: The statements, opinions and data contained in all publications are solely those of the individual author(s) and contributor(s) and not of MDPI and/or the editor(s). MDPI and/or the editor(s) disclaim responsibility for any injury to people or property resulting from any ideas, methods, instructions or products referred to in the content.

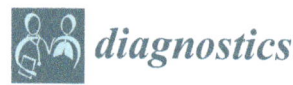

Review

Motion Capture Technologies for Ergonomics: A Systematic Literature Review

Sani Salisu [1,2,*], Nur Intan Raihana Ruhaiyem [1,*], Taiseer Abdalla Elfadil Eisa [3], Maged Nasser [4], Faisal Saeed [5] and Hussain A. Younis [1,6]

1 School of Computer Sciences, Universiti Sains Malaysia, Gelugor 11800, Malaysia; hussain.younis@uobasrah.edu.iq
2 Department of Information Technology, Federal University Dutse, Dutse 720101, Nigeria
3 Department of Information Systems-Girls Section, King Khalid University, Mahayil 62529, Saudi Arabia; teisa@kku.edu.sa
4 Computer & Information Sciences Department, Universiti Teknologi PETRONAS, Seri Iskandar 32610, Malaysia; maged.m.nasser@gmail.com
5 DAAI Research Group, Department of Computing and Data Science, School of Computing and Digital Technology, Birmingham City University, Birmingham B4 7XG, UK; faisal.saeed@bcu.ac.uk
6 College of Education for Women, University of Basrah, Basrah 61004, Iraq
* Correspondence: sani.salisu@fud.edu.ng (S.S.); intanraihana@usm.my (N.I.R.R.)

Abstract: Muscular skeletal disorder is a difficult challenge faced by the working population. Motion capture (MoCap) is used for recording the movement of people for clinical, ergonomic and rehabilitation solutions. However, knowledge barriers about these MoCap systems have made them difficult to use for many people. Despite this, no state-of-the-art literature review on MoCap systems for human clinical, rehabilitation and ergonomic analysis has been conducted. A medical diagnosis using AI applies machine learning algorithms and motion capture technologies to analyze patient data, enhancing diagnostic accuracy, enabling early disease detection and facilitating personalized treatment plans. It revolutionizes healthcare by harnessing the power of data-driven insights for improved patient outcomes and efficient clinical decision-making. The current review aimed to investigate: (i) the most used MoCap systems for clinical use, ergonomics and rehabilitation, (ii) their application and (iii) the target population. We used preferred reporting items for systematic reviews and meta-analysis guidelines for the review. Google Scholar, PubMed, Scopus and Web of Science were used to search for relevant published articles. The articles obtained were scrutinized by reading the abstracts and titles to determine their inclusion eligibility. Accordingly, articles with insufficient or irrelevant information were excluded from the screening. The search included studies published between 2013 and 2023 (including additional criteria). A total of 40 articles were eligible for review. The selected articles were further categorized in terms of the types of MoCap used, their application and the domain of the experiments. This review will serve as a guide for researchers and organizational management.

Keywords: MBased systems; MLess systems; IMS systems; EMG; shoulder; hands

Citation: Salisu, S.; Ruhaiyem, N.I.R.; Eisa, T.A.E.; Nasser, M.; Saeed, F.; Younis, H.A. Motion Capture Technologies for Ergonomics: A Systematic Literature Review. *Diagnostics* **2023**, *13*, 2593. https://doi.org/10.3390/diagnostics13152593

Academic Editor: Jamballi G. Manjunatha

Received: 5 July 2023
Revised: 25 July 2023
Accepted: 2 August 2023
Published: 4 August 2023

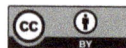

Copyright: © 2023 by the authors. Licensee MDPI, Basel, Switzerland. This article is an open access article distributed under the terms and conditions of the Creative Commons Attribution (CC BY) license (https://creativecommons.org/licenses/by/4.0/).

1. Introduction

Human body motion tracking is currently one of the most expanding research areas. The term "motion capture" (MoCap) has been defined by different scholars depending on their respective research area. MoCap relates to the recording of the movement of objects or people. Various researchers [1–5] have identified two popular optical MoCap systems: marker-based (MBased) and marker-less (MLess) MoCap systems. Both systems have been used by many researchers to assess the ergonomic risks of industrial workers by capturing their body kinematics using smart cameras and transforming the information into three-dimensional (3D) data. However, researchers have extensively argued on which among the main MoCap systems is the best in terms of user satisfaction. Several studies have indicated that MBased MoCap is considerably accurate [6–10]. Other studies [5,11–15] have viewed that MLess MoCap is markedly appropriate. Among non-optical MoCap systems, inertial measurement unit (IMU) has been discussed as the best [16–20].

Medical diagnosis plays a crucial role in the field of healthcare, as it involves identifying and determining the nature of diseases or conditions in patients. Traditionally, medical diagnosis heavily relied on the expertise and experience of healthcare professionals. However, with the advancements in technology and the emergence of artificial intelligence (AI), there has been a significant transformation in the way diagnoses are made. AI-based medical diagnosis utilizes machine learning algorithms to analyze vast amounts of patient data, including medical records, imaging scans and genetic information, to assist healthcare professionals in accurate and timely diagnoses. This introduction explores the applications, benefits and challenges of AI in medical diagnosis, highlighting its potential to improve patient outcomes and revolutionize healthcare practices.

A number of systematic literature reviews and surveys on MoCap systems have been published, e.g., marker-less motion capture systems as a training device in neurological rehabilitation [21], the accuracy of motion capture systems for sport applications [22] and motion capture technology in industrial applications [23]. All of these reviews only considered single MoCap systems for either small groups or specific applications. Hence, presenting a systematic literature review on all MoCap systems is highly needed. Consequently, the purpose of this study is to assist researchers, healthcare practitioners and industrial managers to identify suitable MoCap systems in various applications of their need. For this, the present literature review was conducted to investigate (i) the most used MoCap system on ergonomics, (ii) their application and (iii) the target population and most-used body segments using the preferred reporting items for systematic reviews and meta-analysis (PRISMA) approach.

This systematic literature review is presented to address the research questions which include:

RQ1 Which brand is the most frequently used device in the MBased systems category?
RQ2 What is the main advantage of the Microsoft Kinect MoCap system compared to other systems in the MLess system category?
RQ3 What are some notable features and advantages of Xsens, CaptivL7000, IGS-180 and other systems that fall in to the IMU category?

The article is organized as follows: Section 2 describes the related literature of MoCap systems and a brief note on ergonomics. Section 3 presents the method used for the systematic literature review. Section 4 describes the results obtained from the method adopted. Section 5 gives the details about MoCap systems and the answers for the research questions are presented. Section 6 is the target population. Section 7 discusses and interprets the findings of the selected papers in the review. In Section 8, conclusions are drawn.

2. Related Literature on Motion Capture Systems

Effort has been exerted by many researchers using MoCap techniques to obtain workers' data in their working environment and use such data in applying ergonomic principles to worker guidelines to reduce the risk of musculoskeletal disorder and improve productivity.

Ref. [24] used the Vicon 14 MX optical MoCap system to assess the potential risk of developing knee musculoskeletal disorder caused by residential roofing and determined that an awkward posture during sloppy roofing may have a significant impact on developing this disorder. MoCap was also used to analyze the relationship among body loads, experience and working procedure [25]. The outcome suggested that experienced workers adopt working techniques that are different from those of less experienced workers. MLess MoCap was reported to be the most cost-effective, efficient and easy to use [26–28], and demonstrated promising outcomes in occupational safety [29] and gait analysis [30]. IMU has been used by many researchers to diagnose the biomechanical overload of manual material handling workers [31] and analyze the motion of a healthy human wrist joint [32].

MoCap systems are used in several applications, such as sports, range of motion (ROM), ergonomics, health care, entertainment and advertisements.

Ergonomics

Ergonomics is the scientific study of the relationship between man and his working environments. Numerous researchers and professionals have defined the term based on their respective areas of focus but they eventually turn out to have the same meaning. Research has shown that occupational safety and health administration (OSHA) support is highly required to reinforce workers' knowledge in ergonomics and safety practices [33]. The inherent danger in hazardous occupations (e.g., construction, manufacturing, transportation, warehousing, mining, quarrying and healthcare services) and emergency services (e.g., firefighters, law enforcement and the military) results in substantial risks of occupational injuries [21,33]. Fitri and Halim [34] explained that most prevalent ergonomic-related injuries are musculoskeletal in nature, specifically caused by repetition, overload and an awkward posture in carrying out work. The musculoskeletal system (MSS) comprises the bones of the skeleton, muscles, cartilage, tendons, ligaments, joints and other connective tissues that support and bind tissues and organs. The MSS is responsible for providing shape, support, stability and locomotion to the body. Work-related musculoskeletal disorder (WMSD) is a painful disorder that affects workers' MSS. Ref. [35] indicated that WMSD is a condition that affects the MSS and leads to pain and disabilities. MoCap data are essential for applying ergonomic principles to the guidelines for workers to reduce the risk of musculoskeletal disorder and improve productivity. However, obtaining accurate data is difficult owing to the nature of the working environment, heavy equipment used by workers, wearing personal protective equipment (PPE) and the limitations of MoCap systems.

3. Materials and Methods

This review used four different databases (i.e., Scopus, Web of Science, Google Scholar and PubMed) to search for relevant published articles or research in the field of applications of MoCap systems in ergonomics, healthcare and rehabilitation. The search queries used include some keywords and their combination to search for the relevant published papers within the publication years from 2013 to 2023: MoCap systems, MoCap technology, upper limb, lower limb, spine, ergonomics, gait, movement, kinematics, diagnosis and measurement. Given that our aim was to conduct a comprehensive review of research papers that suit the requirement of our study, a slight difference in the search strategies was adopted knowing the differences in the search capabilities of the selected databases. Title and abstract searches were performed in PubMed and Scopus from the beginning, while full text search was adopted in Web of Science and Google Scholar.

The articles obtained were scrutinized by reading the abstracts and titles to determine their inclusion eligibility. Those with insufficient or irrelevant information were excluded from the screening.

The full text of the searched papers were examined separately to determine the relevant information to enable their inclusion or exclusion. Furthermore, most of the references cited in the selected articles or papers were identified and used to retrieve more relevant papers for the review. To create clean and standard documents (i.e., no noise, no duplicates) retrieved from the different databases or sources, the following additional selection and rejection criteria were adopted.

- Articles should be original or reviews, written in English, and published in English journals or conferences.
- Any relevant articles published or in press between January 2013 and December 2023.
- The main focus being on MoCap applications on the ergonomics of human activities.

4. Results

The computerized literature search resulted in 40 selected published studies on the application of MoCap systems in healthcare, rehabilitation and ergonomics, specifically discussing different human MoCap systems. A total of 1006 articles were first identified, with 24 duplicate articles discovered and excluded ($n = 1006 - 24 = 982$). A total of 98 articles were selected from ($n = 982$) after screening the title/abstract for further evaluation. Thereafter, 58 articles were further excluded following full-text reading, thereby resulting in the selection and analysis of only 40 relevant articles for the review. Figure 1 summarizes the stages of the article search and inclusion/exclusion process. The computerized literature search resulted in 40 published articles on the application of MoCap in ergonomics, healthcare and rehabilitation, particularly discussing different human MoCap systems. These systems are listed in this article. Given that most MoCap systems used in the selected literature are either MBase, MLess or IMU, these tables are titled MBased systems, MLess systems and IMU systems, respectively, with column titles as operational system, operational software, body segment used, number of body segment, measurement error and the domain of the experiments. The application of each MoCap system used is explained in the following section.

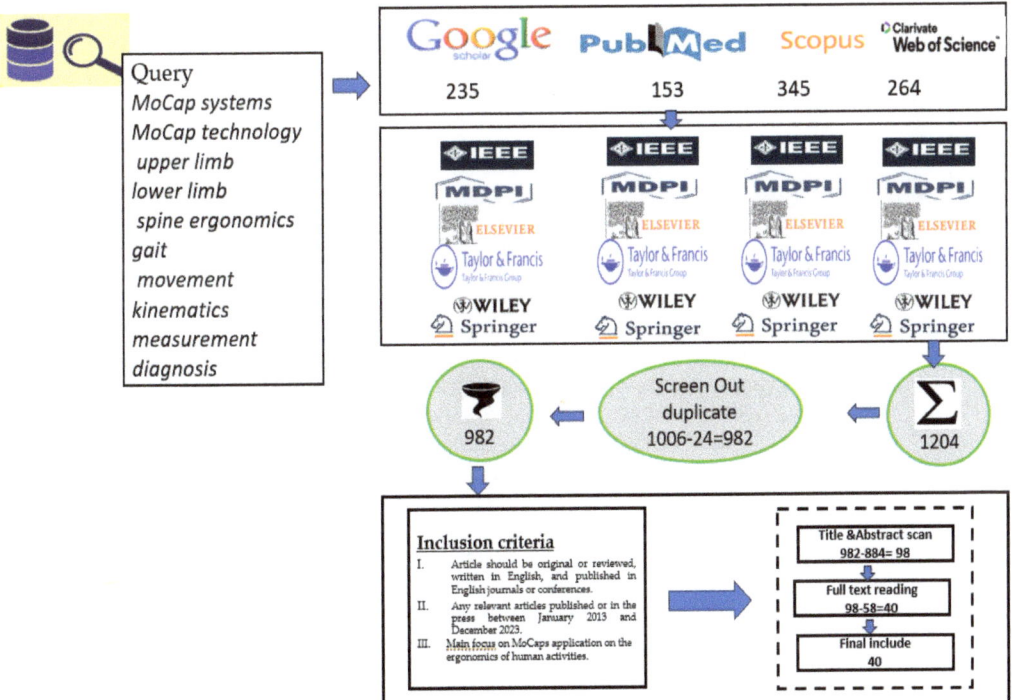

Figure 1. Selection of Studies, Search Query and Inclusion Criteria.

4.1. Distribution of Articles by Nationality of Authors

Figure 2 shows that 19 different countries used motion capture systems on healthcare, rehabilitation and ergonomic analysis in their studies. The selection was made by observing the countries where the studies were conducted. The distribution of 40 selected articles by the nationality of the authors shows that the United States of America has the highest number of published articles (seven), followed by Canada and Spain with four articles each. France and Germany published three articles each, while Brazil, Denmark, Japan, Belgium and Netherlands published two articles, respectively. Only one published article is found in Australia, Czech Republic, England, China, India, Indonesia, Italy, Republic of Korea and Sweden, respectively.

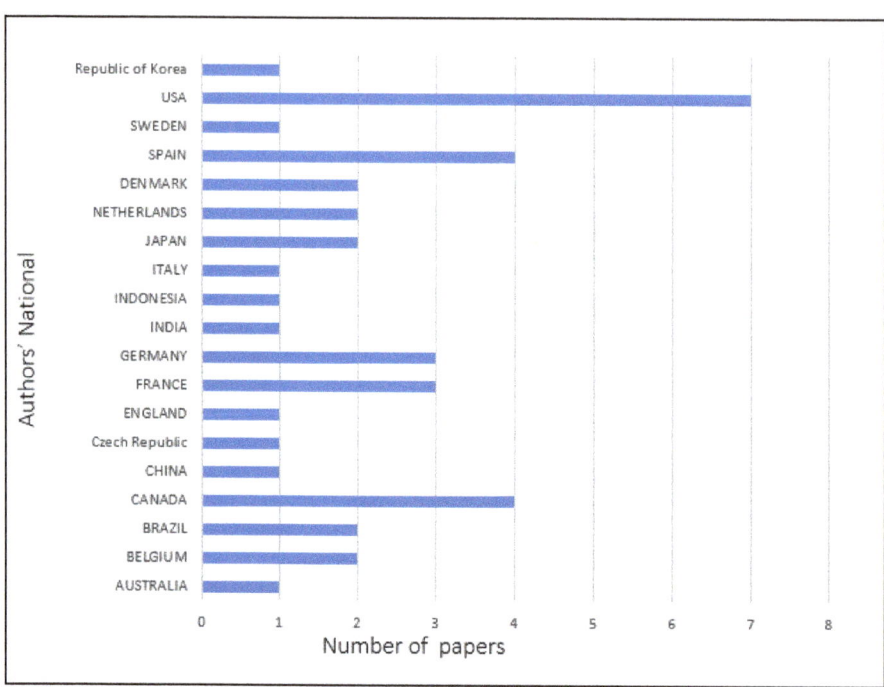

Figure 2. Distribution of selected papers by authors' nationalities.

4.2. Distribution of Articles by Year of Publication

Figure 3 presents the distribution of articles by year of publication from 2013 to 2023, respectively. The number of included articles and their published year in the studies are described as follows. The year 2020 had the highest number of published articles ($n = 10$) which covers 25% of the total published articles in the study. This was followed by the year 2019 with six articles, covering 15% of the total published articles, followed by five articles published in the year 2022, covering 12.5%. Four articles were published in 2018 which covers 10% of the total published articles. Three articles were published in 2015, 2021 and 2023, respectively, covering 22.5% all together. Further, two articles were published in 2013, 2014 and 2017, respectively, which gives the total of 15% of all the published articles. No published article was found in the year 2016, hence 0% for the year 2016 is recorded.

4.3. Distribution of Article by Publishing Company

Figure 4 shows the distribution of the selected articles used by their publishing companies. These selected articles are published by six different publishing companies which include IEEE (New York, NY, USA), MDPI (Basel, Switzerland), Elsevier (Amsterdam, The Netherlands), Springer (Berlin/Heidelberg, Germany), Taylor and Francis (Philadelphia, PA, USA) and Wiley (Hoboken, NJ, USA). The description of this distribution is as follows. From the figure, Elsevier published the highest number of articles used ($n = 12$), nine articles are published in both MDPI and Springer, five articles are published under IEEE, while two articles are published under Taylor and Francis and one article is published under Wiley.

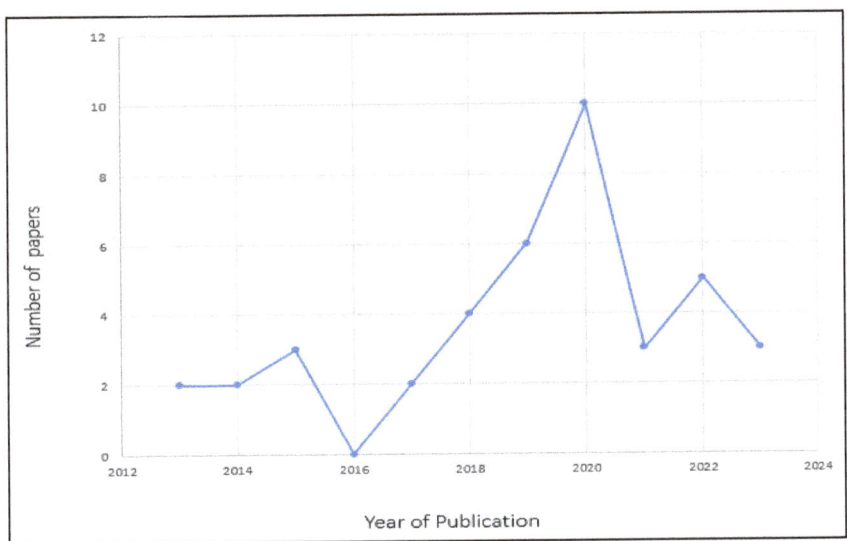

Figure 3. Distribution of selected papers by year of publication.

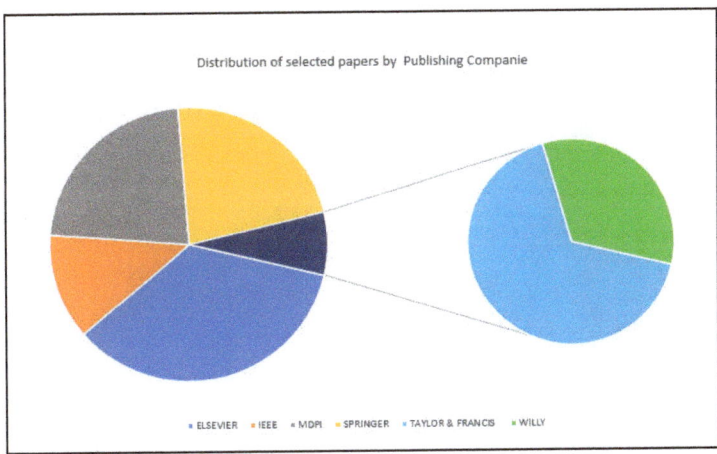

Figure 4. Distribution of selected papers by publishing companies.

5. Types of MoCap System

Different types of motion capture systems were used in the literature as shown in Tables 1–3. These motion capture systems are categorized into the MBased, MLess and IMU systems.

5.1. RQ1 Which Brand Is the Most Frequently Used Device in the MBased Systems Category?

For MBased systems, Vicon is the most frequently used device. Vicon MX3, MX13 and MX20 in the MX series and Vicon T-20 and T-40 are used in the T-series. Meanwhile, Vicon V16 and V5 are used in the V-series. MX represents the megapixels of the camera, such as MX-3+ (0.325 mega pixels). In the T-series, T-160 stands for 16-megapixel cameras, while the Vicon V family represents the vantage, indicating capture at high speed. A 3D MoCap system involves multiple high-definition cameras that are accurate, capable of capturing 370 frames per second at full frame resolution and can capture speeds of 2000 frames per second. Another MBased system used is CMOS. The system hardware was built using off-the-shelf components and the system can run at a rate of 63 frames per second. OptiTrack Flex3 is another system used in this category and consists of a small volume motion camera and is likewise affordable. This system uses six infrared cameras and spherical retroreflective markers of 14 mm diameter to output the marker information as XYZ data. Another MBased system used is OptoTrak. Eight OptoTrak motion tracking cameras were used to capture the 3D motion data of pelvis, hip and knee joints at 100 Hz. The system was used to validate the Kinect V2, used as the main system. The results of another study obtained from PhaseSpace were used to compare the results obtained by using the Kinect systems. Eight infrared PhaseSpace cameras were positioned around the capture space of approximately 4 m × 4 m. Moreover, the system provides the 3D position of LED markers with sub-millimeter accuracy and a frequency of up to 960 HZ. PhaseSpace enabled real-time data capture with under 10 ms latency. Table 1 summarizes the MBased systems.

Table 1. Mbased systems.

Study	Operational System	Operational Software	Body Segments	Number of Segment	Measurement Error	Domain of Experiment
[36]	Vicon T-40	MAS	Hand	1	MAE 5.75 mm	Ergonomics
[37]	Simple\camera	Kinematic inverse	Leg (Hip and Knee)	2	AVE 1.66 and 0.46	Ergonomics
[38]	CMOS and Kinect	Jack software	Whole body	Whole body	Nil	Ergonomics
[39]	ViconTH and iEMG	GraphPad StatMate 2.0	Upper Extremity (shoulder and elbow	2	Nil	Rehabilitation
[40]	PhaseSpace and Kinect1 and 2	PhaseSpace Recap2	Whole body	29 joints	76 mm and 87 mm	Ergonomics
[41]	Opti Track Flex3	Motive: Body	Upper body (hand and head)	2	Small	Ergonomics
[42]	Vicon (Oxford Metrics, Oxford, UK	ULMV 1.0	Upper Extremity	3	Nil	Rehabilitation
[43]	IR cameras, Xtion 3D sensor, and H4 Audio	Nexus 2.5	Head and hand	2	10 ms	Rehabilitation
[44]	Vicon MX13 and Xsens MTw	Nexus 2.0	Full body	all	Nil	Ergonomics

5.2. RQ2 What Is the Main Advantage of the Microsoft Kinect MoCap system Compared to Other Systems in the MLess System Category?

Under this category, Microsoft Kinect is the most frequently used MoCap system. It is an infrared MoCap device used for interactive computer games aimed for the Xbox 360 game console. Originally designed to replace the standard game controller, the device enables users to control and interact with the virtual reality environment through infrared cameras and depth sensors. This system can provide full-body 3D motion detection in real time. Microsoft Kinect is inexpensive, portable and easy to set up [45,46]. Move 4D is another MLess MoCap. Move 4D is a 3D human body motion scanner, modular photogrammetry-based 4D scanning system and consists of a set of 12 synchronized modules to scan full bodies with texture in motion. This system can capture up to 180 frames per second with a resolution of 2 mm. Table 2 presents the summary of MLess systems.

Table 2. MLess system.

Study	Operational System	Operational Software	Body Segment	Number of Segments	Measurement Error	Domain of Experiment
[47]	Microsoft Kinect	Microsoft SDK	Upper limb	4	Nil	Ergonomics
[12]	Microsoft Kinect and OpenSim	Open-Sim	Upper Extremity	4	Nil	Clinical
[48]	Kinect V2 and Vicon MX3	Nexus 2.5 and Microsoft SDK	Upper body	2	0.011 and 0.024	Ergonomics
[49]	Microsoft Kinect V2	Video annotation software, ELAN	Whole body	25 joints	Nil	Clinical
[50]	Kinect V2 and Optotrak	OpenTLD	Lower-Extremity	2	0.95 and 0.27	Clinical
[51]	Microsoft Kinect V2	OpesPose	Lower limb	1	Nil	Clinical
[5]	Microsoft Kinect V2, Captiv L7000	iPi soft	Upper-Extremity	2	<5.0	Ergonomics
[28]	Microsoft Kinect V2	Microsoft SDK	Lower limb	3	<5.0	Clinical
[52]	Move 4D	Move 4D	Whole body	1	Nil	Ergonomics

5.3. RQ3 What Are Some Notable Features and Advantages of Xsens, CaptivL7000, IGS-180 and Other Systems That Fall into the IMU Category?

Xsens was used more than any other system in this category. This system is a full-body MoCap system that integrates directly into the subject pipeline. It enables users to perform the capturing in all environments, as well as being known for easy calibration, real-time visualization, easy play back and capable of exporting and processing 3D data. CaptivL7000 is also an inertia system used under this category. This system is a flexible research software package for the synchronization of video and multiple measurements from TEA sensors and interfaced third-party hardware and measurement devices. IGS-180 is also used in this category. This system is Synergia's professional level MoCap system, offering highly accurate and rich nuanced MoCap data. Moreover, this system is easy to use and does not need cameras capable of data capture at any given location, and there is no concern of occlusion or marker swapping. Thereafter, the MoCap system used is IMU, which uses accelerometers to capture more data on joint impact, limb movement and limb loads. In addition, this system is lightweight, easy to use, flexible and reliable. This system likewise enables field-based inertial measurements of impact and loads up to 200 g. It can capture the highest speed and highest impact sporting movements. An APDM Opal V2 inertial sensor is also used in one of the selected studies. Its sensors are placed on the subject body according to the manufacturer's guidelines. Subjects were asked to walk on the GAITRite mat while wearing an APDM OpalV2 on each foot. Data were recorded simultaneously from the GAITRite and IMU systems [53]. Oqus300 is a MoCap device used in the experiment to capture seven retro-reflective markers that define the participants' trunk segment. Another inertial system used is wireless sensor network (WSN). A human MoCap system based on inertial sensors and suitable for 3D reconstruction was designed to capture human posture data in the study. Ref. [54] added that "A WSN typically has little or no infrastructure. It consists of several sensor nodes (few tens to thousands) working together to monitor a region to obtain data about the environment". The IMS systems are summarized in Table 3.

Table 3. IMU systems.

Study	Operational System	Operational Software	Body Segment	Number of Segments	Measurement Error	Domain of Experiment
[55]	IMUs	Mobile OS	Upper body	5	Nil	Ergonomic
[56]	Xsens MTw and Vicon V612	Xsens MTw	Lower limb	1	<1° and <3°	Clinical
[17]	IGS-180 and Vicon (MX20,	Nexus 1.8.2	Whole body	6	1.1°–5.1°	Clinical
[57]	Xsens MVN Link and Oqus 300 (IMC)	Xsens MVN studio 4.2.4	Lower body	1	>40%	Ergonomics
[58]	IMU and OMC	D-Flow	Lower limb	1	Nil	Rehabilitation
[59]	IMU (Xsens) and EMG	Xsens MTV studio pro.	Upper limb	4	Nil	Ergonomics
[60]	3IMUs and Vicon OXG	MTws Xsens	Lower limb	2	Nil	Clinical
[18]	IMUs and Vicon V5	Free IMU-GUI	Lower limb joints angles	1	0.63 and 1.2	Clinical
[61]	OptiTrack and EMG	OptiTrack	Upper-Extremity	2	Nil	Ergonomics
[62]	EMG and IMU	JMP software	Upper-Extremity	1	Nil	Ergonomics
[63]	APDM Opal V2	Moveo Explorer	Torso, Arms and Legs	3	Nil	Clinical
[64]	Wireless sensor network (WSN)	Truemotion	Whole body	1	Nil	Clinical

6. Target Population

Different target populations with ergonomic problems were involved in the studies. The majority of the studies ($n = 15$) targeted the general population [17,18,28,39,40,44,50,52,58,60,64–68], twelve of which targeted the working population [5,38,47,48,55,59,61,62,69–72]. Six studies targeted the healthcare population [12,41,42,51,56,73], while other studies ($n = 4$) targeted sports persons [36,57,63,74]. Only one study [75] targeted university students. The remaining two studies targeted gesture and communication professionals [43,49]. Table 4 showcases the MoCaps system diagnosing different disorders from different populations.

Table 4. MoCaps System for Diagnostics.

Study	System	Sampling Frequency	Target Population	Sample Size	Diagnostic Outcomes
[39]	ViconTH and iEMG	200 HZ	General population	25	Lead clinicians to a more specific assessment and better intervention in upper extremity rehabilitation
[48]	Kinect V2 and Vicon MX3	Vicon100 HZ/Kinect30 HZ	Police, Traffic and Aircraft marshals	1	Kinect is an effective tool in tracking upper body motion
[38]	CMOS and Kinect	-	Assembly Operators In Aerospace Manufacturing	-	For fostering operation of an aircraft fuselage
[51]	Microsoft Kinect	30 HZ	Dementia Patients	14	The system can be used as a tool for monitoring of Parkinson's in residential setting
[43]	IR cameras, Xtion 3D sensor and H4 Audio	100 HZ, 30 HZ and 44.1-KHZ	Deaf Translators	3	Used to investigate implicit detection of speech gesture

Table 4. Cont.

Study	System	Sampling Frequency	Target Population	Sample Size	Diagnostic Outcomes
[41]	OptiTrak Flex 3	100 HZ	Surgeon	20	May improve skill acquisition and reduce physical stress during laparoscopic surgery
[36]	Vicon T-40	200 HZ	Swimmers	-	The system is accurate and feasible
[57]	Xsens MVT Link and Oqus 300	240 HZ and 120 HZ	Sportsmen	11	Using Inertia system, trunk speed is more accurate during walking than in transition period
[47]	Microsoft Kinect	30 HZ	Factory Operators	-	Kinect sensor is comparable to the Vicon system
[12]	Microsoft Kinect and OpenSim	-	Manual Wheelchair Users	-	The system is easy to use by clinicians
[65]	Vicon T20 and Vicon Bonita Video	-	General population	10	Allows a quantitative assessment of lower limb motion in the sagittal plane
[49]	Microsoft Kinect V2	-	Gesture and Communication professional	-	Can be useful to clinicians and researchers
[28]	Microsoft Kinect V2	30 HZ	General population	22	Kinect detects kinematic abnormalities of the trunk during slow walking on a flat land easier than on the treadmill
[42]	Vicon (Oxford Metrics, Oxford, UK)	100 HZ	People with Spinal muscular atrophy	17	Used for evaluating the need for clinical intervention
[5]	Microsoft Kinect V2 and Captiv L7000	30 HZ and 128 HZ	Manual operators in the industry	12	Kinect V2 accuracy reduced when occlusion occurs
[17]	IGS-180 and Vicon (MX20, T40)	60 HZ and 100 HZ	General population	20	The accuracy of joint kinematics can be affected when pairing a module unlike segment kinematics T
[18]	IMUs and ViconV5	128 HZ and 200 HZ	General population	7	IMU system is applicable in unconstrained rehabilitative contexts
[63]	APDM Opal V2	128 HZ	Female Gymnasts	8	The relationship between back pain and gymnastics training load/intensity is still not clear
[56]	Xsens MTw and Vicon V612	60 HZ and 120 HZ	Transfemoral amputees	1	The deviation of knee extension angle is found to be about 1
[50]	Kinect V2 and Optotrak	100 HZ and 100 HZ	General population	-	RGB data stream of Kinect sensor is efficient in estimating joint kinematics and unsuitable for measuring local dynamic stability
[40]	PhaseSpace (Impuls X2) and Kinect 1 and 2	480 HZ and 30 HZ	General population	10	Kinect 2 is more robust and accurate tracking of human pose as compared to Kinect 1
[55]	IMUs	100 HZ	Manual Workers in an Industry	12	The tool used can reduce the risk of musculoskeletal disorders in industrial settings
[64]	Wireless sensor network (WSN)	120 HZ	General population	240 sets of data	The system can meet the needs of doctors for real time monitoring of patients' physiological parameters during clinical health monitoring
[44]	Vicov MX13 and Xsens MTw	100 HZ and 60 HZ	General population	12	Not suitable in real life situations

Table 4. Cont.

Study	System	Sampling Frequency	Target Population	Sample Size	Diagnostic Outcomes
[61]	OptiTrack and EMG	120 HZ and 100 HZ	Firefighters and Emergency Medical Service	14	The system will reduce the biomechanical loads experienced by EMS providers when lifting and moving the patients
[52]	Move 4D	-	General population	-	The application is used for biomechanical analysis purposes
[62]	IMU and EMG	1500 HZ	Industrial Workers	14	Can be used to improve workplace design, injuries and enhance workers' productivity
[58]	IMU and OMC	200 HZ	General population	3	Sensor network shows high accuracy in capturing significant gait parameters and features
[60]	3IMUs and Vicon OXG	100 HZ	General population	10	IMUs can be used to lower limb joint angle during straight walking
[59]	IMU (Xsens) and EMG	120 HZ and 2000 HZ	Banana production industrial workers	3	Bunches position, tools used by the workers and repetition movement led to musculoskeletal risk.
[66]	TTL-Pulse	200 HZ	General Population	15	Evaluating the performance of a motion capture device for diagnosing the risk of musculoskeletal disorder when doing physical activities
[75]	BR- BEWE TW		University students	425	Frequent risk of musculoskeletal disorder
[67]	Microsoft Kinect V2 and Vicon Bonita	100 HZ and 200 HZ	General Population	1	Potential health risks of the participants
[74]	QualisysAB,	100 HZ	Sport	16	To diagnose the kinematic differences among female Futsal players
[69]	MoCap suit—Axis Studio	90 HZ and 60 HZ	Operators working in automotive production	20	To predict the effect of bad working place on operators
[70]	IMUs	100 HZ	Workers form textile industry	93	To diagnose workers with lateral epicondylitis
[73]	Flexi 13, OptiTrack	100 HZ	Healthcare	10	Diagnosis and treatment of shoulder pain in rehabilitation homes
[71]	XSens MVN Link	240 HZ	Manual Workers	9	Diagnose the prevalence of work-related musculoskeletal disorders among the manual materials handlers.
[68]	STT-IWS, STT Systems and San Sebastian	100 HZ	General population	14	For effective diagnosis, assessment and treatment of spinal disorders
[72]	15 IMU	60 HZ	Workers on repetitive workstation circle	1	Compute the joint risks for every posture and output the total risk for the assessed workstation

7. Discussion

Choosing the right MoCap systems for ergonomic applications can be very difficult. Tables 1–3 may serve as a guide for researchers in making the right selection. Based on the result of this review, the majority of MoCap systems used in the selected articles were IMU-based (covering about 40%), while the camera-based systems (MBased and MLess) covered the remaining 60%, most likely due to the operational and processing cost and other technical challenges.

Outcomes revealed that the best selection of MoCap systems is mainly by the type of application. For example, quality control is achieved mainly via the use of the IMU system, while improving productivity via MBased and MLess systems. Another factor that warrants the use of MoCap systems is the environment; in uncontrolled environments, an IMU system is the best option, because the units can assess the performance of the subject throughout the experiment. However, in a controlled setting, e.g., laboratories, MBased and MLess systems will perform more accurately.

People's wellbeing and safety was found to be the most common area of research in MoCap systems. For instance, all the studies in the selected articles focused on either ergonomic, clinical or rehabilitation research.

Other findings from this review revealed that when MoCap is combined with EMG, the musculoskeletal assessment of the subject was improved as well as the number of muscles to be analyzed; for example, biceps, triceps and forearm extensor strength muscle torques were measured with 0.2–2.000 as the measuring range [42] and EMG was used to investigate the physiological demand of right arm muscles involved in the bunch removal task [59]. It is obvious that neither MLess nor MoCap were combined with EMG in any of the selected articles. Table 4 is showing the outcomes of the diagnosis of the subjects using the selected motion capture systems as presented above. AI-based medical diagnosis offers improved accuracy, efficiency and accessibility, but ethical and privacy concerns must be addressed.

This review article is not perfect as it is attached with some limitations. There are many published articles relevant to MBase, MLess and IMU that may not be included in the review, to reserve future reproducibility. However, utilizing the PRISMA approach allowed us to identify a reasonable number of studies compared to some recent systematic literature reviews.

8. Conclusions

This systematic literature review has underscored how MoCap systems are utilized by researchers and organizational management to solve the issues of musculoskeletal disorder. The research was mainly driven by three experimental domains which include ergonomic, clinical and rehabilitation applications. In conclusion, the use of various technologies such as Kinect, IMU systems, sensor networks and motion capture devices has shown promising results in the field of medical diagnosis. These tools provide accurate and feasible assessments of various musculoskeletal parameters and can aid in diagnosing and monitoring conditions such as upper extremity rehabilitation, Parkinson's, back pain, joint kinematics and work-related musculoskeletal disorders. However, challenges related to accuracy, occlusion, real-life applicability and privacy concerns need to be addressed for wider implementation. Overall, these technologies hold great potential in improving diagnosis, assessment and treatment in the field of medical diagnostics and workplace ergonomics.

The IMU system is the most-used MoCap system for such applications, as it relatively satisfies all the usability goals including the cost-effectiveness and displays minimal impact on the application domains of this research. Furthermore, the IMU system has long developed its performance in terms of low power utilization, logical partitioning and portability for easy body activity monitoring.

IMU systems may likely become the substitute of highly accurate but expensive MBased and MLess MoCap systems, especially with the current advancement that is making it smarter with built-in functions and embedded algorithms, such as deep learning and Kalman filters, that will process the data retrieved by IMU systems for more accuracy.

Moreover, systems need to be portable to interfere less with the subjects and workplace, while real-time assessments should go with health and safety applications to influence the acceptance and implementation of such technologies by researchers and organizational management.

MBased MoCap systems, such as vicon-T40 and PhaseSpace, come at a high cost and present high accuracy for some body activities and tracking tasks, but only in a controlled environment (e.g., laboratories). Attempts must be made to improve its usability. MLess MoCap systems, such as the Kinect series, are very low-cost compared to MBased MoCap systems, which also show high performance accuracy for specific classification and activity tracking tasks; nevertheless, efforts should be made to develop the tracking of more complex activities in real-time scenes. Finally, the ergonomic research domain has the highest number of articles in the selected publications.

Author Contributions: Writing—original draft, conceptualization, S.S.; methodology, formal analysis: S.S., H.A.Y., T.A.E.E., M.N. and F.S.; writing—review and editing, N.I.R.R., T.A.E.E., M.N., H.A.Y. and F.S.; supervision, N.I.R.R.; project administration, funding acquisition: T.A.E.E. All authors have read and agreed to the published version of the manuscript.

Funding: Deanship of Scientific Research at King Khalid University funded this work through a large group Research Project under grant number (RGP2/52/44).

Institutional Review Board Statement: Not applicable.

Informed Consent Statement: Not applicable.

Data Availability Statement: Not applicable.

Acknowledgments: The authors extend their appreciation to the Deanship of Scientific Research at King Khalid University for funding this work through a large group Research Project under grant number (RGP2/52/44).

Conflicts of Interest: The authors declare no conflict of interest.

References

1. Fernandez, I.G.; Ahmad, S.A.; Wada, C. Inertial Sensor-Based Instrumented Cane for Real-Time Walking Cane Kinematics Estimation. *Sensors* **2020**, *20*, 4675. [CrossRef] [PubMed]
2. Ferrari, E.; Gamberi, M.; Pilati, F.; Regattieri, A. Motion Analysis System for the Digitalization and Assessment of Manual Manufacturing and Assembly Processes. *IFAC-PapersOnLine* **2018**, *51*, 411–416. [CrossRef]
3. Hood, S.; Ishmael, M.K.; Gunnell, A.; Foreman, K.B.; Lenzi, T. A Kinematic and Kinetic Dataset of 18 Above-Knee Amputees Walking at Various Speeds. *Sci. Data* **2020**, *7*, 150. [CrossRef]
4. Perrott, M.A.; Pizzari, T.; Cook, J.; McClelland, J.A. Comparison of Lower Limb and Trunk Kinematics between Markerless and Marker-Based Motion Capture Systems. *Gait Posture* **2017**, *52*, 57–61. [CrossRef] [PubMed]
5. Steinebach, T.; Grosse, E.H.; Glock, C.H.; Wakula, J.; Lunin, A. Accuracy Evaluation of Two Markerless Motion Capture Systems for Measurement of Upper Extremities: Kinect V2 and Captiv. *Hum. Factors Ergon. Manuf.* **2020**, *30*, 291–302. [CrossRef]
6. Gagnon, D.; Plamondon, A.; Larivière, C. A Comparison of Lumbar Spine and Muscle Loading between Male and Female Workers during Box Transfers. *J. Biomech.* **2018**, *81*, 76–85. [CrossRef] [PubMed]
7. Kakar, R.S.; Tome, J.M.; King, D.L.; Jin, Z.; Kakar, R.S.; Tome, J.M.; King, D.L. Biomechanical and Physiological Load Carrying Efficiency of Two Firefighter Harness Variations Biomechanical and Physiological Load Carrying Efficiency of Two Firefighter Harness Variations. *Cogent Eng.* **2018**, *5*, 1502231. [CrossRef]
8. Koopman, A.S.; Näf, M.; Baltrusch, S.J.; Kingma, I.; Rodriguez-guerrero, C.; Babic, J. Biomechanical Evaluation of a New Passive Back Support Exoskeleton Torque Source. *J. Biomech.* **2020**, *105*, 109795. [CrossRef]
9. Kumada, H.; Takada, K.; Terunuma, T.; Aihara, T. Monitoring Patient Movement with Boron Neutron Capture Therapy and Motion Capture Technology. *Appl. Radiat. Isot.* **2020**, *163*, 109208. [CrossRef]
10. Świtoński, A.; Josiński, H.; Michalczuk, A.; Wojciechowski, K. Quaternion Statistics Applied to the Classification of Motion Capture Data. *Expert Syst. Appl.* **2021**, *164*, 113813. [CrossRef]
11. Colyer, S.L.; Evans, M.; Cosker, D.P.; Salo, A.I.T. A Review of the Evolution of Vision-Based Motion Analysis and the Integration of Advanced Computer Vision Methods Towards Developing a Markerless System. *Sport. Med.-Open* **2018**, *4*, 24. [CrossRef] [PubMed]
12. Rammer, J.; Slavens, B.; Krzak, J.; Winters, J.; Riedel, S.; Harris, G. Assessment of a Markerless Motion Analysis System for Manual Wheelchair Application. *J. Neuroeng. Rehabil.* **2018**, *15*, 96. [CrossRef] [PubMed]
13. Maletsky, L.P.; Sun, J.; Morton, N.A. Accuracy of an Optical Active-Marker System to Track the Relative Motion of Rigid Bodies. *J. Biomech.* **2007**, *40*, 682–685. [CrossRef] [PubMed]
14. Colombo, G.; Regazzoni, D.; Rizzi, C. Markerless Motion Capture Integrated with Human Modeling for Virtual Ergonomics. In Proceedings of the 4th International Conference, DHM 2013, Held as Part of HCI International 2013, Las Vegas, NV, USA, 21–26 July 2013; Volume 8026, pp. 314–323. [CrossRef]

15. Schmitz, A.; Ye, M.; Shapiro, R.; Yang, R.; Noehren, B. Accuracy and Repeatability of Joint Angles Measured Using a Single Camera Markerless Motion Capture System. *J. Biomech.* **2013**, *47*, 587–591. [CrossRef] [PubMed]
16. Milosevic, B.; Leardini, A.; Farella, E. Kinect and Wearable Inertial Sensors for Motor Rehabilitation Programs at Home: State of the Art and an Experimental Comparison. *Biomed. Eng. Online* **2020**, *19*, 25. [CrossRef] [PubMed]
17. Lebel, K.; Boissy, P.; Nguyen, H.; Duval, C. Inertial Measurement Systems for Segments and Joints Kinematics Assessment: Towards an Understanding of the Variations in Sensors Accuracy. *Biomed. Eng. Online* **2017**, *16*, 56. [CrossRef]
18. Calibrations, S.; Lebleu, J.; Gosseye, T.; Detrembleur, C.; Mahaudens, P.; Cartiaux, O.; Penta, M. Lower Limb Kinematics Using Inertial Sensors during Locomotion: Accuracy and Reproducibility of Joint Angle Calculations with Di Ff Erent. *Sensors* **2020**, *20*, 715.
19. Kobsar, D.; Charlton, J.M.; Tse, C.T.F.; Esculier, J.; Graffos, A.; Krowchuk, N.M.; Thatcher, D.; Hunt, M.A. Validity and Reliability of Wearable Inertial Sensors in Healthy Adult Walking: A Systematic Review and Meta-Analysis. *J. Neuroeng. Rehabil.* **2020**, *3*, 62. [CrossRef]
20. Bortolini, M.; Faccio, M.; Gamberi, M.; Pilati, F. Motion Analysis System (MAS) for Production and Ergonomics Assessment in the Manufacturing Processes. *Comput. Ind. Eng.* **2020**, *139*, 105485. [CrossRef]
21. Chander, H.; Garner, J.C.; Wade, C.; Knight, A.C. Postural Control in Workplace Safety: Role of Occupational Footwear and Workload. *Safety* **2017**, *3*, 18. [CrossRef]
22. van der Kruk, E.; Reijne, M.M. Accuracy of Human Motion Capture Systems for Sport Applications; State-of-the-Art Review. *Eur. J. Sport Sci.* **2018**, *18*, 806–819. [CrossRef] [PubMed]
23. Menolotto, M.; Komaris, D.S.; Tedesco, S.; O'flynn, B.; Walsh, M. Motion Capture Technology in Industrial Applications: A Systematic Review. *Sensors* **2020**, *20*, 5687. [CrossRef]
24. Breloff, S.P.; Dutta, A.; Dai, F.; Sinsel, E.W.; Warren, C.M.; Ning, X.; Wu, J.Z. Assessing Work-Related Risk Factors for Musculoskeletal Knee Disorders in Construction Roofing Tasks. *Appl. Ergon.* **2019**, *81*, 102901. [CrossRef] [PubMed]
25. Ryu, J.; Alwasel, A.; Haas, C.T.; Abdel-Rahman, E. Analysis of Relationships between Body Load and Training, Work Methods, and Work Rate: Overcoming the Novice Mason's Risk Hump. *J. Constr. Eng. Manag.* **2020**, *146*, 04020097. [CrossRef]
26. Clark, R.A.; Mentiplay, B.F.; Hough, E.; Pua, Y.H. Three-Dimensional Cameras and Skeleton Pose Tracking for Physical Function Assessment: A Review of Uses, Validity, Current Developments and Kinect Alternatives. *Gait Posture* **2019**, *68*, 193–200. [CrossRef] [PubMed]
27. Springer, S.; Seligmann, G.Y. Validity of the Kinect for Gait Assessment: A Focused Review. *Sensors* **2016**, *16*, 194. [CrossRef] [PubMed]
28. Tamura, H.; Tanaka, R.; Kawanishi, H. Reliability of a Markerless Motion Capture System to Measure the Trunk, Hip and Knee Angle during Walking on a Flatland and a Treadmill. *J. Biomech.* **2020**, *109*, 109929. [CrossRef] [PubMed]
29. Mehrizi, R.; Peng, X.; Xu, X.; Zhang, S.; Li, K. A Deep Neural Network-Based Method for Estimation of 3D Lifting Motions. *J. Biomech.* **2019**, *84*, 87–93. [CrossRef] [PubMed]
30. Andre, J.; Lopes, J.; Palermo, M.; Goncalves, D.; Matias, A.; Pereira, F.; Afonso, J.; Seabra, E.; Cerqueira, J.; Santos, C. Markerless Gait Analysis Vision System for Real-Time Gait Monitoring. In Proceedings of the 2020 IEEE International Conference on Autonomous Robot Systems and Competitions (ICARSC), Ponta Delgada, Portugal, 15–17 April 2020; pp. 269–274. [CrossRef]
31. Gandolfi, E. *Virtual Reality and Augmented Reality in Europe*; Springer International Publishing: Berlin/Heidelberg, Germany, 2018; Volume 2, ISBN 978-3-030-01789-7.
32. Wirth, M.A.; Fischer, G.; Verdú, J.; Reissner, L.; Balocco, S.; Calcagni, M. Comparison of a New Inertial Sensor Based System with an Optoelectronic Motion Capture System for Motion Analysis of Healthy Human Wrist Joints. *Sensors* **2019**, *19*, 5297. [CrossRef]
33. Waldman, H.S.; Smith, J.E.W.; Lamberth, J.; Fountain, B.J.; McAllister, M.J. A 28-Day Carbohydrate-Restricted Diet Improves Markers of Cardiometabolic Health and Performance in Professional Firefighters. *J. Strength Cond. Res.* **2019**, *33*, 3284–3294. [CrossRef]
34. Fitri, M.; Halim, A. Initial Ergonomic Risk Assessment on Unrolling and Rolling Fire Hose Activity Among Firefighters at Putrajaya Fire and Rescue Station. *Hum. Factors Ergon. J.* **2019**, *4*, 53–56.
35. Perruccio, A.V.; Yip, C.; Power, J.D.; Canizares, M.; Badley, E.M. Brief Report: Discordance Between Population Impact of Musculoskeletal Disorders and Scientific Representation: A Bibliometric Study. *Arthritis Care Res.* **2019**, *71*, 56–60. [CrossRef] [PubMed]
36. Monnet, T.; Samson, M.; Bernard, A.; David, L.; Lacouture, P. Measurement of Three-Dimensional Hand Kinematics during Swimming with a Motion Capture System: A Feasibility Study. *Sport. Eng.* **2014**, *17*, 171–181. [CrossRef]
37. Yunardi, R.T. Winarno Marker-Based Motion Capture for Measuring Joint Kinematics in Leg Swing Simulator. In Proceedings of the 2017 5th International Conference on Instrumentation, Control, and Automation (ICA), Yogyakarta, Indonesia, 9–11 August 2017; pp. 13–17. [CrossRef]
38. Puthenveetil, S.C.; Daphalapurkar, C.P.; Zhu, W.; Leu, M.C.; Liu, X.F.; Gilpin-Mcminn, J.K.; Snodgrass, S.D. Computer-Automated Ergonomic Analysis Based on Motion Capture and Assembly Simulation. *Virtual Real.* **2015**, *19*, 119–128. [CrossRef]
39. Ricci, F.P.F.M.; Santiago, P.R.P.; Zampar, A.C.; Pinola, L.N.; de Cássia Registro Fonseca, M. Upper Extremity Coordination Strategies Depending on Task Demand during a Basic Daily Activity. *Gait Posture* **2015**, *42*, 472–478. [CrossRef] [PubMed]
40. Wang, Q.; Kurillo, G.; Ofli, F.; Bajcsy, R. Evaluation of Pose Tracking Accuracy in the First and Second Generations of Microsoft Kinect. In Proceedings of the 2015 International Conference on Healthcare Informatics, Dallas, TX, USA, 21–23 October 2015; pp. 380–389. [CrossRef]

41. Takayasu, K.; Yoshida, K.; Mishima, T.; Watanabe, M.; Matsuda, T.; Kinoshita, H. Upper Body Position Analysis of Different Experience Level Surgeons during Laparoscopic Suturing Maneuvers Using Optical Motion Capture. *Am. J. Surg.* **2019**, *217*, 12–16. [CrossRef]
42. Janssen, M.M.H.P.; Peeters, L.H.C.; De Groot, I.J.M. Quantitative Description of Upper Extremity Function and Activity of People with Spinal Muscular Atrophy. *J. Neuroeng. Rehabil.* **2020**, *17*, 126. [CrossRef]
43. Nirme, J.; Haake, M.; Gulz, A.; Gullberg, M. Motion Capture-Based Animated Characters for the Study of Speech–Gesture Integration. *Behav. Res. Methods* **2020**, *52*, 1339–1354. [CrossRef]
44. Pavei, G.; Salis, F.; Cereatti, A.; Bergamini, E. Body Center of Mass Trajectory and Mechanical Energy Using Inertial Sensors: A Feasible Stride? *Gait Posture* **2020**, *80*, 199–205. [CrossRef]
45. Kang, Y.S.; Chang, Y.J. Using a Motion-Controlled Game to Teach Four Elementary School Children with Intellectual Disabilities to Improve Hand Hygiene. *J. Appl. Res. Intellect. Disabil.* **2019**, *32*, 942–951. [CrossRef]
46. Sin, H.; Lee, G. Additional Virtual Reality Training Using Xbox Kinect in Stroke Survivors with Hemiplegia. *Am. J. Phys. Med. Rehabil.* **2013**, *92*, 871–880. [CrossRef] [PubMed]
47. Haggag, H.; Hossny, M.; Nahavandi, S.; Creighton, D. Real Time Ergonomic Assessment for Assembly Operations Using Kinect. In Proceedings of the 2013 UKSim 15th International Conference on Computer Modelling and Simulation, Cambridge, UK, 10–12 April 2013; pp. 495–500. [CrossRef]
48. Schlagenhauf, F.; Sreeram, S.; Singhose, W. Comparison of Kinect and Vicon Motion Capture of Upper-Body Joint Angle Tracking. *IEEE Int. Conf. Control Autom. ICCA* **2018**, *2018*, 674–679. [CrossRef]
49. Trujillo, J.P.; Vaitonyte, J.; Simanova, I.; Özyürek, A. Toward the Markerless and Automatic Analysis of Kinematic Features: A Toolkit for Gesture and Movement Research. *Behav. Res. Methods* **2019**, *51*, 769–777. [CrossRef] [PubMed]
50. Chakraborty, S.; Nandy, A.; Yamaguchi, T.; Bonnet, V.; Venture, G. Accuracy of Image Data Stream of a Markerless Motion Capture System in Determining the Local Dynamic Stability and Joint Kinematics of Human Gait. *J. Biomech.* **2020**, *104*, 109718. [CrossRef] [PubMed]
51. Sabo, A.; Mehdizadeh, S.; Ng, K.D.; Iaboni, A.; Taati, B. Assessment of Parkinsonian Gait in Older Adults with Dementia via Human Pose Tracking in Video Data. *J. Neuroeng. Rehabil.* **2020**, *17*, 97. [CrossRef] [PubMed]
52. Parrilla, E.; Ruescas, A.V.; Solves, J.A.; Ballester, A.; Nacher, B.; Alemany, S.; Garrido, D. *A Methodology to Create 3D Body Models in Motion*; Springer International Publishing: Berlin/Heidelberg, Germany, 2021; Volume 1206, ISBN 9783030510633.
53. Muthukrishnan, N.; Abbas, J.J.; Krishnamurthi, N. A Wearable Sensor System to Measure Step-Based Gait Parameters for Parkinson's Disease Rehabilitation. *Sensors* **2020**, *20*, 6417. [CrossRef] [PubMed]
54. Yick, J.; Mukherjee, B.; Ghosal, D. Wireless Sensor Network Survey. *Comput. Netw.* **2008**, *52*, 2292–2330. [CrossRef]
55. Vignais, N.; Miezal, M.; Bleser, G.; Mura, K.; Gorecky, D.; Marin, F. Innovative System for Real-Time Ergonomic Feedback in Industrial Manufacturing. *Appl. Ergon.* **2013**, *44*, 566–574. [CrossRef] [PubMed]
56. Seel, T.; Raisch, J.; Schauer, T. IMU-Based Joint Angle Measurement for Gait Analysis. *Sensors* **2014**, *14*, 6891–6909. [CrossRef] [PubMed]
57. Fleron, M.K.; Ubbesen, N.C.H.; Battistella, F.; Dejtiar, D.L.; Oliveira, A.S. Accuracy between Optical and Inertial Motion Capture System for Assessing Trunk Speed during Preferred Gait and Transition Period. *Sports Biomech.* **2018**, *18*, 366–377. [CrossRef]
58. Abdelhady, M.; Van Den Bogert, A.J.; Simon, D. A High-Fidelity Wearable System for Measuring Lower-Limb Kinetics and Kinematics. *IEEE Sens. J.* **2019**, *19*, 12482–12493. [CrossRef]
59. Merino, G.; da Silva, L.; Mattos, D.; Guimarães, B.; Merino, E. Ergonomic Evaluation of the Musculoskeletal Risks in a Banana Harvesting Activity through Qualitative and Quantitative Measures, with Emphasis on Motion Capture (Xsens) and EMG. *Int. J. Ind. Ergon.* **2019**, *69*, 80–89. [CrossRef]
60. Nazarahari, M.; Rouhani, H. Semi-Automatic Sensor-to-Body Calibration of Inertial Sensors on Lower Limb Using Gait Recording. *IEEE Sens. J.* **2019**, *19*, 12465–12474. [CrossRef]
61. Lavender, S.A.; Sommerich, C.M.; Bigelow, S.; Weston, E.B.; Seagren, K.; Pay, N.A.; Sillars, D.; Ramachandran, V.; Sun, C.; Xu, Y.; et al. A Biomechanical Evaluation of Potential Ergonomic Solutions for Use by Firefighter and EMS Providers When Lifting Heavy Patients in Their Homes. *Appl. Ergon.* **2020**, *82*, 102910. [CrossRef] [PubMed]
62. Mcdonald, A.C.; Tsang, C.; Meszaros, K.A.; Dickerson, C.R. International Journal of Industrial Ergonomics Shoulder Muscle Activity in Off-Axis Pushing and Pulling Tasks. *Int. J. Ind. Ergon.* **2020**, *75*, 102892. [CrossRef]
63. Pimentel, M.N.; Potter, M.N.; Carollo, J.J.; Howell, D.R.; Sweeney, E.A. Peak Sagittal Plane Spine Kinematics in Female Gymnasts with and without a History of Low Back Pain. *Clin. Biomech.* **2020**, *76*, 105019. [CrossRef] [PubMed]
64. Gao, L.; Zhang, G.; Yu, B.; Qiao, Z.; Wang, J. Wearable Human Motion Posture Capture and Medical Health Monitoring Based on Wireless Sensor Networks. *Meas. J. Int. Meas. Confed.* **2020**, *166*, 108252. [CrossRef]
65. Castelli, A.; Paolini, G.; Cereatti, A.; Croce, U. Della 2015—A 2D Markerless Gait Analysis Methodology: Validation on Healthy Subjects—2D Markerless Technique Is Proposed to Perform Lower Limb Sagittal Plane Kinematic Analysis Using Single Video Camera. Subject-Specific, Multisegmental Model of Lower Limb W. *Comput. Math. Methods Med.* **2015**, *2015*, 186780.
66. Needham, L.; Evans, M.; Wade, L.; Cosker, D.P.; McGuigan, M.P.; Bilzon, J.L.; Colyer, S.L. The Development and Evaluation of a Fully Automated Markerless Motion Capture Workflow. *J. Biomech.* **2022**, *144*, 111338. [CrossRef]
67. Brunner, O.; Mertens, A.; Nitsch, V.; Brandl, C. Accuracy of a Markerless Motion Capture System for Postural Ergonomic Risk Assessment in Occupational Practice. *Int. J. Occup. Saf. Ergon.* **2022**, *28*, 1865–1873. [CrossRef]

68. Michaud, F.; Lugrís, U.; Cuadrado, J. Determination of the 3D Human Spine Posture from Wearable Inertial Sensors and a Multibody Model of the Spine. *Sensors* **2022**, *22*, 4796. [CrossRef] [PubMed]
69. Kubr, J.; Ho, P. Scopus—Detalles Del Documento—Diseño Ergonómico de Un Lugar de Trabajo Utilizando Realidad Virtual y Un Traje de Captura de Movimiento. *Appl. Sci.* **2022**, *12*, 2150.
70. Michaud, F.; Pazos, R.; Lugrís, U.; Cuadrado, J. The Use of Wearable Inertial Sensors and Workplace-Based Exercises to Reduce Lateral Epicondylitis in the Workstation of a Textile Logistics Center. *Sensors* **2023**, *23*, 5116. [CrossRef] [PubMed]
71. Muller, A.; Mecheri, H.; Corbeil, P.; Plamondon, A.; Robert-Lachaine, X. Inertial Motion Capture-Based Estimation of L5/S1 Moments during Manual Materials Handling. *Sensors* **2022**, *22*, 6454. [CrossRef]
72. Marín, J.; Marín, J.J. Forces: A Motion Capture-Based Ergonomic Method for the Today's World. *Sensors* **2021**, *21*, 5139. [CrossRef]
73. Seol, J.; Yoon, K.; Kim, K.G. Mathematical Analysis and Motion Capture System Utilization Method for Standardization Evaluation of Tracking Objectivity of 6-DOF Arm Structure for Rehabilitation Training Exercise Therapy Robot. *Diagnostics* **2022**, *12*, 3179. [CrossRef]
74. Ferrández-Laliena, L.; Vicente-Pina, L.; Sánchez-Rodríguez, R.; Orantes-González, E.; Heredia-Jimenez, J.; Lucha-López, M.O.; Hidalgo-García, C.; Tricás-Moreno, J.M. Diagnostics Using the Change-of-Direction and Acceleration Test (CODAT) of the Biomechanical Patterns Associated with Knee Injury in Female Futsal Players: A Cross-Sectional Analytical Study. *Diagnostics* **2023**, *13*, 928. [CrossRef]
75. Mainjot, A.K.; Oudkerk, J.; Bekaert, S.; Dardenne, N.; Streel, S.; Koenig, V.; Grenade, C.; Davarpanah, A.; Donneau, A.F.; Forthomme, B.; et al. Bruxism as a New Risk Factor of Musculo-Skeletal Disorders? *J. Dent.* **2023**, *135*, 104555. [CrossRef] [PubMed]

Disclaimer/Publisher's Note: The statements, opinions and data contained in all publications are solely those of the individual author(s) and contributor(s) and not of MDPI and/or the editor(s). MDPI and/or the editor(s) disclaim responsibility for any injury to people or property resulting from any ideas, methods, instructions or products referred to in the content.

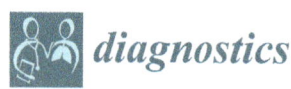

Systematic Review

Postural Control Measurements to Predict Future Motor Impairment in Preterm Infants: A Systematic Review

Jennifer Bosserman [1], Sonia Kelkar [2], Kristen D. LeBlond [3], Jessica Cassidy [2] and Dana B. McCarty [2,4,*]

1. Physical Medicine and Rehabilitation, Johns Hopkins Hospital, Baltimore, MD 21205, USA; jbosser3@jh.edu
2. Department of Health Sciences, University of North Carolina at Chapel Hill School of Medicine, Chapel Hill, NC 27599, USA
3. Physical Therapy and Occupational Therapy, Duke Health, Durham, NC 27705, USA
4. North Carolina Children's Hospital, Chapel Hill, NC 27599, USA
* Correspondence: dana_mccarty@med.unc.edu

Abstract: Preterm infants are more likely to demonstrate developmental delays than fullterm infants. Postural measurement tools may be effective in measuring the center of pressure (COP) and asymmetry, as well as predicting future motor impairment. The objective of this systematic review was to evaluate existing evidence regarding use of pressure mats or force plates for measuring COP and asymmetry in preterm infants, to determine how measures differ between preterm and fullterm infants and if these tools appropriately predict future motor impairment. The consulted databases included PubMed, Embase, Scopus, and CINAHL. The quality of the literature and the risk of bias were assessed utilizing the ROB2: revised Cochrane risk-of bias tool. Nine manuscripts met the criteria for review. The postural control tools included were FSA UltraThin seat mat, Conformat Pressure-Sensitive mat, Play and Neuro-Developmental Assessment, and standard force plates. Studies demonstrated that all tools were capable of COP assessment in preterm infants and support the association between the observation of reduced postural complexity prior to the observation of midline head control as an indicator of future motor delay. Postural measurement tools provide quick and objective measures of postural control and asymmetry. Based on the degree of impairment, these tools may provide an alternative to standardized assessments that may be taxing to the preterm infant, inaccessible to therapists, or not sensitive enough to capture motor delays.

Keywords: postural control; center of pressure; preterm infant; force plate; postural measurement

1. Introduction

There is a risk of motor impairment in all preterm infants born <37 weeks of gestation; however, the risk is highest in infants born moderately preterm (32–34 weeks of gestation) at 20.6% and very preterm (<32 weeks of gestation) at 36.1% [1,2]. When comparing fullterm and preterm infants, the risk of motor impairment ranges from 2 to 7% compared to 54–64%, respectively [3]. There are notable differences between the movement patterns of preterm and fullterm infants. Preterm infants demonstrate a lower quality of spontaneous movements, with descriptions such as low fluency, less variety, and impaired sequencing [4]. Preterm infants are also more likely to display abnormal or absent fidgety movements, ref. [5,6] which is a highly sensitive indicator of future motor impairment at 12 weeks of age. Preterm infants also lack postural complexity, defined as the use of a variety of postural control strategies, as compared to healthy term infants [7].

Preterm infants are more likely to display body and head asymmetry and show preference for extension patterns than fullterm infants [6]. These asymmetrical patterns may be attributed to the development of increased power in the extensor muscle groups in preterm infants. Increased muscle power [8] results in the hyperextended posture commonly observed in preterm infants. This posture further leads to difficulties in maintaining midline orientation [8].

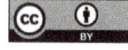

Citation: Bosserman, J.; Kelkar, S.; LeBlond, K.D.; Cassidy, J.; McCarty, D.B. Postural Control Measurements to Predict Future Motor Impairment in Preterm Infants: A Systematic Review. *Diagnostics* **2023**, *13*, 3473. https://doi.org/10.3390/diagnostics13223473

Academic Editors: Mario Cesarelli, Francesco Amato and Carlo Ricciardi

Received: 22 September 2023
Revised: 15 November 2023
Accepted: 17 November 2023
Published: 18 November 2023

Copyright: © 2023 by the authors. Licensee MDPI, Basel, Switzerland. This article is an open access article distributed under the terms and conditions of the Creative Commons Attribution (CC BY) license (https://creativecommons.org/licenses/by/4.0/).

The neonatal intensive care unit (NICU) environment is not optimal for neonatal neuromotor development for a variety of reasons, including noise levels, lighting, and other noxious stimuli, as well as suboptimal musculoskeletal support [9]. Preterm infants are vulnerable to the effects of gravity on alignment, posture, mobility, respiratory abilities, and the shaping of the musculoskeletal system [10,11]. Without the intrauterine environment facilitating a flexed posture and limiting extremity movement, preterm infants succumb to the weight of gravity and begin to favor an extended posture. In an attempt to gain postural stability in the absence of uterine wall restraint [10,11], preterm infants often extend their trunk and extremities further into the flat surface they are placed upon, resulting in commonly described postures of exaggerated cervical lordosis and hyperextension [10]. This combination of the effects of gravity and hyperextended posture leads to weak and overstretched muscles of the anterior neck and trunk, interferes with purposeful self-soothing movements directed towards the midline, and contributes to developmental delay [12].

Extended posture and associated asymmetries in movement can result in head or positional preferences. The prevalence of such positional asymmetries ranges from 45 to 79% of preterm infants [13,14]. Head turn preferences in preterm infants are associated with suboptimal reflexes, decreased maturation of gross motor movements, and the development of torticollis and deformational plagiocephaly during infancy [13,14]. These impairments, if not fully addressed, further contribute to delays with increasing infant age, including impaired fine motor skills, asymmetrical gait patterns, and postural asymmetries [13,15].

Moderate to severe neuromotor and sensory disabilities are highly prevalent in extremely and very preterm infants born between 22 and 34 weeks of gestation [16], requiring early assessment and intervention. Preterm infants born 24–31 weeks of gestation remain in the NICU for a range of 34–123 days [17]. Due to increased risk of motor delay, these infants often receive physical and/or occupational therapy services during hospitalization. Current evidence supports parent- and therapist-delivered motor intervention to improve motor and cognitive developmental outcomes in preterm infants [18], and immediate, ongoing therapy services after hospital discharge to reduce the risk of developmental delays; however, there is often a delay in the initiation of therapy services after NICU discharge [19,20], especially if no significant motor impairment or diagnosis has been documented using a standardized or objective measure. Standardized assessments vary based on the appropriate age for administration, domains of function tested (e.g., motor, neurobehavior), applications, and predictive validity. Few standardized assessments are sensitive enough to detect developmental delays for infants at or near term-equivalent age [21,22], which is often the age of the infant at the time of NICU discharge.

Standardized infant assessments also vary greatly by administration requirements, with many necessitating costly training programs to learn and administer testing [23]. While these training programs are in place for the essential purpose of ensuring reliable and valid results for clinical and research applications, the rigorous requirements are often out of reach for therapists and the NICUs they serve due to a lack of continuing education funds and travel requirements. In the absence of extended time for clinicians to attend training programs and funding to pay for such programs, it is prudent to identify objective measures that indicate potential delay that can be used, assessed, and understood by a variety of clinicians and researchers. Quantitative measurements such as center of pressure (COP) and variability of movement have been shown to be predictive of motor impairment or delay in preterm infants [24], but these measures are not currently used in the clinical setting to identify infants at risk for movement delay.

Pediatric therapist researchers are advocating for the expanded use of technology in clinical settings to detect early motor delay [25]. Postural measurement tools, including portable pressure-sensitive mats and force plates, may be effective in measuring COP in preterm infants, and therefore useful for detecting early delays in high-risk infant populations [24]. Additionally, the use of wearable sensors, including inclusive clothing, exoskeletons, and smart tracking devices, are being examined in high-risk infant populations to determine potential ways that this technology can assist with understanding how specific movement characteristics may enhance or detract from the infant's developmental trajectory [25].

The use of such technologies expands opportunities for the use of artificial intelligence to assist in the early and accurate diagnosis of neuromotor disabilities. Gaining a better understanding of the role of early postural control deviations as measured by force plates or sensors allows researchers to use these technologies to build algorithms that detect and quantify movements associated with future motor impairments [26].

The purpose of this review was to evaluate the existing evidence regarding the use of technology, specifically, pressure mats or force plates, to measure both linear and non-linear measures of postural control and movement in preterm infants. We also evaluated how those measures differ in preterm and fullterm infants and how these differences may predict future motor impairment or disability in this population.

2. Methods

The following inclusion criteria were used to select studies: (1) articles include infants born at or prior to 37 weeks, (2) measurements were collected in supine, (3) measurements were collected using a pressurized mat or mattresses, and (4) articles were in reference to humans. Exclusion criteria included the following: (1) a study population of infants born after 37 weeks of gestation, (2) measurements taken in positions other than supine, or (3) articles with reference to animals. We did not include gray literature or dissertations.

The protocol for the review was drafted using the Preferred Reporting Items for Systematic Reviews and Meta-analysis Extension (PRISMA) [27] and was registered to the Open Science Framework (OSF, registration DOI number: 10.17605/OSF.IO/G82WK) [28]. The objective of this systematic review was to answer the question: "In preterm infants, can center of pressure (COP) measurements and variability of movement measurements in supine help determine the risk of motor delay in infancy?". A search strategy using keywords was developed by the primary author (JB) in consultation with a university librarian and included "("Infant, Newborn" [MeSH] OR "Premature Birth" [MeSH] OR Neonatal [tiab]) AND ("Postural Balance" [MeSH] OR "Pressure, Mat*" [tiab] OR "Multi-sensor" [tiab] OR "Force Plate" [tiab])". Four databases were searched in September 2023 (PubMed, Embase, Scopus, and CINAHL). One investigator (JB) used MeSH headings and text words to complete the search. Results were imported to Covidence [29], a systematic review production tool for title/abstract/full-text review and data abstraction.

Two reviewers (JB, SK) independently reviewed and extracted papers that met the inclusion criteria for full text review through methods consistent with the PRISMA guidelines [30]. Any disagreement about inclusion was discussed amongst the reviewers (JB, SK), and the senior author (DM) made the final determination. Papers that passed the full-text review were evaluated with an extraction table based on recommendations from the Cochrane Collaboration [31] and included the following characteristics: study aims, study design, data sources, study population, outcome measures, data analysis strategy, postural measurement tool, results, implications, strengths, and limitations. Data extracted were then reviewed using a descriptive approach to summarize key findings.

The quality of the literature and risk of bias were rated utilizing the ROB2, revised Cochrane risk-of-bias tool, for randomized trials [32] for each included study. Independent assessments were completed by two reviewers (JB and DM), and full agreement was reached after discussion.

3. Results

3.1. Study Selection

The initial keyword search identified nine hundred and one studies. Two hundred and fifty-three of these were excluded as duplicate studies from multiple databases. The remaining six hundred and forty-eight studies underwent title and abstract screening based on the inclusion and exclusion criteria. A full-text review for eligibility was completed for twenty-six full-text studies, and nine met all eligibility criteria (Figure 1).

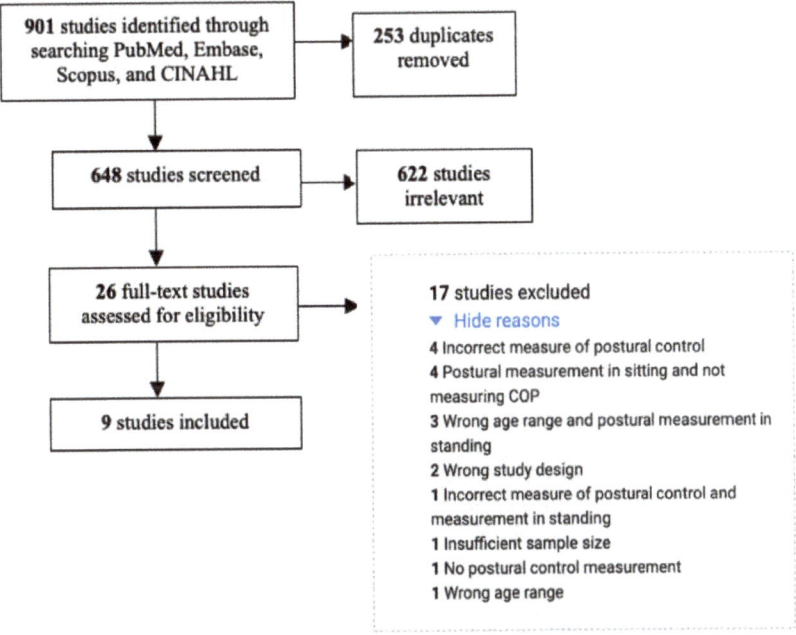

Figure 1. Study selection process.

3.2. Characteristics of the Included Literature

Of the included studies, six were prospective cohort studies [7,24,33–36], two were cross-sectional studies [37,38], and one was a case study [39]. The characteristics of these studies are noted in Table 1. All studies were conducted in the United States [7,24,33,37–39], Norway [34,35], or Poland [34].

Table 1. Study characteristics.

First Author, Year	Aim	Study Design	Study Population	Postural Measurement Tool	Outcome
Dusing et al., 2009 [39]	To determine whether infants born at full term and infants born preterm differ in their COP movement variability characteristics, evaluated both linearly and nonlinearly while positioned supine.	Cross-Sectional Study	47% fullterm	FSA UltraThin Seat Mat	Infants born pre-term exhibited larger root-mean-squared values in the caudal–cephalic direction than infants born full-term.
Dusing et al., 2005 [38]	To compare trunk position in supine of infants born preterm and at term. A secondary purpose was to determine the feasibility of using pressure data to assess trunk position.	Cross-Sectional Study	45% fullterm	FSA UltraThin Seat Mat	Infants born preterm differ in their trunk positions immediately after birth as demonstrated by decreased time spent in flexion or neutral.
Dusing et al., 2016 [36]	To fill knowledge gaps on the development of adaptive postural control in infants born preterm	Cohort Study (Prospective Observational Study)	0% fullterm	Conformat Pressure-Sensitive Mat	Infants born preterm did not alter the postural variability in the caudal–cephalic direction in response to a visual stimulus prior to 4 months of age. They were able to adapt postural variability in the medial–lateral direction at 2.5 months of age.

Table 1. *Cont.*

First Author, Year	Aim	Study Design	Study Population	Postural Measurement Tool	Outcome
Dusing et al., 2014 [7]	To investigate group differences in postural variability between infants born preterm and at risk for developmental delays or disability and infants born full term with typical development, during the emergence of early behaviors	Cross-Sectional Study	55% fullterm	Conformat Pressure-Sensitive Mat	Measures of early postural complexity are helpful in the development of interventions during the first months of life to prevent the delay in postural control strategies in preterm infants.
Dusing et al., 2014 [39]	To describe how changes in postural control during development may relate to action and perception in 3 infants born preterm with brain injury	Case Study	0% fullterm	Conformat Pressure-Sensitive Mat	Excessive postural complexity and reduced postural complexity alter the infants' abilities to act on the world around them and use perceptual information to modify their actions.
Fallang et al., 2003 [34]	To discuss the clinical and neurophysiological data of postural behavior	Cohort Study (Prospective Observational Study)	25% fullterm	Force plate	Preterm infants show a relatively immobile postural behavior and maximum velocity of COP was substantially lower than full-term infants.
Fallang et al., 2005 [35]	To investigate whether parameters of nonoptimal reaching and reduced COP behavior at an early age are associated with dysfunctional neuromotor and behavioral development at school age.	Cohort Study (Retrospective Observational Study)	19% fullterm	Force plate	In preterm infants who do not develop CP, a lack of successful reaching at 4 months and an inadequate quality of reaching at 6 months (corrected age) are sensitive markers of clinically significant forms of brain dysfunction.
Kniaziew-Gomoluch et al., 2023 [36]	To assess reliability and validity of force plates to measure posture in preterm infants	Cohort Study (Prospective Observational Study)	0% fullterm	Force plate	Comparative analysis between the groups of infants with normal FMs and abnormal FMs in supine showed significant differences for all parameters that described spontaneous COP displacement.
Prosser et al., 2022 [24]	To investigate the ability of biomechanical measures of early postural control to distinguish infants with future impairment in motor control.	Cohort Study (Prospective Observational Study)	53% fullterm	Play and Neuro-Developmental Assessment (PANDA) gym	Quantitative methods of measuring postural control in infants born preterm and who are still hospitalized are feasible and show promise for early detection of motor impairment.

Key: COP = center of pressure; FM = Fidgety Movements.

3.3. Participants

All studies included infants born preterm (<37 weeks of gestation). The majority of studies (*n* = 6) also included a control group of fullterm infants with typical motor control (Table 1) [7,24,33–35]. Other participant characteristics reported were variable and are included below in the results section.

3.4. Quality Assessment

The results of the quality assessment can be seen in Table 2. Due to the nature of the infant population and study designs, blinding and random allocation did not occur. This resulted in all nine studies receiving the rating of "high concern" for Domain 1, risk of bias associated with the randomization process, as well as Overall Risk of Bias, per the scoring criteria [32]. Two studies [34,36] also received "high concern" in other domains due to deviation from the intended intervention.

Table 2. Quality assessment utilizing the ROB2: revised Cochrane risk-of bias tool.

ROB2 Quality Ratings Areas of Quality Assessed	Fallang et al., 2003 [33]	Fallang et al., 2005 [34]	Dusing et al., 2005 [38]	Dusing et al., 2009 [37]	Dusing et al., 2014 [7]	Dusing et al., 2014 [39]	Dusing et al., 2016 [36]	Prosser et al., 2022 [24]	Kniaziew-Gomoluch et al., 2023 [36]
Domain 1 Risk-of-bias-judgement: Risk of bias arising from the randomization process	High Concern	High Concern	High Concern	High Concern	High Concern	High Concern	High Concern	High Concern	High Concern
Domain 2 Risk-of-bias-judgement: Risk of bias due to deviations from the intended interventions (effect of assignment to intervention)	High Concern	High Concern	Low Concern	Low Concern	Low Concern	Low Concern	Some Concern	Low Concern	Some Concern
Domain 3 Risk-of-bias-judgement: Missing outcome data	High Concern	Some Concern	Some Concern	Low Concern	Low Concern	Low Concern	Some Concern	Some Concern	Low Concern
Domain 4 Risk-of-bias-judgement: Risk of bias in measurement of the outcome	Low Concern	Some Concern	Low Concern	Low Concern	Low Concern	Low Concern	Low Concern	Low Concern	Low Concern
Domain 5 Risk-of-bias-judgement: Risk of bias in selection of the reported result	High Concern	Some Concern	Low Concern	Low Concern	Low Concern	Low Concern	Low Concern	Some Concern	Low Concern
Overall Risk of Bias	High Concern	High Concern	High Concern	High Concern	High Concern	High Concern	High Concern	High Concern	High Concern

3.5. Postural Control Measurement Systems and Measures of Postural Control

Postural control tools and measurement parameters varied between studies as seen in Table 1. Two studies utilized the FSA UltraThin seat mat (Vista Medical Ltd., Manitoba, MB, Canada) [37,38] to measure the maximum pressure value, the ratio of head and pelvis to trunk pressure, and COP. The Conformat Pressure-Sensitive mat (Tekscan Inc., Norwood, MA, USA) was utilized in three studies [7,33,39] to measure COP, the magnitude and complexity of movement, head control, and reaching ability. The Play and Neuro-Developmental Assessment (PANDA) gym (Penn Center for Innovation, Philadelphia, PA, USA) [24] was used to measure limb and trunk kinematics and COP measurements. Lastly, three studies used standard force plates by AMTI (Advanced Medical Technologies Inc, Watertown, MA or Kistler (Kistler Instrument Corp., Amherst, NY, USA) [34–36] to measure postural adjustments with reaching and COP displacement.

Both linear and non-linear measures of postural control were used in the reviewed studies. Linear measures such as path length quantify the amount of COP variability [40]. Generally, in the adult population, high variability in COP is interpreted as postural instability, whereas lower COP variability indicates greater postural control; however, the studies reviewed for this manuscript noted greater COP variability in healthy fullterm control infants as compared to preterm infants, who demonstrated less complexity in movement [24].

Non-linear metrics, which incorporate time into COP variability, were also used for postural control analysis. These non-linear metrics quantify the amount of randomness, fluctuation, and unpredictability during dynamic movement [40]. As observed in linear postural metrics, preterm infants actually demonstrated smaller amounts of entropy, or randomness, than fullterm infants, indicating less variability of complex movement [38].

3.5.1. FSA UltraThin Seat Mat

The Force Sensing Array (FSA) UltraThin seat mat is a pressure-sensitive mat that is commonly used in wheelchair seating systems. The FSA seat mat includes a 4D pressure mapping system [41] that measures the total duration of trunk flexion, extension, or neutral positioning, determined according to the total number of frames the infant's trunk was in for each position and multiplying the total consecutive frames by the sampling period (200 ms) [37]; approximate entropy, a ratio that estimates the randomness, fluctuation, and unpredictability of time-series data [39]; and root mean square values, the standard deviation of the displacement of the COP in the caudal–cephalic and medial–lateral directions [42,43].

In a cohort of 33 infants aged 38.30–42.30 weeks corrected age, researchers found that term infants (mean gestational age of 38.9 weeks) spent significantly 81% of the awake segment in flexion or neutral ($p = 0.027$), and only 74.91% of preterm infants (mean gestational age of 31.9 weeks) spent the awake segment in flexion or neutral ($p = 1.52$) [37]. In a cohort of 32 infants at 41–43 weeks corrected age, preterm infants exhibited larger root mean square values (preterm = 1.11 cm, term = 0.83 cm; $p = 0.01$) and smaller approximate entropy values (preterm = 1.11, term = 1.19; $p = 0.02$) in the caudal–cephalic direction than term infants [38]. Authors concluded that smaller approximate entropy and larger root mean square values in preterm infants suggest less complex, repetitive movement, and less stable posture in the caudal–cephalic direction [38].

3.5.2. Conformat Pressure-Sensitive Mat

A Conformat Pressure-Sensitive mat is a portable and lightweight seating and positioning system often used for wheelchair pressure mapping, which provides information on pressure distribution and the center of force trajectory [7]. Dusing et al. used the Conformat Pressure-Sensitive mat to measure the root mean square and approximate entropy values (as defined in the previous section) in the caudal–cephalic and medial–lateral directions [7,33,39].

Results from a cohort of three infants 2–6 months old demonstrated an interaction between condition and age, in the caudal–cephalic direction of postural variability ($p = 0.03$), and that preterm infants demonstrated low complexity movements in the caudal–cephalic direction, ref. [39] indicating that decreased postural complexity before the development of midline head control may be an indicator of future motor delay.

3.5.3. The PANDA Gym

The Play And NeuroDevelopmental Assessment (PANDA) includes an array of toys with sensors in them, a camera-based computer vision system, and a mat structure covered in carbon fiber [24]. This gym also includes a PVC pipe above the platform for toy suspension and to support the video system [24]. In a cohort of 15 infants aged 3–11 months old, the PANDA gym measured seven variables including path length, the total distance an object moved from its initial position to its final position; ExcursionX/Y, with ExcursionX being the farthest distance in the medial–lateral direction, or side-to-side shifting, and ExcursionY being the farthest distance in the caudal–cephalic direction, or vertical shifting; and ElipseArea, the scatter of COP in the X and Y directions [24].

Vertical displacement (ExcursionY) was significantly lower in the preterm group compared to the term group (difference = 3.65 cm, 95% confidence interval (CI): 0.13–7.17 cm, $p = 0.043$), demonstrating a smaller distance traveled in the caudal–cephalic direction, with minimal vertical shifting [24]. The COP variability (EllipseArea) was significantly lower in the preterm vs. term group (difference = 2.3 cm, 95% CI: 1.06–4.84 cm, $p = 0.038$). These results indicate less movement variability in preterm infants, specifically in the caudal–cephalic direction. The total distance traveled (path length) was significantly higher in the preterm group compared to the fullterm group for three conditions (no toy 153.4 vs. 101.3 cm, $p = 0.0054$; bilateral reach 146.1 vs. 87.5 cm, $p = 0.0088$; and unilateral reach 176.6 vs. 112.2 cm, $p = 0.0005$), demonstrating increased movement from the initial position to the final position in preterm infants. Lastly, in the group that was identified as having impaired motor control at 2 years of age, as determined from a medical record review, path length was found to be higher in all conditions (no toy 155.6 vs. 115.9 cm, $p = 0.033$; bilateral reach 158.4 vs. 100.1 cm, $p = 0.003$, and unilateral reach 223.1 vs. 122.2 cm, $p < 0.0001$) [24].

3.5.4. Force Plates

A multi-axis force plate is capable of measuring all dynamic motion sequences, including abruptly changing forces [40]. In two studies [32,33], total body COP was analyzed from force plates using several parameters, including the path length (as defined above), the length and duration of the movement path/time, the number of directional changes in COP displacement, and the maximum velocity (Vmax): the maximum speed in which the infant moves in the cranial–caudal and medial–lateral directions [34,35].

Findings from a long-term follow-up study conducted by Fallang et al. [35] showed that in fifty-two 4-month-old infants, a lower maximum velocity of COP and smaller displacement of COP in the medial–lateral direction were related to coordination problems at 6 years of age ($p = 0.04$). At 4 and 6 months, performance below the 15th percentile on the Movement ABC at 6 years was associated with a lower Vmax of COP in the medial–lateral direction at 4 months ($p = 0.02$) and 6 months ($p = 0.03$) and a lower number of cranial–caudal oscillations (4 months $p = 0.02$, 6 months $p = 0.01$) [35]. In a related study, Fallang et al. found that the total body COP in preterm infants differed from fullterm infants due to a smaller COP distance travelled during reaching in both the cranial–caudal and medial–lateral directions, demonstrating relatively immobile postural behavior [34].

A recent study by Kniaziew-Gomoluch et al. [36] used force plates to examine postural control in 37 preterm infants born between 24 and 33 weeks of gestation at 12–14 weeks corrected age. Infants simultaneously were video-recorded for the General Movements Assessment. Researchers found significant differences in all parameters of spontaneous COP displacement between infants with normal fidgety movements and those without fidgety movements ($p < 0.05$). Using the Intraclass Correlation Coefficient for test–retest data, all parameters measured in supine were considered to have moderate to good reliability [36].

4. Discussion

While there is still much to learn about the quantitative measurement of postural control in preterm infants, the available evidence demonstrates that tools such as force plates and pressure mats are feasible for the measurement of infant postural control and asymmetry. Further, these tools identified differences in preterm infant movement as compared to fullterm infant movement. Quantitative measurements of trunk positioning during spontaneous activity may be a reasonable and useful measure to identify infants at high risk for motor impairment or disability and those who are not [24,36,37]. In opposition to how postural complexity is interpreted in adults, several studies indicate that reduced postural complexity in infants before development of midline head control may indicate future motor delay [7,33,37,38]. Evidence also suggests that these postural control measures are sensitive to the later development of neuromotor dysfunction. One study found associations between postural control parameters at 4 and 6 months and motor scores at 6 years of age [35], and another study found that postural control parameters were significantly different between groups of preterm infants with normal and abnormal fidgety movements—an early predictor of cerebral palsy [36].

Postural measurements have been used most consistently in research applications, but the results from this systematic review demonstrate potential for clinical application to support early identification of infants with motor delay—potentially as early as term-equivalent age. Specific atypical measurements of postural control that have been associated with future motor impairment include COP path length, COP extent, variety of movement, and speed of movement, especially in the caudal–cephalic direction [24,38]. Sensitive measures that predict future motor impairment and characterize some preterm infant movement characteristics include predictable and repetitive COP movement in the caudal–cephalic direction, a relatively immobile posture, a lack of successful reaching by 4 months, and inadequate reaching quality at 6 months in supine [7,34,36].

Currently, many preterm infants do not qualify for early intervention services when assessed based on state-by-state qualification standards for Part C of the Individuals with Disabilities Education Improvement Act [44]. Additionally, the available standardized assessments may not be sensitive enough to capture the extent of an infant's delay prior to NICU discharge. Because standardized assessments generally quantify the infant's capacity to exert postural control in specific developmental positions, but do not always quantify the quality and characteristics of the infant's movement, subtle postural differences may be missed [21]. For example, in a recently published study, Wang et al. discusses that the General Movement Assessment (GMA) can identify absent or abnormal fidgety movements and has 98% sensitivity for the diagnosis of cerebral palsy at 12 weeks [36], but a limitation of this assessment is the absence of a measurement tool used to quantify these movements [21]. The Motor Optimality Score (MOS), a detailed scoring of the GMA, is currently in the early stages of reliability testing [45] but requires advanced GMA certification to administer. Based on the recent findings of Kniaziew-Gomoluch et al. [36], COP parameters as measured by force plates are sensitive enough to detect differences between infants who demonstrate normal fidgety and abnormal fidgety movements.

Of the measurement tools described in this review, perhaps the most promising for future clinical use is the PANDA gym [24]. With its portable design and ongoing research using machine learning to develop algorithms to produce measurements and relevant scores, the PANDA gym has the potential for widespread use in various clinical settings to diagnose early movement dysfunction. While early validity assessments of this mat system are promising, additional reliability, validity, and sensitivity to change testing should be conducted prior to clinical applications. Additionally, findings from Kniaziew-Gomoluck et al. [36], demonstrate a correlation between force plate-measured postural control parameters and absent fidgety movements between 12–14 weeks post-term, indicating a potential clinical usefulness for early cerebral palsy detection [36,46]. COP path length, which is measured via the PANDA gym and force plates, consistently differed between fullterm and preterm infants in the studies we reviewed and appear to be early indicators of motor delay [36]. Most studies did not address whether force plate and pressure mat technologies can be easily disinfected between uses in the highly vulnerable preterm infant population; however, the carbon fiber core dragon plate used in the PANDA gym can be easily cleaned with soap and water or disinfectant wipes between use [24]. This plate is covered with foam padding or a blanket for infant comfort for single patient use to decrease the spread of infection.

Limitations of this study include the acknowledgement that the use of pressure-sensitive mats and force plates in the clinical setting may not be easily attained due to the high cost of equipment and maintenance requirements; however, with more advanced technology, newer devices are becoming available that may increase affordability and portability necessary for clinical spaces. We also acknowledge that a shift in clinical practice and eligibility standards would be necessary to use atypical postural control measurements to quantify motor delays. Furthermore, clinicians would need additional training to collect and interpret these data in a meaningful and objective way.

This study provides ample evidence for the use of pressure mats and force plates to measure postural control, asymmetry, and variability of movement in preterm infants, but future research is needed to employ this globally. Future research should focus on the validity, predictive ability, sensitivity to change over time, and quantification of severity necessary to detect future motor impairments [24]. Further, infants should be assessed over a shorter time period to improve the test–retest reliability of these methods [33]. A longitudinal follow-up of high-risk infants and those who later develop motor impairment would also be useful in determining which infants can adapt to changing task demands based on postural control in early infancy [4]. Studies presented in this systematic review support the association between the observation of reduced postural complexity prior to the observation of midline head control as an indicator of future motor delay [7,33,37,38]. This observation should be verified utilizing larger sample sizes with a long-term follow-up. Future research is also necessary to determine critical periods of time in which postural complexity has a greater impact on development and optimal variability of movement, as well as which occupational therapy and physical therapy interventions best mitigate the risk of delay [37]. Based on the risk-of-bias assessment for the manuscripts assessed in this study, the blinding of researchers or the separation of tasks for collecting and reducing the data should be considered in the methodology of future studies.

5. Conclusions

There is a need to identify impairments in early posture and movement complexity in order to avoid delays in post-NICU therapy services. Altered posture and movement in preterm infants limits the infants' ability to explore the world around them, perform variable movements, use perceptual information to modify movement, and practice a variety of postural control strategies [33]. Postural measurement tools such as force plates and pressure-sensitive mats provide quick and objective measures of COP and asymmetry, and, based on the degree of impairment in postural control and movement, may indicate future motor impairment, providing an alternative to the application of standardized assessments for the quantification of developmental delay.

Author Contributions: Conceptualization, D.B.M.; methodology, D.B.M. and J.B.; validation, D.B.M., J.B. and S.K.; formal analysis, D.B.M., J.B. and S.K.; investigation, J.B. and S.K.; resources, J.C. and K.D.L.; data curation, J.B.; writing—original draft preparation, J.B.; writing—review and editing, J.B., D.B.M., K.D.L. and J.C.; visualization, J.B.; supervision, D.B.M. and J.C.; project administration, D.B.M. All authors have read and agreed to the published version of the manuscript.

Funding: This research received no external funding.

Data Availability Statement: Data are contained within the article.

Acknowledgments: The authors would like to thank the UNC Chapel Hill Division of Physical Therapy, Department of Health Sciences for its resource support during the development and execution of this project.

Conflicts of Interest: The authors declare no conflict of interest.

References

1. Van Hus, J.W.; Potharst, E.S.; Jeukens-Visser, M.; Kok, J.H.; Van Wassenaer-Leemhuis, A.G. Motor impairment in very preterm-born children: Links with other developmental deficits at 5 years of age. *Dev. Med. Child. Neurol.* **2014**, *56*, 587–594. [CrossRef]
2. Bélanger, R.; Mayer-Crittenden, C.; Minor-Corriveau, M.; Robillard, M. Gross Motor Outcomes of Children Born Prematurely in Northern Ontario and Followed by a Neonatal Follow-Up Programme. *Physiother. Can.* **2018**, *70*, 233–239. [CrossRef]
3. Spittle, A.J.; Cameron, K.; Doyle, L.W.; Cheong, J.L. Victorian Infant Collaborative Study Group. Motor Impairment Trends in Extremely Preterm Children: 1991–2005. *Pediatrics* **2018**, *141*, e20173410. [CrossRef]
4. Kakebeeke, T.H.; von Siebenthal, K.; Largo, R.H. Movement quality in preterm infants prior to term. *Biol. Neonate* **1998**, *73*, 145–154. [CrossRef]
5. Fjørtoft, T.; Evensen, K.A.I.; Øberg, G.K.; Songstad, N.T.; Labori, C.; Silberg, I.E.; Loennecken, M.; Møinichen, U.I.; Vågen, R.; Støen, R.; et al. High prevalence of abnormal motor repertoire at 3 months corrected age in extremely preterm infants. *Eur. J. Paediatr. Neurol.* **2016**, *20*, 236–242. [CrossRef]
6. Örtqvist, M.; Einspieler, C.; Marschik, P.B.; Ådén, U. Movements and posture in infants born extremely preterm in comparison to term-born controls. *Early Hum. Dev.* **2021**, *154*, 105304. [CrossRef]
7. Dusing, S.C.; Izzo, T.A.; Thacker, L.R.; Galloway, J.C. Postural complexity differs between infant born full term and preterm during the development of early behaviors. *Early Hum. Dev.* **2014**, *90*, 149–156. [CrossRef]
8. de Groot, L. Posture and motility in preterm infants. *Dev. Med. Child. Neurol.* **2000**, *42*, 65–68. [CrossRef]
9. Williams, K.G.; Patel, K.T.; Stausmire, J.M.; Bridges, C.; Mathis, M.W.; Barkin, J.L. The neonatal intensive care unit: Environmental stressors and supports. *Int. J. Environ. Res. Public Health* **2018**, *15*, 60. [CrossRef]
10. Sweeney, J.K.; Gutierrez, T. Musculoskeletal implications of preterm infant positioning in the NICU. *J. Perinat. Neonatal Nurs.* **2002**, *16*, 58–70. [CrossRef]
11. Byrne, E.; Garber, J. Physical therapy intervention in the neonatal intensive care unit. *Phys. Occup. Ther. Pediatr.* **2013**, *33*, 75–110. [CrossRef]
12. Byrne, E.; Campbell, S.K. Physical therapy observation and assessment in the neonatal intensive care unit. *Phys. Occup. Ther. Pediatr.* **2013**, *33*, 39–74. [CrossRef]
13. Dunsirn, S.; Smyser, C.; Liao, S.; Inder, T.; Pineda, R. Defining the nature and implications of head turn preference in the preterm infant. *Early Hum. Dev.* **2016**, *96*, 53–60. [CrossRef]
14. Nuysink, J.; van Haastert, I.C.; Eijsermans, M.J.C.; Koopman-Esseboom, C.; van der Net, J.; de Vries, L.S.; Helders, P.J. Prevalence and predictors of idiopathic asymmetry in infants born preterm. *Early Hum. Dev.* **2012**, *88*, 387–392. [CrossRef]

15. Konishi, Y.; Mikawa, H.; Suzuki, J. Asymmetrical head-turning of preterm infants: Some effects on later postural and functional lateralities. *Dev. Med. Child. Neurol.* **1986**, *28*, 450–457. [CrossRef]
16. Pierrat, V.; Marchand-Martin, L.; Arnaud, C.; Kaminski, M.; Resche-Rigon, M.; Lebeaux, C.; Bodeau-Livinec, F.; Morgan, A.S.; Marret, S.; Ancel, P.-Y.; et al. Neurodevelopmental outcome at 2 years for preterm children born at 22 to 34 weeks' gestation in France in 2011: EPIPAGE-2 cohort study. *BMJ* **2017**, *358*, j3448. [CrossRef]
17. Seaton, S.E.; Barker, L.; Draper, E.S.; Abrams, K.R.; Modi, N.; Manktelow, B.N. Estimating neonatal length of stay for babies born very preterm. *Arch. Dis. Child. Fetal Neonatal Ed.* **2019**, *104*, F182–F186. [CrossRef] [PubMed]
18. Khurana, S.; Kane, A.E.; Brown, S.E.; Tarver, T.; Dusing, S.C. Effect of neonatal therapy on the motor, cognitive, and behavioral development of infants born preterm: A systematic review. *Dev. Med. Child. Neurol.* **2020**, *62*, 684–692. [CrossRef] [PubMed]
19. McManus, B.M.; Richardson, Z.; Schenkman, M.; Murphy, N.; Morrato, E.H. Timing and Intensity of Early Intervention Service Use and Outcomes Among a Safety-Net Population of Children. *JAMA Netw. Open* **2019**, *2*, e187529. [CrossRef] [PubMed]
20. Nwabara, O.; Rogers, C.; Inder, T.; Pineda, R. Early therapy services following neonatal intensive care unit discharge. *Phys. Occup. Ther. Pediatr.* **2017**, *37*, 414–424. [CrossRef]
21. Wang, J.; Siddicky, S.F.; Johnson, T.; Kapil, N.; Majmudar, B.; Mannen, E.M. Supine lying center of pressure movement characteristics as a predictor of normal developmental stages in early infancy. *Technol. Health Care* **2022**, *30*, 43–49. [CrossRef]
22. Noble, Y.; Boyd, R. Neonatal assessments for the preterm infant up to 4 months corrected age: A systematic review. *Dev. Med. Child. Neurol.* **2012**, *54*, 129–139. [CrossRef] [PubMed]
23. Pineda, R.; McCarty, D.B.; Inder, T. Neurological and Neurobehavioral Evaluation. In *Neonatalology Questions and Controversies: Neurology (Neonatology: Questions & Controversies)*, 4th ed.; Perlman, J.M., Inder, T., Eds.; Elsevier: Amsterdam, The Netherlands, 2023.
24. Prosser, L.A.; Aguirre, M.O.; Zhao, S.; Bogen, D.K.; Pierce, S.R.; Nilan, K.A.; Zhang, H.; Shofer, F.S.; Johnson, M.J. Infants at risk for physical disability may be identified by measures of postural control in supine. *Pediatr. Res.* **2022**, *91*, 1215–1221. [CrossRef] [PubMed]
25. Lobo, M.A.; Hall, M.L.; Greenspan, B.; Rohloff, P.; Prosser, L.A.; Smith, B.A. Wearables for Pediatric Rehabilitation: How to Optimally Design and Use Products to Meet the Needs of Users. *Phys. Ther.* **2019**, *99*, 647–657. [CrossRef] [PubMed]
26. Panchal, J.; Sowande, O.F.; Prosser, L.; Johnson, M.J. Design of pediatric robot to simulate infant biomechanics for neurodevelopmental assessment in a sensorized gym. In Proceedings of the 2022 9th IEEE RAS/EMBS International Conference for Biomedical Robotics and Biomechatronics (BioRob), Seoul, Republic of Korea, 21–24 August 2022. [CrossRef]
27. Liberati, A.; Altman, D.G.; Tetzlaff, J.; Mulrow, C.; Gøtzsche, P.C.; Ioannidis, J.P.A.; Clarke, M.; Devereaux, P.J.; Kleijnen, J.; Moher, D. The PRISMA statement for reporting systematic reviews and meta-analyses of studies that evaluate healthcare interventions: Explanation and elaboration. *BMJ* **2009**, *339*, b2700. [CrossRef] [PubMed]
28. Open Science Framework. Can Center of Pressure Measurement PredictFuture Motor Impairment in Preterm Infants? A Systematic Review. *OSF* 2022. Available online: http://osf.io/28afw (accessed on 19 September 2023).
29. Veritas Health Innovation. *Covidence Systematic Review Software*; Veritas Health Innovation: Melbourne, Australia, 2023.
30. Rethlefsen, M.L.; Page, M.J. PRISMA 2020 and PRISMA-S: Common questions on tracking records and the flow diagram. *J. Med. Libr. Assoc.* **2022**, *110*, 253–257. [CrossRef]
31. Chapter 5: Collecting Data | Cochrane Training. Available online: https://training.cochrane.org/handbook/current/chapter-05 (accessed on 19 September 2023).
32. Sterne, J.A.C.; Savović, J.; Page, M.J.; Elbers, R.G.; Blencowe, N.S.; Boutron, I.; Cates, C.J.; Cheng, H.-Y.; Corbett, M.S.; Eldridge, S.M.; et al. RoB 2: A revised tool for assessing risk of bias in randomised trials. *BMJ* **2019**, *366*, l4898. [CrossRef]
33. Dusing, S.C. Postural variability and sensorimotor development in infancy. *Dev. Med. Child. Neurol.* **2016**, *58* (Suppl. 4), 17–21. [CrossRef] [PubMed]
34. Fallang, B.; Saugstad, O.D.; Grøgaard, J.; Hadders-Algra, M. Kinematic quality of reaching movements in preterm infants. *Pediatr. Res.* **2003**, *53*, 836–842. [CrossRef]
35. Fallang, B.; Øien, I.; Hellem, E.; Saugstad, O.D.; Hadders-Algra, M. Quality of reaching and postural control in young preterm infants is related to neuromotor outcome at 6 years. *Pediatr. Res.* **2005**, *58*, 347–353. [CrossRef]
36. Kniaziew-Gomoluch, K.; Szopa, A.; Łosień, T.; Siwiec, J.; Kidoń, Z.; Domagalska-Szopa, M. Reliability and repeatability of a postural control test for preterm infants. *Int. J. Environ. Res. Public Health* **2023**, *20*, 1868. [CrossRef] [PubMed]
37. Dusing, S.C.; Kyvelidou, A.; Mercer, V.S.; Stergiou, N. Infants born preterm exhibit different patterns of center-of-pressure movement than infants born at full term. *Phys. Ther.* **2009**, *89*, 1354–1362. [CrossRef] [PubMed]
38. Dusing, S.; Mercer, V.; Yu, B.; Reilly, M.; Thorpe, D. Trunk position in supine of infants born preterm and at term: An assessment using a computerized pressure mat. *Pediatr. Phys. Ther.* **2005**, *17*, 2–10. [CrossRef]
39. Dusing, S.C.; Izzo, T.; Thacker, L.R.; Galloway, J.C. Postural complexity influences development in infants born preterm with brain injury: Relating perception-action theory to 3 cases. *Phys. Ther.* **2014**, *94*, 1508–1516. [CrossRef]
40. Mehdizadeh, H.; Khalaf, K.; Ghomashchi, H.; Taghizadeh, G.; Ebrahimi, I.; Sharabiani, P.T.A.; Mousavi, S.J.; Parnianpour, M. Effects of cognitive load on the amount and temporal structure of postural sway variability in stroke survivors. *Exp. Brain Res.* **2018**, *236*, 285–296. [CrossRef] [PubMed]
41. State of New Mexico, New Mexico. Available online: https://newmexico.networkofcare.org/aging/assistive/detail.aspx?id=13393&cid=0&cn=&org=vista-medical-ltd (accessed on 16 May 2023).

42. Delgado-Bonal, A.; Marshak, A. Approximate entropy and sample entropy: A comprehensive tutorial. *Entropy* **2019**, *21*, 541. [CrossRef] [PubMed]
43. Biomechanics and Life Sciences I Kistler. Available online: http://www.kistler.com/INT/en/biomechanics-and-life-sciences/C00000187 (accessed on 19 September 2023).
44. McCarty, D.B.; Letzkus, L.; Attridge, E.; Dusing, S.C. Efficacy of Therapist Supported Interventions from the Neonatal Intensive Care Unit to Home: A Meta-Review of Systematic Reviews. *Clin. Perinatol.* **2023**, *50*, 157–178. [CrossRef]
45. Örtqvist, M.; Marschik, P.B.; Toldo, M.; Zhang, D.; Fajardo-Martinez, V.; Nielsen-Saines, K.; Ådén, U.; Einspieler, C. Reliability of the Motor Optimality Score-Revised: A study of infants at elevated likelihood for adverse neurological outcomes. *Acta Paediatr.* **2023**, *112*, 1259–1265. [CrossRef]
46. Kniaziew-Gomoluch, K.; Szopa, A.; Kidoń, Z.; Siwiec, A.; Domagalska-Szopa, M. Design and Construct Validity of a Postural Control Test for Pre-Term Infants. *Diagnostics* **2022**, *13*, 96. [CrossRef] [PubMed]

Disclaimer/Publisher's Note: The statements, opinions and data contained in all publications are solely those of the individual author(s) and contributor(s) and not of MDPI and/or the editor(s). MDPI and/or the editor(s) disclaim responsibility for any injury to people or property resulting from any ideas, methods, instructions or products referred to in the content.

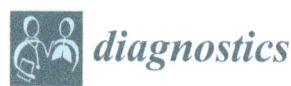 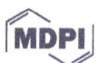

Systematic Review

The E-Textile for Biomedical Applications: A Systematic Review of Literature

Giuseppe Cesarelli [1,2,†], **Leandro Donisi** [2,3,†], **Armando Coccia** [2,4], **Federica Amitrano** [2,4,*], **Giovanni D'Addio** [2,‡] and **Carlo Ricciardi** [2,4,‡]

1. Department of Chemical, Materials and Production Engineering, University of Naples "Federico II", 80125 Naples, Italy; giuseppe.cesarelli@unina.it
2. Bioengineering Unit, Institute of Care and Scientific Research Maugeri, 82037 Pavia, Italy; leandro.donisi@unina.it (L.D.); armando.coccia@unina.it (A.C.); gianni.daddio@icsmaugeri.it (G.D.); carloricciardi.93@gmail.com (C.R.)
3. Department of Advanced Biomedical Sciences, University of Naples "Federico II", 80131 Naples, Italy
4. Department of Electrical Engineering and Information Technologies, University of Naples "Federico II", 80125 Naples, Italy
* Correspondence: federica.amitrano@unina.it
† These authors contributed equally to this work.
‡ These authors contributed equally to this work.

Abstract: The use of e-textile technologies spread out in the scientific research with several applications in both medical and nonmedical world. In particular, wearable technologies and miniature electronics devices were implemented and tested for medical research purposes. In this paper, a systematic review regarding the use of e-textile for clinical applications was conducted: the Scopus and Pubmed databases were investigate by considering research studies from 2010 to 2020. Overall, 262 papers were found, and 71 of them were included in the systematic review. Of the included studies, 63.4% focused on information and communication technology studies, while the other 36.6% focused on industrial bioengineering applications. Overall, 56.3% of the research was published as an article, while the remainder were conference papers. Papers included in the review were grouped by main aim into cardiological, muscular, physical medicine and orthopaedic, respiratory, and miscellaneous applications. The systematic review showed that there are several types of applications regarding e-textile in medicine and several devices were implemented as well; nevertheless, there is still a lack of validation studies on larger cohorts of subjects since the majority of the research only focuses on developing and testing the new device without considering a further extended validation.

Keywords: e-textile; health monitoring; diagnosis; wearable; biomedical engineering; sEMG; ECG; smart garments; motion analysis; IMUs

Citation: Cesarelli, G.; Donisi, L.; Coccia, A.; Amitrano, F.; D'Addio, G.; Ricciardi, C. The E-Textile for Biomedical Applications: A Systematic Review of Literature. *Diagnostics* **2021**, *11*, 2263. https://doi.org/10.3390/diagnostics11122263

Academic Editors: Markos G. Tsipouras and Ayman El-Baz

Received: 22 September 2021
Accepted: 29 November 2021
Published: 3 December 2021

Publisher's Note: MDPI stays neutral with regard to jurisdictional claims in published maps and institutional affiliations.

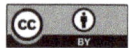

Copyright: © 2021 by the authors. Licensee MDPI, Basel, Switzerland. This article is an open access article distributed under the terms and conditions of the Creative Commons Attribution (CC BY) license (https://creativecommons.org/licenses/by/4.0/).

1. Introduction

Wearable technology includes devices that consumers can comfortably wear and use for extended periods of time in an unobtrusive way, like clothing or accessories, with the aim of collecting the data of users' personal health or, more generally, of interfacing with the user. The predominant category of wearable devices in the current market consists of, by far, smart accessories including smartwatches, wristbands, smart glasses, and various clothing clip-ons [1]. These accessories typically rely on existing miniature sensors and electronics enclosed in compact items that can be worn. However, their structure makes them rigid and nonflexible and, consequently, not ideal for the development of more advanced wearable systems that need larger contact and interface with user's body. The integration of micro- and nano-electronics in textile substrates can be relevant for the development of more ergonomic smart materials, which are broadly known as electronic textiles (e-textiles). Through e-textile technology, a wide spectrum of functions, found in rigid and nonflexible electronic products nowadays, can be potentially developed on a textile substrate [2].

This attractive opportunity aroused a great deal of interest in wearable e-textile devices. The market of wearable technologies has a compound annual growth rate of 15.5%, which is expected to further continue thanks to the rapid improvements in technology and miniature devices, as well as mobile computing. In a recent market forecast the industry of wearable devices is estimated to grow to more than $US155 billion by 2027 [3], with the involvement of many big companies which are multiplying their research efforts to shift from the wearable electronic hardware to the more comfortable e-textiles.

The growing demand from consumers is encouraging manufacturers to produce and sell billions of wearable electronic products, covering various sectors of the market, including health and wellness, military and defense, space exploration, fashion, and entertainment. Healthcare is identified as one of the most promising market, piloted by the increasing desire of consumers to continually monitor their own health and by the interest of healthcare professionals to have more health data at their disposal to better examine a larger cohort of patients.

The comfort, ease-of-use, and ubiquity offered by smart biomedical clothes potentially represent key factors for the continuous long-term clinical monitoring. The integration of these innovative devices in Internet of Things (IoT) networks, exploiting simple but efficient wireless solutions, makes it possible to establish smart systems for remote health monitoring, allowing patients to continue to stay at home rather than in expensive healthcare facilities. One of the main purposes of a wearable health monitoring system is to ensure continuous, noninvasive, and seamless surveillance of health and physical well-being, enabling people to lead independent and active lives in their familiar home environment [4]. This is a great advantage especially for patients with chronic diseases and/or with mobility difficulties. The use of wearable monitoring systems underlines two other benefits for users: firstly, it reduces the influence and stress that the clinical environment exerts on patient's performance [5]; secondly, the great amount of data gathered with this system can be processed using Artificial Intelligence (AI) algorithms to detect a possible worsening of a patient's clinical situation [6].

From the public health system perspectives, the development of smart wearable biomedical systems has the potential to offer advanced services to patients, combining the frequently worn material with the most technologically advanced, sensing, processing and communicating capabilities [7], and, at the same time, to support health cost reduction by facilitating early hospital discharges. Nevertheless, the great perspectives illustrated clash with the technological limitations that hinder the large-scale production and diffusion of market-ready garments or textiles. These technological challenges justify the remarkable research efforts, which are evidenced by the large number of research prototypes and innovative solutions proposed in the scientific literature.

The main issues to be addressed in the design and fabrication of e-textile systems concern breathability, flexibility, and "washability", which are fundamental features for comfortable user experience and must be maintained even after integration of the electronic components. Power supply is also a very critical challenge for e-textile devices. Common rechargeable batteries are usually used, though they increase the weight of the devices and are incompatible with the flexibility and washing requirements of textile integration. To overcome these limitations, different functional materials were designed to have different features and approach the goal of self-powered textiles [8]. However, technological innovations should be implemented while ensuring a safe degree of reliability for device performances in comparison with the standard methods commonly used in clinical environment [9].

In addition to technological problems, regulatory issues regarding patient safety, privacy, and data management also represent obstacles to the large commercial diffusion of e-textiles [10,11]. More efforts are needed to develop algorithms to ensure highly secured communication channels in existing low-power, short-range wireless platforms [4].

In summary, it is undeniable that the development of smart textiles requires a multidisciplinary approach in which knowledge and skills in both industrial sciences—e.g., chemistry, design, and fabrication of smart materials—and Information and Communication Technologies (ICT)—e.g., microelectronics and circuit design and fabrication—are fundamentally integrated with a deep understanding of textile arts [2]. Therefore, this review explores the progress in smart e–textiles design and manufacturing, with a focus on biomedical sensors and devices developed for healthcare monitoring. The main aim is to provide a complete overview of the state-of-the-art in this promising area, investigating the various applications and the different approaches and solutions proposed by research groups working on these themes. Indeed, to the best of authors' knowledge, this is the first systematic review summarizing the research on e-textile for medical applications. Therefore, the choice will be to apply broad criteria for the papers to perform a wider selection and include as many types of papers as possible.

2. Materials and Methods

The query was conducted on Scopus and Pubmed databases starting from 2010 until 2020 using the words "e-textile", "textronics", "textile-electronics" and "monitoring"; 262 articles were found in this time range (23 of them were duplicated). Only English articles were considered, and reviews, conference reviews, book chapters, and books were excluded, thereby reaching 208 papers. Afterwards, all the papers were screened firstly through title and abstract, and then through full text, reaching 71 papers, which were included in this systematic review. Figure 1 shows the whole workflow.

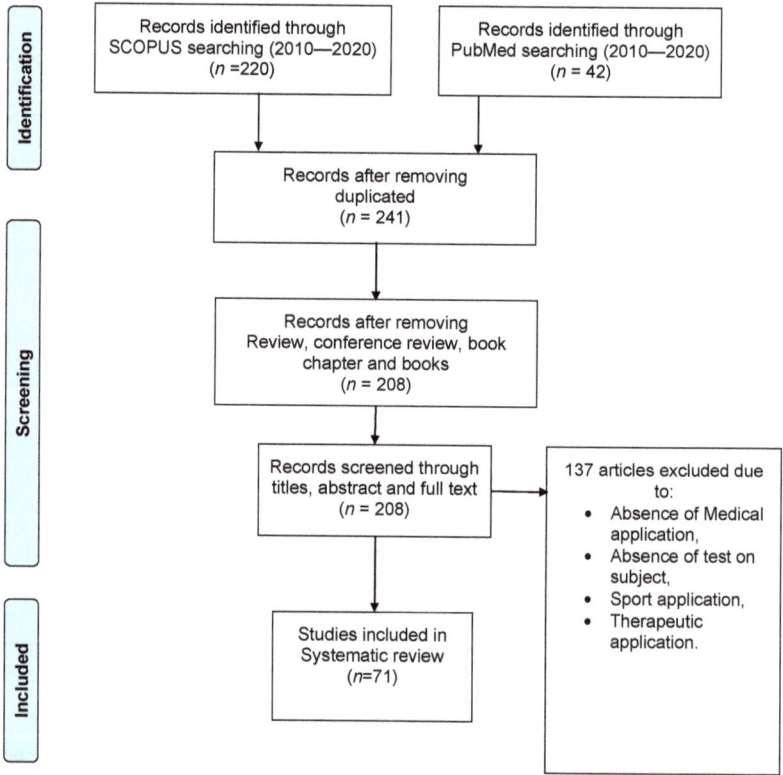

Figure 1. Flow chart for selecting papers from Scopus and Pubmed databases.

The articles were categorized into conference papers and articles, Industrial Bioengineering (IB), and ICT domains. Figure 2 depicts the proportions.

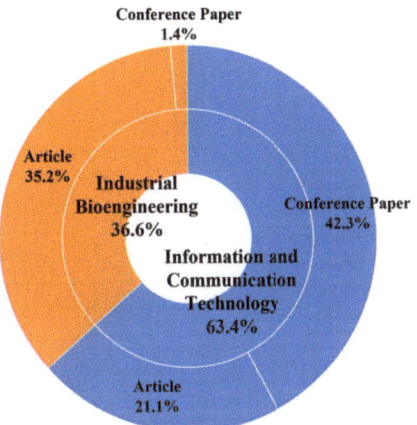

Figure 2. Distribution of papers according to ICT and IB categories, conference papers, and articles.

3. Results

In Table 1 references to the articles included in this review are grouped according to the type of acquired data. The researches are also organized in macro-categories regarding the biomedical field of potential diagnosis. In Table S1 the readers can find more accurate insights regarding each of the articles briefly discussed in the next subsections, where, differently, we propose at the end of each subsection summary tables highlighting, in the first instance, "Aim", "Dataset" and "Acquired data" for each of the articles investigated.

Table 1. Number of instances for each acquired data, data type, and potential diagnosis combined with related references.

Biomedical Field	Acquired Data	Instances
Cardiac	ECG	21 [12–32]
	Heart rate	3 [24,25,33]
	Blood pulse	7 [27,34–39]
	LEVOP	1 [40]
Muscular	EMG	10 [16,19,21,41–47]
	Pressure signal from muscles	1 [48]
Physiatry/Orthopaedics	Finger flexion angles	4 [37,49–51]
	Acceleration data	4 [30,52–54]
	Angle of inclination	2 [24,25]
	Motion signals	6 [19,21,34,55–57]
	Elbow flexion angles	2 [58,59]
	Knee flexion angle	3 [51,58,60]
	Scapular flexion angles	1 [60]
	Angular velocity signal	1 [61]
	Plantar pressures	1 [61]
	Sleep posture	1 [41]
	FS and LL indexes	1 [62]
	Back movements	1 [63]
	Spinal cord bending angles	1 [38]
	Strain signals	4 [53,54,64,65]

Table 1. Cont.

Biomedical Field	Acquired Data	Instances
Respiratory	Respiratory rate	7 [15,30,41,66–69]
	Breath pressure	2 [48,70]
	Breath signal	6 [32,35,36,38,39,71]
Other Themes	EOG	3 [72–74]
	EDA	4 [14,16,75,76]
	Skin temperature	8 [15,24,25,30,35,36,77,78]
	Biomedical microwave sensing	1 [79]
	Pharynx motion	2 [37,49]
	Cheek motion	1 [37]
	Sodium and lactate concentration in human sweat	1 [80]
	Sweat Volume	2 [59,78]
	Resistance signals	1 [81]
	Alert of the volume of leaked urine	1 [82]
	Hydrogen peroxide concentration	1 [32]

Abbreviations. ECG: Electrocardiogram; EDA: Electrodermal Activity; EMG: Electromyography; EOG: Electrooculography; FS: Forward Shift; LEVOP: Lower Extremity Venous Occlusion Plethysmography; LL: Lateral Lean.

3.1. The Applications in Cardiology

The first line of Table 1 summarized in a concise and schematic form the principal acquired data—in the field of cardiology diagnostics—using e-textile systems.

The electrocardiography signal—called equivalently electrocardiogram (ECG)—was over the years one of the most appropriate tools to diagnose in advance and, consequently, to try to prevent the clinical complications caused by chronic and cardiovascular diseases [83,84]; in recent years, wearable sensors proved to be possible novel alternatives for the ECG acquisition [9], because the e-textiles (used as ECG diagnostic systems) indicated to address—or potentially address—several of the advantages highlighted in Section 1 [83].

The researches in this field are summarized in Table 2. In this 10-year report of papers, the first prototype of ECG e-textile system was presented by Wu et al. [23]. The authors fabricated a cloth electrode into which multiwalled carbon nano-tubes (MWCNTs) were randomly distributed into the fabric, of which one side was connected and fastened with traditional silver/silver chloride (Ag/AgCl) electrodes. The ECG acquisition performed on a single healthy control (HC) demonstrated the novel cloth electrode showed similar performances to the traditional Ag/AgCl electrodes, which might be potentially replaced for the daily and long-term monitoring of the ECG [23]. Similar studies were performed by Acar and Le and the respective coworkers [20,22], which also tested the e-textiles by applying the electrodes on smart garments. In particular, Acar et al. fabricated nylon graphene oxide (GO)-coated fibers, which were later embedded in an elastic armband; the evaluations on a single HC showed a 96% correlation between the ECG waveforms acquired with graphene textile electrodes and the conventional Ag/AgCl ones [22]. More accurate statistical data, on the other hand, were presented by Le et al. to compare the performances of silver-based textile electrodes (embedded in a smart bra) and Ag/AgCl gel counterparts [20]. A similar bra was designed and fabricated by Shathi et al. [27] which proved their reduced GO/poly(3,4-ethyelenedioxythiophne polystyrene sulfonate) (PEDOT:PSS) electrodes showed an improved ECG signal response in both wet and dry conditions; additionally, their e-textile electrodes demonstrated an improved flexibility, bendability, and stretchability when compared with that of conventional electrodes. The manufactured ones—integrated in the sports bra—were the final product of a fabrication study in which even other kinds of e-textile electrodes were analyzed [26]. Sinha et al. [16] fabricated and analyzed in the same period similar PEDOT:PSS-coated electrodes, demonstrating the capability of such devices to record ECG—and, in addition, electrodermal activity (EDA) and electromyography (EMG)—for a single HC in both dry and wet conditions.

Another interesting approach to fabricate e-textiles for ECG monitoring was proposed by Li et al. [18]. The authors designed and fabricated an e-textile solution combining the advantages of both the Japanese Kirigami pattering and the inkjet printing strategy demonstrating an ECG stable signal acquisition on a single HC with more than 100% strain of electrodes. Micro/nano fabrication strategies could be considered as a potential solution even for the fabrication of electrical interconnects/stretchable conductive adhesives (SCA). Specifically, a mixture, composed by Ag particles, MWCNTs and silicone rubber, was prepared and SCA electrodes were fabricated depositing such mixture on a polydimethylsiloxane (PDMS) layer, later integrated with a same layer deposited onto an elastic bandage [31]. From the outcomes of the investigations, the authors showed the ECG signal resulted both of good quality and thoroughly stable both for multiple patients' configurations (even after the SCA-equipped elastic bandage was washed) if compared with the results obtained with commercial counterparts. Liang et al. [32] recently presented the preliminary results of a similar research. Specifically, they worked to develop a stable and biocompatible composite ink—a dispersion of silk sericine-MWCNTs—which could be processed using well-consolidated printing processes (e.g., inkjet printing). The authors demonstrated the ink could be used, even though a straightforward dying process, to fabricate conductive fibers/yarns and textiles "with desired mechanoelectrical properties" [32]. The integration of such conductive textiles (even breathable and reusable) on a compression shirt allowed to collect fine structures of the ECG signals in dry state, demonstrating the potential applicability of these smart clothes in healthcare (i.e., monitoring human biosignals). Another solution based on micro/nanofabrication strategies was proposed by Yao et al. [19] who manufactured silver nanowire/thermoplastic polyurethane (AgNW/TPU) electrodes to be later integrated on commercial patches. The authors demonstrated these devices were capable to acquire EGC—in dry state—of a quality comparable to the commercial gel electrodes; moreover, they did not find signal degradation up to 50% strain and 100 cycles. As shown in Table 2, in addition to ECG, even EMG and body motion signals were collected. Similar signals were analyzed even by Jin et al. [21] who used an e-textile sportswear in which an EMG sensor, a strain sensor, and a fluoroelastomer conductor, reinforced with polyvinylidene fluoride (PVDF) nanofibers, were integrated. The system showed the possibility to acquire ECG signal, and even the others, without significant degradation during a 1 h exercise of an HC.

In the last few years, although the research on ECG monitoring in the field of wearable e-textiles seems still in a preliminary stage, few authors tried to develop slightly more complex e-textile solutions. For instance, in 2013 Kuroda et al. [13] proposed two prototypes of e-textile sensing vests, where different combinations of conductive and nonconductive yarns were investigated. The first prototype demonstrated the Japanese NISHIJIN production process was suitable to acquire a clean ECG signal as well as the second more advanced prototype (albeit fabricated—for an eventual mass production—using a different manufacturing technique), although some limitations in the ECG acquisition appeared [13]. In the same period, Catarino et al. [12] investigated the capabilities of a novel shirt prototype; specifically, three electrodes were knitted with Elitex for a double purpose: firstly, to allow the integration of electrical connections in the textile substrate, and secondly, to fix the electrodes in specific areas of the shirt prototype. Even if the ECG signals demonstrated different in case of either dry or wet electrodes, the authors claimed the results were of acceptable quality (considering conventional gel electrodes performances) and a tailor-made design of the shirt (according to the target patient) could potentially maximize the ECG acquisition performance [12]. Similar findings were presented even by Zięba et al. [29]. The authors showed a custom-made laminar textile electrode made of a silver woven fabric to be potentially integrated in a shirt and a sock, following predesigned configurations. The authors demonstrated (on a single HC) that the electroconductive material showed negligible difference with conventional electrodes and could be effectively used to potentially fabricate e-textile integrated shirts and/or socks. More recently, Tao et al. [30] integrated on a flexible printed circuit board (later, in turn, integrated on a sportswear shirt) an EGC sensor, connected, in turn, to a textile electrode by conductive threads. The authors validated the system demonstrating the effective ECG acquisition, even after 30 washing cycles when the print circuit board was integrated on a sportswear fabric using 4 mm thick PDMS.

The literature on e-textile applications for ECG acquisition showed even approaches for which the signal acquisition was only one of the milestones. For instance, Lopez et al. [24,25] designed and presented a medical Information Technology (IT) platform—based on multiple subsystems—for patients' localization and monitoring. The authors proposed as a healthcare monitoring subsystem for ECG acquisition a Nylon/Lycra shirt into which two e-textile electrodes were integrated. The results—after acquiring ECG on 5 patients with cardiological diseases—showed ECG was of a higher quality (also in dry state) when the subjects were still, while the signal slightly worsened when sudden movements took place. However, the authors demonstrated the use of a conductive gel and/or mechanisms to reduce motion artifacts could improve signal quality [24]. Similar conclusions were presented further in their more recent article [25]. Similarly, Ferreira et al. [15] designed and presented the Baby Night Watch IT platform to monitor infants potentially affected by Sudden Infant Death Syndrome. In this study, a chest belt, into which electrodes and silver coated polyamide yarns were integrated, was chosen as healthcare monitoring subsystem, demonstrating a comparable performance with counterpart commercial products in terms of ECG measurements. In particular, both the custom-made and the commercial chest belts demonstrated capable to acquire very robust heart rate pulses when infants did not move and were lying on their back, while the authors found several missing heart beat pulses when infants were more active.

Finally, a few research groups also performed experiments on a relatively significant number of subjects (if compared to the already cited contributions). For instance, Postolache et al. [14] presented a wheelchair prototype where e-textiles, namely, electrodes made of fibers coated by conductive polymer and silver, were integrated in correspondence of the armrests. The data acquired by 7 HC demonstrated the proposed platform showed results comparable to that of the commercial counterparts. A similar number of HC were object of ECG acquisitions in the study of Arquilla et al. [28]. The authors manufactured a set of three electrodes—made of nylon coated by silver nanoparticles—stitched on a nonextensive fabric backing. Two minutes of ECG acquisitions on 8 HC demonstrated once again the capabilities of e-textile electrodes, showing their potential applicability across a wide range of anthropometries and skin types and signal invariance during stretch, bend, or wash tests. The most important diagnostic example, however, was such proposed by Fouassier et al. [17]. Specifically, the authors designed and manufactured a t-shirt prototype—into which electrodes made of silver yarns and hydrogel pads were integrated—aimed at working as a 12-lead ECG acquisition system. This solution allowed, to the best of the authors' knowledge, short-duration 12-lead ECG acquisitions with quality levels comparable to conventional Holter recordings on 30 HC for 4 different analyzed positions.

Often, in the context of cardiac field, diagnostic data can be acquired also using simpler and/or different strategies. For instance, Lopez et al. [24,25] were also able to acquire simultaneously and show (on their IT platform) the hearth rate from 5 patients with cardiological diseases, using the same shirt used for ECG acquisition. Later, Dabby et al. [33] showed similar conclusions using another e-textile prototype; specifically, they demonstrated their e-textile solutions (bras, shirts, and shorts) demonstrated capable to acquire a heart rate signal comparable to a commercial chest strap. Equivalently, even Tao et al. [30] solution demonstrated capable to monitor the heart rate (calculated from the RR interval data of ECG signal).

Blood pulse, namely, pulse rate, is another potential diagnostic data that e-textiles can collect from patients. The first examples presented in this 10-year report of papers are those showed by Frydrysiak et al. [35,36]. The authors, partially inspired by their previous study [29], presented a solution to acquire the pulse signal from elderly people using a shirt into which the textile electrodes were integrated by different configurations. Analogously to Lopez et al. and Ferreira et al., the pulse acquisition was only one of the milestones of the presented textronics system, whose aim was even to collect other data (e.g., patients' breathing rhythm) which are made available in real time for a potentially advanced subject monitoring. Quite recently, the research on blood pulse monitoring has gained increasing importance, as testified by the growing number of contributions appeared in the literature. For instance, Jang et al. [38] developed a composite fiber sensor which was later sewed in an electric armband applied, in turn, on an artificial arm with varied blood pressures. The experiment on this artificial setup demonstrated the system was capable to distinguish rachial artery pulses with varying blood pressure and pulse rate. Another recent solution was described in [37]. The authors presented a three-dimensional, composite spacer textile pressure/strain sensor, mainly designed for human motion detection purposes, which could even be used to monitor the arterial pulse pressure when the system was attached to one of the wrists of HCs. The results suggest the device could detect different pulse trends, which are linked to different pathologies and/or complications related to behavioral risk factors. Similar measurements were carried out by Shathi et al. [27], who acquired the pulse rate of a single HC demonstrating their e-textile electrode, in direct contact with the female volunteer's wrist, showed a pulse response in nearly accordance with normal kits; some deflections/distortions in pulse rate were found during running. Similar results were presented even by Fan et al. [39]. They proposed a triboelectric all-textile sensor array (TATSA), a composite textile made of stainless steel fibers inserted into several pieces of one-ply Terylene yarns, which was conveniently embedded into several clothes such as wristbands, fingerstalls, socks, and chest straps. The TATSA proved not only to acquire a good quality, namely, in line with the signals acquired with other devices and solutions, pulse rate, but even the possibility to acquire and highlight differences in pulses depending on the measuring position (the authors applied TATSA on neck, wrist, fingertip, and ankle) and subjects' ages, demonstrating the straightforward applicability of the solution to different populations. Simultaneously, Tang et al. [34] designed and manufactured a nonwoven fabric e-textile prototype, which demonstrated capable to effectively monitor blood pulse. Finally, in recent years, to the authors' best knowledge, the last diagnostic solution in the field of cardiology, by means of e-textiles, was oriented to record lower extremity venous occlusion plethysmography (LEVOP). To this aim, Goy et al. [40] developed and fabricated a custom-made battery powered plethysmograph, connected on the one side to an oscilloscope, and on the other side on a set of different e-textile electrodes. The authors conducted LEVOP recordings on 5 HC demonstrating all the three set of the proposed e-textiles materials can be used for LEVOP recordings, showing additionally a statistical in-depth analysis related to the recorded signals from the different materials.

In conclusion, from the systematic analysis conducted, it was demonstrated the design and fabrication of e-textile solutions for biomedical applications gained considerable attention in recent years, and the promising results suggest a potential interest in further research. Maybe, to obtain a definitive answer regarding the direct practical applicability of these e-textile solutions, more studies involving larger cohort of subjects (healthy and pathological) are still required. However, as readers can ascertain reading the next subsections, currently this field seems to be the most advanced in this sense.

Table 2. Insights regarding cardiac literature: authors, aim, dataset, and acquired data.

Authors	Aim	Dataset	Acquired Data
Lopez et al. (2010a) [24]	Describing a novel healthcare IT platform for localization and monitoring within hospital environments	5 PP	ECG; Heart rate; Angle of inclination; Activity index; Body temperature; Patient's location; Battery level; Alert code
Lopez et al. (2010b) [25]	Presenting a medical IT platform platform based on Wireless Sensor Networks and e-textile for patients' localization and monitoring	5 PP	ECG; Heart rate; Angle of inclination; Activity index; Body temperature; Patient's location; Battery level; Alert code
Wu et al. (2010) [23]	Presenting a novel cloth electrode for ECG monitoring	1 HC	ECG
Zieba et al. (2011) [29]	Creating new sensorical clothing structures to measure human physiological signals in a non-invasive way	1 HC	ECG
Catarino et al. (2012) [12]	Designing and fabricating textile integrated electrodes for ECG continuous health monitoring for disabled or elderly people	1 HC	ECG
Kuroda et al. (2013) [13]	Prototyping an ECG sensing e-textile vest	1 HC	ECG
Goy et al. (2013) [40]	Fabricating e-textiles to monitor LEVOP	5 HC	LEVOP
Postolache et al. (2014) [14]	Presenting a wheelchair architecture equipped with e-textiles for ECG and SKC sensing	7 HC	ECG; EDA
Ferreira et al. (2016) [15]	Presenting the design and fabrication of SWSs to prevent infants' SIDS	HC [#]	Body temperature; Respiratory rate; ECG
Frydisiak & Tesiorowski (2016a) [35]	Designing a smart textronic shirts for the health monitoring of elderly people	HC [#]	Blood Pulse; Breath Signal; Skin Temperature
Frydisiak & Tesiorowski (2016b) [36]	Designing a smart textronic shirts for the health monitoring of elderly people	HC [#]	Blood Pulse; Breath Signal; Skin Temperature
Dabby et al. (2017) [33]	Presenting a new method for building wearable electronic and textile sensor systems directly integrated in garments to detect the heart rate	1 HC	Heart Rate
Acar et al. (2018) [22]	Developing a single-arm ECG armband embedded with flexible graphene textiles for ECG data acquisition	1 HC	ECG
Tao et al. (2018) [30]	Presenting a novel system—made up of a washable and wearable smart textile shirt, smartphone app and software desktop—for the acquisition of ECG signal, breathing rate, acceleration data for activity recognition and skin temperature	5 HC [ML] HC [#]	ECG; Skin temperature; Respiratory rate; Acceleration data
Li et al. (2019) [18]	Fabricating e-textiles depositing conducting materials thorough inkjet printing on conventional textiles for monitoring purposes	1 HC	ECG
Yao et al. (2019) [19]	Designing and fabricating multifunctional e-textiles with mechanical and functional properties comparable with typical textiles for monitoring applications	1 HC	ECG; EMG (arm); Motion signals
Le et al. (2019) [20]	Comparing differences in ECG registration between silver-based textile electrodes and silver/silver-chloride gel electrodes, both integrated in a smart bra	1 HC	ECG
Jin et al. (2019) [21]	Fabricating a metal–elastomer–nanofibers conductive material for long-term monitoring	1 HC	ECG; EMG (bicep muscle); Motion signals

Table 2. *Cont.*

Authors	Aim	Dataset	Acquired Data
Kim et al. (2019) [37]	Developing an all-textile based pressure/strain sensor for physiological signals using 3D spacer textile	HC #	Blood Pulse (wrist and neck); Finger flexion angles; Cheek motion; Pharynx motion
Ko et al. (2019) [31]	Designing SCAs for various applications	1 HC	ECG
Jang et al. (2019) [38]	Preparing a highly sensitive fiber-type strain sensor with a broad range of strain by introducing a single active layer onto the fiber	1 HC	Blood Pulse; Spinal Cord Bending Angles; Breath Signal
Fouassier et al. (2019) [17]	Comparing the quality of the ECG signal registered using both a 12-lead Holter and a novel smart 12-lead ECG acquisition T-shirt	30 HC	ECG
Sinha et al. (2020) [16]	Fabricating PEDOT:PSS coated electrodes to record EMG, ECG and EDA	4 HC ^{emg} 1 HC ^{eda} 1 HC ^{ecg}	EDA; ECG; EMG (biceps, triceps, tibialis, and quadriceps)
Tang et al. (2020) [34]	Fabricating machine-washable e-textiles with high strain sensitivity and high thermal conduction for monitoring applications	1 HC	Motion signals; Blood pulse
Arquilla et al. (2020) [28]	Using sewn textile electrodes for ECG monitoring	8 HC	ECG
Shathi et al. (2020a) [26]	Presenting a highly flexible and wearable e-textile for smart clothing and ECG detection	1 HC	ECG
Shathi et al. (2020b) [27]	Developing e-textile electrodes for the detection of high-quality biomedical signals	1 HC	ECG; Blood pulse
Liang et al. (2020) [32]	Developing a stable and biocompatible silk sericine carbon nanotubes (CNT) ink and demonstrating its versatile applications in flexible electronics for monitoring human biosignals	HC #	ECG, Breath Signal; Hydrogen peroxide concentration
Fan et al. (2020) [39]	Developing TATSA for precise epidermal physiological signal monitoring	1 HC 1 PP	Blood Pulse; Breath Signal

number of subjects not provided; ^{ecg}: Electrocardiographic acquisitions; ^{eda}: Electrodermal Activity acquisitions; ^{emg}: Electromyographic acquisitions; ^{ML}: Machine Learning training set. **Abbreviations**. ECG: Electrocardiogram; EDA: Electrodermal Activity; EMG: Electromyography; HC: Healthy Controls; IT: Information Technology; LEVOP: Lower Extremity Venous Occlusion Plethysmography; PEDOT:PSS: Poly(3,4-Ethylenedioxythiophne) Polystyrene Sulfonate); PP: Pathological Patients; SCAs: Stretchable Conductive Adhesives; SIDS: Sudden Infant Death Syndrome; SKC: Skin Conductivity; TATSA: Triboelectric All-Textile Sensor Array; SWSs: Smart Wearable Systems.

3.2. The Applications in the Muscular Setting

Surface Electromyography (sEMG) is a noninvasive methodology to measure muscle activity using surface electrodes placed on the skin overlying a muscle or a group of muscles [85]. This technique is widely used in rehabilitation research, sport sciences, kinesiology, and ergonomics [86]. Electrodes for sEMG are mostly combined with electrode gel to reduce the electrode-skin impedance [87]. Nevertheless, in recent decades, e-textile sensors, fabrics which are given sensing properties of different physical nature, such as capacitive, resistive, optical and solar, are increasingly spreading due to their wearable nature [88]. The researches in this field are summarized in Table 3. Ozturk and Yapici [43] proposed wearable graphene textile electrodes to monitor muscular activity showing their feasibility to acquire sEMG signals. They performed a benchmarking study with wet Ag/AgCl electrodes showing good agreement between the two technologies of electrodes in terms of signal-to-noise ratio (SNR) and signal morphology with correlation values up to 97% for sEMG signals acquired from the biceps brachii muscle. The same authors, in line with the previous conference paper [43], presented a research article [42] in which they underlined deeply the use of graphene-coated fabrics as textile electrodes in sEMG acquisition, considering not only the biceps brachii muscle but also triceps brachii and quadriceps femoris muscles. They performed a benchmarking study between the proposed textile electrodes and commercial wet Ag/AgCl ones for each muscle in terms of the skin-electrode impedance (SEI), SNR, and cross correlation reaching results within the range of commercial Ag/AgCl electrodes. The results demonstrated that graphene-coated textile fabrics could represent a valid alternative to gelled Ag/AgCl electrodes and therefore they could be used to develop wearable and smart garments. A similar work was conducted by Awan et al. [44] who investigated the use of a graphene-based electromyograph fabric sensor as a comparable alternative to commercial Ag/AgCl wet electrodes. The authors demonstrated that textile electrodes outperformed the standard Ag/AgCl electrodes in terms of SNR. Additionally, they, after tests on 8 HC, underlined graphene-based smart fabrics can potentially represent a viable alternative to non-reusable Ag/AgCl electrodes for high-quality EMG monitoring. Other authors proposed wearable devices to monitor EMG signals through textile electrodes; as first example, Nijima et al. [46] proposed a wearable EMG sensor for monitoring masticatory muscles with PEDOT:PSS textile electrodes with the aim to monitor daily activities such as diet, sleep bruxism, and human motor control. The same authors in a more recent work [45] used the above-mentioned prototype to monitor muscle fatigue related to the muscles of the limbs, starting from the acquisition of temporal muscles, based on the assumption that there is a strong correlation between frowning and jaw clenching muscle activity and the physical efforts made when exercising. Choudhry et al. [48] designed textile-based piezoresistive sensors developed using flexible conductive threads stitched on fabric. They embedded the sensor inside a garment to measure small pressure changes exerted by human muscles. Other authors proposed multifunctional e-textiles to monitor several vital signals, EMG signals included. As described in Section 3.1, Yao et al. [19] developed an integrated textile patch comprising four dry electrophysiological electrodes, a capacitive strain sensor, and a wireless heater for electrophysiological monitoring, motion tracking, and thermotherapy, respectively. Jin et al. [21] showed their solution demonstrated its feasibility for continuous long-term monitoring of ECG, EMG signal and motion during 1 h of weight-lifting excercises without significant degradation of signal quality. As third example, Sinha et al. [16] showed how PEDOT:PSS coated electrodes, integrated in a spandex t-shirt, were effectively able to record simultaneously EMG, ECG, and EDA in dry state. The authors concluded this solution could represent a tool for continuous and simultaneous measurement of vital signals in at-risk patients. Samy et al. [41] employed five EMG electrodes: three were attached to subject's chin to detect its muscle movement, which can be indicative of teeth grinding (bruxism), sleep apnea, and other sleep disorders, while the other two electrodes were attached to the legs, between the knee and the ankle, to record leg movement. Finally, Farina et al. [47] proposed the use of Smart Fabric and Interactive Textile system as an alternative solution for recording high-density EMG signals for myoelectric control. They designed a sleeve covering the upper and lower arm containing 100 electrodes arranged in four grids of 5×5 electrodes for EMG. The textile electrodes were realized with stainless steel yarns and they had a diameter of 10 mm and an interelectrode distance of 20 mm. The proposed method for interfacing myoelectric prostheses with the neuromuscular system by integrating electrodes in garments proved its feasibility, allowing for high accuracy in EMG classification.

From the analysis carried out on this topic it is possible to conclude that several technologies and materials were proposed for the realization of electrodes in e-textile able to acquire EMG signals. Future investigation on enriched study population both normal and pathological will confirm the potential the utility of textile electrodes in clinical practice to replace well-known pregelled electrodes.

Table 3. Insights regarding literature in muscular setting: authors, aim, dataset, and acquired data.

Authors	Aim	Dataset	Acquired Data
Farina et al. (2010) [47]	Proposing a novel way for interfacing myoelectric prostheses with the neuromuscular system by integrating electrodes in garments	3 HC	EMG
Samy et al. (2014) [41]	Performing sleep stage analysis with a contact-free unobtrusive system	7 HC	Respiratory rate and its variability; Leg EMG from pressure images; Sleep posture
Niijima et al. (2017) [46]	Designing and fabricating an EMG-integrated sensors cap to register EMG data of the masticatory muscles for monitoring ADL	1 HC [1] 3 HC [2]	EMG (temporal muscles)
Niijima et al. (2018) [45]	Assessing the feasibility of estimating biceps fatigue using an e-textile headband	10 HC	EMG (temporal muscles)
Ozturk & Yapici (2019) [43]	Studying the performance of graphene textiles in muscular activity monitoring (acquisition of surface EMG signals from biceps brachii muscle), comparing the outcome with Ag/AgCl electrodes	1 HC	EMG (biceps brachii)
Awan et al. (2019) [44]	Presenting the fabrication of graphene-based e-textile for EMG monitoring, comparing sensing performance with commercial Ag/AgCl wet electrodes	8 HC	EMG (arm)
Yao et al. (2019) [19]	Designing and fabricating multifunctional e-textiles with mechanical and functional properties comparable with typical textiles for monitoring applications	1 HC	ECG; EMG (arm); Motion signals
Jin et al. (2019) [21]	Fabricating a metal—elastomer—nanofibers conductive material for long-term monitoring	1 HC	ECG; EMG (bicep muscle); Motion signals
Choudhry et al. (2020) [48]	Fabricating piezoresistive sensors—and studying their washability—to monitor breathing and muscular activity	1 HC	Breath pressure signal of the ribcage; Pressure signal from biceps femoris muscle
Sinha et al. (2020) [16]	Fabricating PEDOT:PSS coated electrodes to record EMG, ECG and EDA	4 HC [emg] 1 HC [eda] 1 HC [ecg]	EDA; ECG; EMG (biceps, triceps, tibialis, and quadriceps)
Ozturk & Yapici (2020) [42]	Investigating the performance of conductive graphene textiles as surface EMG electrodes, later integrated in textile electrodes as pedometer	4 HC	sEMG

[1] experiment 1; [2] experiment 2; [ecg]: Electrocardiographic acquisitions; [eda]: Electrodermal Activity acquisitions; [emg]: Electromyographic acquisitions. **Abbreviations**. ADL: Activities of Daily Living; ECG: Electrocardiogram; EDA: Electrodermal Activity; EMG: Electromyography; HC: Healthy Controls; PEDOT:PSS: Poly(3,4-Ethyelenedioxythiophne) Polystyrene Sulfonate).

3.3. The Applications in Orthopaedics

Recently, the development and the spread of Inertial Measurement Units (IMUs) for spatiotemporal and kinematic assessment has represented an innovative progress in the field of biomechanics and wearable sensors. Indeed, wearable sensors based on IMUs are spreading in the biomedical field showing good performances [89–91] compared to their gold standards. Moreover, considering that the working principle of IMUs is based on the measurement of inertia, IMUs can be applied anywhere without a reference [92] and integrated with textile technology [93]. The research in this field is summarized in Table 4. Bartalesi et al. [53], indeed, developed a wearable system that integrates and fuses information gathered from textile-based piezoresistive sensor arrays and triaxial accelerometers, which demonstrated able to perform a real time estimation of the local curvature and the length of the spine lumbar arch. The authors performed a comparative study between their system and a stereophotogrammetric system, showing a very low error when reconstructing the lumbar arch length of a single HC. Considering the same idea (namely, merging several technologies), Li et al. [58] presented a method to integrate and package a triaxial accelerometer within a textile as to create an e-textile fully integrated within the weave structure of the fabric itself, making it invisible to the wearer. The integrated e-textile based accelerometer sensor system placed on arm and knee joints was used to identify the activity type, such as walking or running, through the calculation of the joint bending angles. They performed a benchmarking analysis between the proposed device and the related gold standard, showing good agreement with an error lower than 1%. Amitrano et al. [61] proposed a new wearable e-textile based system for biomedical signals remote monitoring able to acquire angular velocities of the lower limbs. Specifically, the system equips an IMU and textile pressure sensors made of EeonTex, namely a conductive and nonwoven microfiber with piezo-resistive functionality, which were placed correspondingly between the ankle and the plantar zone of the considered (3) HCs, respectively. The proposed system finds wide application in the field of remote monitoring and telemedicine.

Other research groups proposed wearable systems for remote monitoring; for instance, Lorussi et al. [60] proposed a wearable system to remotely monitor musculoskeletal disorders. The system is composed of IMUs, e-textile sensors and a decision support system included in a dedicated app able to assist the patient in performing personalized rehabilitation exercises designed by a physician/therapist, remotely and in real-time (also through alerts). Raad et al. [55] proposed a wearable smart glove for remote monitoring of rheumatoid arthritis patients monitoring finger flexions while patients performed several activities at home. The e-textile glove used flex and force sensors and an Arduino platform to transmit motion data to the physiotherapists through a mobile phone, on which a dedicated app is installed. Other authors proposed a complete platform for healthcare monitoring. As described in Section 3.1, Lopez et al. [25] proposed a novel healthcare IT platform capable of monitoring several physiological parameters, such as electrocardiogram (ECG), heart rate, body temperature, and the capability to track the location of a group of patients within hospital environments through the combination of e-textiles and wireless sensors. The same authors, in another work [24], proposed a medical IT platform, based on wireless sensor networks and e-textiles, which supports indoor location-aware services as well as monitors physiological parameters, such as ECG, heart rate, and body temperature. Tao et al. proposed a totally flexible and washable textronic device able to acquire several types of biological data. The data containing vital physiological signs, skin temperature, and activity motions were transferred via low-energy Bluetooth technology to a smart phone and then via 4G or Wi-Fi into a remote data server to realize a continuously Web-based monitoring system. Other researchers proposed wearable devices that are completely textile and do not integrate devices such as IMUs. In this context, Della Toffola et al. [54] proposed a wearable system for long-term monitoring of knee kinematics: compliance with the use of knee sleeve is monitored by using an e-textile sensor that measures the knee sleeve fabric stretch, thus allowing to infer whether the subjects under test wears the knee sleeve. Garcia Patino et al. [63] proposed a compact textile-based wearable platform to track trunk movements when the considered user bends forward. The smart garment developed for this purpose was prototyped with an inductive sensor formed by sewing a copper wire into an elastic fabric in a zigzag pattern. Heo et al. [50] proposed a flexible glove sensor—which included stretchable and flexible PDMS films—to monitor upper extremity prosthesis functions. Other researchers studied new arrangements of materials for biomedical applications, Jin et al. [21] studied a highly durable nanofiber-reinforced metal elastomer composite consisting of metal fillers, an elastomeric binder matrix, and electro-spun PVDF nanofibers to enhance both cyclic stability and conductivity, showing a good continuous long-term monitoring of ECG, EMG signal, and motions during weightlifting exercises without significant degradation of signal quality. Li et al. [64] fabricated a textile-based stretchable sensor by using an electronic dyeing method; the conductive textile showed good flexibility and adaptable strain-electric response. The authors demonstrated the excellent performances for monitoring and analysis of several human activities. Tang et al. [34] reported the functionalized conductive, sensitive, wearable, and washable vacuum pressure sensor based on carbon nanotubes (CNTs), e-textile with unique nanostructures growth on the non-woven fabric by using the novel, and facile nano-soldering method. They proved that CNTs e-textile sensor has a good linearity, high sensitivity and low power consumption. Moreover, they showed the good repeatability, washability, durability, and super-hydrophobic performance of the CNTs underling its feasibility to realize smart clothes. Yao et al. [19] presented mechanically and electrically robust integration of nanocomposites with textiles by laser scribing and heat press lamination showing a good washability and good electromechanical performance up to 50% strain. They underlined the potential utility of these new materials and methods in healthcare, activity tracking, rehabilitation, sports, medicine, and human-machine interactions. Finally, Ye et al. [51] reported a scalable dip-coating strategy to construct conductive silk fibers showing their feasibility to be woven into fabrics, resulting in textiles sensitive to physical stimuli such as: force, strain, and temperature.

Park et al. [65] proposed a dynamically stretchable high-performance supercapacitor fabricated with MWCNT/MoO3 for powering an integrated sensor in an all-in-one textile system to detect various bio signals. This system sewed into cloth both t-shirt and glove successfully detects strain due to joint movement and the wrist pulse.

Zhang et al. [57] designed a fabric E-textile for tracking active motion signals. The fiber-shaped coaxial tribo-sensor is fabricated with silver yarn and polytetrafluoroethylene yarn, which allows for integrating well with cloths at large scales due to its satisfactory breathability, good washability, and desirable flexibility.

Jang et al. [38] proposed a highly sensitive fiber-type strain sensor with a broad range of strain by introducing a single active layer onto the fiber. The sensors were sewn into electrical fabric bands, which are integrable to a wireless transmitter to monitor waveforms of pulsations, respirations, and various postures of level of bending a spinal cord. About the last issue, the authors developed an electronic band-type posture corrector (E-posture-corrector) with the fiber sensor to continuously measure resistive changes to bending angles of a human spinal cord.

Kiaghadi et al. [59] presented the design of Tribexor, an end-to-end sensing system that leverages triboelectric textiles to measure joint motions and sweating behavior showing that the sensor has high performance in natural conditions by benchmarking the accuracy of sensing several kinematic metrics as well as sweat level.

Other authors focused on activity recognition and monitoring. Fevgas et al. [52], indeed, presented a platform and a methodology for rapid prototype development of e-textile applications for human activity monitoring to address the problems of human movement and gesture monitoring, posture recognition and fall detection. Kim et al. [37] proposed a carbon nanotube ink drop-coated textile resistive pressure sensor on a typical three-dimensional spacer textile able to detect human health and motion. The resulting 3D spacer textile pressure sensor unit showed a wide range of sensing performance of 200 kPa–50 kPa, which facilitates the detection of physiological signals, such as acoustic vibrations and hand motion. Vu et al. [56] introduced a new approach to classify human body movements, by using textile sensors, embedded into fabrics, using AI to recognize different standard human motions (e.g., walking, jumping, running, and sprinting) starting from features extracted from strain signals. The last authors proposed also another work [49] in which they presented an e-textile strain sensor integrated on a glove to monitor angles of finger motions. They also proved the feasibility of this sensor placing it onto the skin of the neck to record the pharynx motions when speaking, coughing and swallowing. Samy et al. [41] proposed an unobtrusive framework for sleep stage identification based on a high-resolution, pressure-sensitive e-textile bed sheet able to acquire information related to body movement, posture, and body orientation. Finally, Hayashi et al. [62] proposed a smart wheelchair, composed of e-textile pressure sensors placed on the seat and back support, able to monitor the patients posture on the basis of quantitative sitting-posture scores.

The articles related to this section show how the integration of IMUs for movement assessment in e-textile garments is a consolidated practice. By means of the integration of algorithms, it is possible to compute several kinematic parameters starting from acceleration or angular velocities. Moreover, the kinematic information can be acquired thanks to the capability of some materials described in some articles to change their intrinsic resistance when they are stretched showing their feasibility in the movement assessment.

Table 4. Insights regarding orthopaedic literature: authors, aim, dataset, and acquired data.

Authors	Aim	Dataset	Acquired Data
Bartalesi et al. (2010) [53]	Designing, developing, and testing a wearable system to perform the real time estimation of the local curvature and the length of the spine lumbar arch	1 HC	Acceleration data; Strain signals
Lopez et al. (2010a) [24]	Describing a novel healthcare IT platform for localization and monitoring within hospital environments	5 PP	ECG; Heart rate; Angle of inclination; Activity index; Body temperature; Patient's location; Battery level; Alert code
Lopez et al. (2010b) [25]	Presenting a medical IT platform platform based on Wireless Sensor Networks and e-textile for patients' localization and monitoring	5 PP	ECG; Heart rate; Angle of inclination; Activity index; Body temperature; Patient's location; Battery level; Alert code
Fevgas et al. (2010) [52]	Presenting a platform and a methodology for the rapid prototype development of e-textile applications for human activity monitoring	3 HC	Acceleration data
Della Toffola et al. (2012) [54]	Presenting a wearable system for long-term monitoring of knee kinematics in the home and community settings	1 HC	Acceleration data; Strain signals
Samy et al. (2014) [41]	Performing sleep stage analysis with a contact-free unobtrusive system	7 HC	Respiratory rate and its variability; Leg EMG from pressure images; Sleep posture
Hayashi et al. (2017) [62]	Using smart wheelchairs to monitor posture	3 HC	FS index and LL index
Li et al. (2017) [64]	Presenting an electronic dyeing method to fabricate wearable silver-based e-textile sensors for human motion monitoring and analysis	1 HC	Strain signals at heel, lower and upper knee
Vu & Kim (2018) [56]	Introducing a new approach to classify human body movements using textile sensors integrated into smart muscle pants	1 HC	Motion Signals
Lorussi et al. (2018) [60]	Developing a sensing platform constituted by wearable sensors for musculo-skeletal rehabilitation	5 HC	Knee and scapular flexion angles
Tao et al. (2018) [30]	Presenting a novel system—made up of a washable and wearable smart textile shirt, smartphone app and software desktop—for the acquisition of ECG signal, breathing rate, acceleration data for activity recognition and skin temperature	5 HC [ML] HC [#]	ECG; Skin temperature; Respiratory rate; Acceleration data
Kiaghadi et al. (2018) [59]	Developing of a wearable joint sensor	1 HC	Elbow Flexion Angles; Sweat Volume
Kim et al. (2019) [37]	Developing an all-textile based pressure/strain sensor for physiological signals using 3D spacer textile	HC [#]	Blood Pulse (wrist and neck); Finger flexion angles; Cheek motion; Pharynx motion

Table 4. *Cont.*

Authors	Aim	Dataset	Acquired Data
Park et al. (2019) [65]	Evaluation of a dynamically stretchable high-performance supercapacitor for powering an integrated sensor in an all-in-one textile system to detect various biosignals	1 HC	Strain Signals
Zhang et al. (2019) [57]	Developing a fabric E-textile for tracking active motion signals	1 HC	Motion Signals
Jang et al. (2019) [38]	Preparing a highly sensitive fiber-type strain sensor with a broad range of strain by introducing a single active layer onto the fiber	1 HC	Pulse Signals; Spinal Cord Bending Angles; Breath Signal
Ye et al. (2019) [51]	Fabricating e-textile sensors sensible to body and environmental stimuli modifying the surface of natural silks with CNTs	1 HC	Knee flexion angle; Finger flexion angle
Yao et al.(2019) [19]	Designing and fabricating multifunctional e-textiles with mechanical and functional properties comparable with typical textiles for monitoring applications	1 HC	ECG; EMG (arm); Motion signals
Jin et al. (2019) [21]	Fabricating a metal–elastomer–nanofibers conductive material for long-term monitoring	1 HC	ECG; EMG (bicep muscle); Motion signals
Raad et al. (2019) [55]	Proposing a novel Smart Glove for both live and on-demand monitoring	1 HC	Motion signals (hand and finger movement)
Amitrano et al. (2020) [61]	Presenting a novel e-textile smart sock and verifying its performances during gait analysis	3 HC	Angular velocity signals of the ankle; Foot plantar pressures
Vu & Kim (2020) [49]	Fabricating and optimizing the performance of e-textile strain sensors	1 HC	Finger flexion angles; Pharynx motion
Heo et al. (2019) [50]	Introducing, characterizing, and experimenting novel textile strain sensors based on AgNW	1 HC	Finger flexion angles
Li et al. (2020) [58]	Describing a miniature accelerometer solution integrated seamlessly within the fabric of a sleeve to monitor movement	3 HC	Elbow and knee bending angle
Tang et al. (2020) [34]	Fabricating machine-washable e-textiles with high strain sensitivity and high thermal conduction for monitoring applications	1 HC	Motion signals; Blood pulse
Garcia Patino et al. (2020) [63]	Designing a textile-based wearable platform to prevent low back pain	1 HC	Motion signals (Back movements)

number of subjects not provided; ML: Machine Learning training set. **Abbreviations**. AgNW: Silver NanoWire; CNTs: Carbon Nanotubes; ECG: Electrocardiogram; EMG: Electromyography; FS: Forward Shift; HC: Healthy Controls; IT: Inormation Technology; LL: Lateral Lean; PP: Pathological Patients.

3.4. The Applications in the Respiratory Tract

Respiration is a crucial vital function for humans; abnormalities in such a function may have a different origin and can lead to patient deterioration and, ultimately, death. Previous research extensively documented the clinical importance of respiratory rate diagnosis and how precise and routine monitoring is yet to be achieved, on the one side due to intrinsic difficulties (linked both to human and machines limitations) and on the other side because of limited use and/or the small diffusion of advanced respiratory monitoring systems [94,95]. To reach this gap, several methods were proposed and were widely investigated over time [96,97]; among these, several e-textile applications were also proposed. The research in this field is summarized in Table 5.

To the best of the authors' knowledge, Zięba et al. [68] presented the first prototype in this 10-year report of papers. The proposed solution was a textronic shirt with sensorial stripes (namely, a textile knitted sensor made of silver yarns) whose ends were connected to a current amplifier to acquire breathing rhythm. The authors evidenced the device was able to acquire the signal, although some limitations (e.g., sensors positioning) could not be overlooked when the HC was not at rest during the acquisitions. In the same period, the authors [69] presented a similar prototype with a different configuration—and amount—of the sensorial stripes (in this case, the authors embedded 3 stripes upon the chest). Correspondingly, a similar but different prototype—namely, the same textronic shirt equipped with two sensorial stripes localized upon the chest—was proposed to monitor the elderlies' breathing rhythm [35,36]. In the same period, Ramos–Garcia et al. designed and fabricated a Respiratory Inductive Plethysmograph based breathing system aimed at potentially monitoring breathing rate. The proposed system was a polyester/spandex t-shirt on which a stretch e-textile sensor was placed around the HC' chest. The preliminary results indicated the proposed system, which needs further improvements to be properly used for multiple tasks, was capable of effectively monitoring breathing rate of 3 HCs. Another more recent solution was described in [30]. The authors used the same sportswear shirt prototype—already described in Section 3.1 for the ECG acquisition—to detect the respiration rate using the same ECG sensor connected to a different textile electrode. The more recent example in this 10-year report of papers is, to our best knowledge, the solution adopted by Fan et al. [39], who positioned the TATSA around the chest to monitor the respiratory signal. Summing up the promising results related to both the cardiac and the respiratory signals, the authors proceeded even with new experiments assessing a different shirt configuration (designed by embedding two TATSA on the abdomen and wrist positions to monitor both the respiratory and pulse signal, respectively) which allowed to effectively ascertain respiratory—and, as expected, heart rate-related variations—differences in an HC and a patient affected by sleep apnea syndrome.

Another solution to potentially monitor this pathology using e-textile prototypes was described in [66]. Specifically, the authors manufactured an e-textile bed sheet (where the e-textile piezoresistive layer is enclosed between two sheets of conventional fabric layers) aimed to indirectly acquire respiratory rate data; additionally, the authors designed an IT platform capable of accurately (yet noninvasively) processing the acquired data. The analyses performed on 14 HC demonstrated that the overall system was effectively capable to inconspicuously monitor patients' respiratory rate when they slept in supine position. Albeit patients' movements effectively invalidated respiratory rate monitoring, the system demonstrated a valid tool to track diseases (e.g., the already mentioned apnea disease) for which patients movements can be limited. Similar e-textiles and IT platforms were used later from the same research group and other colleagues. On the one hand, Liu et al. [67] conducted new investigations to automatically monitor respiratory rate, considering either the analysis of a restricted patient area (e.g., torso) or different bed configurations (e.g., tilted bed setups); on the other hand, Samy et al. [41] concentrated, as already described in Section 3.2, on new objectives, among which we can mention the sleep stage analysis. In this case, the respiratory rate (even when acquired by the e-textile bedsheet) demonstrated a different output during the different sleep stages of the patients. This finding can help to design and implement the proposed device as an unobtrusive sleep stage identification system, which would help to potentially perform early diagnoses of sleep disorders and chronic diseases. Respiratory rate demonstrated important even in the case of infants sleeping monitoring [66]. It is not by chance if Ferreira et al. [15] investigated—using their custom-made chest belt and the Baby Night Watch IT platform (see also Section 3.1)—respiratory rate variations in infants to monitor eventual Sudden Infant Death Syndrome events; nevertheless, albeit the chest belt represents for all intents and purposes an e-textile system, respiratory rate was acquired by the authors using a triaxial accelerometer integrated in the chest belt, differently from the ECG signal. An e-textile embedded chest belt was developed even by Jang et al. [38]. Specifically, the authors sewed horizontally on the chest belt the same composite fiber sensor (developed even for pulse acquisition), aiming at monitoring respiratory waveforms from an HC in various breathing conditions. The authors claimed the results agree with those found using a commercial breathing sensor and, finally, hypothesized the fiber sensor could be potentially used to fabricate devices capable to evaluate the breathing quantities (for instance, respiration volume, and lung capacities). Another recent e-textile prototype for the potential diagnosis of respiratory signal related diseases was that presented by Choudhry et al. [48], who integrated on a vest a different multilayer sensor around a HC's ribcage area. The preliminary results indicated the system was capable to recognize indirect changes in breath pressure and that the acquired signal was coherent with average adult breaths count. Finally, Lian et al. [70] proposed a multifunctional e-textile material—whose layers were composed of high-density AgNWs and a sensing fabric, respectively—which was used to fabricate a face mask, through which they showed the feasibility to indirectly evaluate variations in breathing rate. This prototype could show potential applications also for healthcare monitoring (e.g., cardiac and respiratory illnesses linked to particulate matter 2.5 penetration in human body); however, to the best of the authors' knowledge, the authors did not consider this particular case as the main application for the multifunctional e-textile. Differently, in the same period another prototype of e-textile mask was presented by Liang et al. [32]. Contrarily from the previous paper, in this case the authors merely sewed the conductive textiles (briefly described in Section 3.1 yet) onto a mask which was capable, thanks to the sensibility of the conductive textile components to ascertain humidity variations which are different during HCs' periodic exhaling and inhaling, of precisely monitoring HCs' breath, which can help to keep under control or avoid pathologies such as lethal sleep apnea.

From the outcome of our investigation it is possible to conclude that, as already seen for the previous subsections, further research is needed validate the direct practical applicability of these e-textile solutions. Nevertheless, since a lower number of publications on this topic—probably a consequence of a scarce research interest by many research group—seem to be available in the literature, the "bench to the bedside" process (and, consequently, the needed temporal range) would be more complicated than the solutions considered in the previously analyzed fields.

Table 5. Insights regarding literature in in respiratory field: authors, aim, dataset and acquired data.

Authors	Aim	Dataset	Acquired Data
Zieba et al. (2012) [68]	Designing a textile knitted sensor to monitor the frequency of human breathing	1 HC	Respiratory rate
Frydisiak & Zieba (2012) [69]	Designing a textile knitted sensor to monitor the frequency of human breathing	HC [#]	Respiratory rate
Huang et al. (2013) [66]	Presenting an e-textile bedsheet to measure human respiratory rate	14 HC	Respiratory rate
Samy et al. (2014) [41]	Performing sleep stage analysis with a contact-free unobtrusive system	7 HC	Respiratory rate and its variability; Leg EMG from pressure images; Sleep posture
Liu et al. (2014) [67]	Presenting an unobtrusive on-bed respiration system	12 HC	Respiratory rate
Ramos-Garcia et al. (2016) [71]	Using a coverstitched stretch sensor in a commercial shirt to monitor respiration	3 HC	Breath signal
Ferreira et al. (2016) [15]	Presenting the design and fabrication of SWSs to prevent infants' SIDS	HC [#]	Body temperature; Respiratory rate; ECG
Frydisiak & Tesiorowski (2016a) [35]	Designing a smart textronic shirts for the health monitoring of elderly people	HC [#]	Blood Pulse; Breath Signal; Skin Temperature
Frydisiak & Tesiorowski (2016b) [36]	Designing a smart textronic shirts for the health monitoring of elderly people	HC [#]	Blood Pulse; Breath Signal; Skin Temperature

Table 5. *Cont.*

Authors	Aim	Dataset	Acquired Data
Tao et al. (2018) [30]	Presenting a novel system—made up of a washable and wearable smart textile shirt, smartphone app and software desktop—for the acquisition of ECG signal, breathing rate, acceleration data for activity recognition and skin temperature	5 HC ^{ML} HC $^{\#}$	ECG; Skin temperature; Respiratory rate; Acceleration data
Jang et al. (2019) [38]	Preparing a highly sensitive fiber-type strain sensor with a broad range of strain by introducing a single active layer onto the fiber	1 HC	Blood Pulse; Spinal Cord Bending Angles; Breath Signal
Choundry et al. (2020) [48]	Fabricating piezoresistive sensors—and studying their washability—to monitor breathing and muscular activity	1 HC	Breath pressure signal of the ribcage; Pressure signal from biceps femoris muscle
Lian et al. (2020) [70]	Fabricating a multifunctional e-textile for multiple applications (such as diagnostics and environmental)	1 HC	Breath pressure signal
Liang et al. (2020) [32]	Developing a stable and biocompatible silk sericine carbon nanotubes (CNT) ink and demonstrating its versatile applications in flexible electronics for monitoring human biosignals	HC $^{\#}$	ECG, Breath Signal; Hydrogen peroxide concentration
Fan et al. (2020) [39]	Developing TATSA for precise epidermal physiological signal monitoring	1 HC 1 PP	Blood Pulse & Breath Signal

$^{\#}$ number of subjects not provided; ^{ML}: Machine Learning training set. **Abbreviations**. ECG: Electrocardiogram; EMG: Electromyography; HC: Healthy Controls; PP: Pathological Patients; SIDS: Sudden Infant Death Syndrome; SWSs: Smart Wearable Systems; TATSA: Triboelectric All-Textile Sensor Array.

3.5. Miscellaneous

The previous subsections have dealt with the main themes on which the applications and developments of e-textile technologies focused. However, there are applications of e-textile even on less common themes, which confirm the wide development of these technologies in the last decade and testify to the variety of purposes to which textile technologies can be applied. In this paragraph, we collected several works that offer applications on 'other themes' different from those described in detail in the previous subsections, widening the horizon of biomedical applications of e-textile technologies. The research presented in this subsection is summarized in Table 6.

Golparvar and Yapici focused their work on the use of e-textiles in the field of electrooculography (EOG), proposing, for the first time, the use of graphene-coated fabric electrodes for electrooculogram acquisition. In [72] they performed a comparative study between conventional Ag/AgCl electrodes and their e-textile electrodes demonstrating high degree of flexibility, elasticity, and the possibility of incorporating the novel electrodes into various types of personal clothing. The following year, the same authors presented two research articles [73,74] in which they designed a devoted unit for textile-based EOG that can achieve on-board noise removal and signal amplification. Moreover, they developed and implemented a controlled automatic blink detection algorithm, able to detect voluntary blinks in real-time. The performances of the device in recording EOG signal during specific eye movement patterns and in detecting voluntary blinks were explored in their works resulting in good agreement with the reference EOG systems based on Ag/AgCl electrodes.

EDA, also known as galvanic skin response (GSR), is another bioelectrical signal, usually recorded with common Ag/AgCl electrodes, which was one of the subject of study and applications of textile-based electrodes and devices. Sinha et al. [16] employed the same PEDOT:PSS based electrodes used for ECG and EMG recording even to collect EDA signal from fingers and wrist. To this aim, they developed a sensing shirt able to simultaneously record the three biosignals, finding potential applications in continuous health monitoring as well as physiotherapy. Similarly, Postolache et al. [14] developed e-textile electrodes for measuring skin conductance using the same materials employed for ECG recording (textile made of fibers coated with conductive polymer and silver). E-textile electrodes were attached to the wheelchair armrests to monitor physiological stress parameters of the wheelchair user in unobtrusive way. Haddad et al. [75] used a different approach to develop EDA electrodes; specifically, they integrated Ag/AgCl uniformly coated yarns within three different textile substrates (100% cotton, 100% nylon, and 100% polyester). The e-textile electrodes were used to record EDA on the distal phalanx of the fingers, and their performances were compared with the standard rigid Ag/AgCl electrodes, resulting in higher stability for e-textile electrodes when changes in skin temperature occurred. Jennifer Healey [76] proposed a different application of GSR measurement, developing a 'GSR sock' by integrating two fabric electrodes from a commercial heart rate monitor strap into a standard sock. The electrodes were placed to make contact with the ball and heel foot of a HC. The experimental testing showed that the sock prototype provided a meaningful measure of GSR activity that can be used unobtrusively in daily monitoring.

Chen et al. [81] applied their expertise in flexible electronics and polymers to develop a fiber-shaped e-textile strain sensor using polyurethane fibers, AgNWs and styrene-butadiene-styrene (SBS) via knitting and simple dip-coating processes. Due to the textile-based structures and hierarchical fibers, the e-textile exhibited good capability of detecting multiple deformation, including tensile strain and pressure, which enables a wide range of biomedical purposes. In particular, the authors proposed different applications in health monitoring such as pulse beating detection, phonation detection, scoliosis correction, and Restless Legs Syndrome (RLS) diagnosis. A similar strain sensor was developed by Vu & Kim [49], using a slightly different manufacturing process: a polyester/spandex fabric was immersed in a single-walled carbon nanotubes (SWCNT) ink, which gives sensing capabilities, and, after squeezing and drying processes, silver pastes were printed onto the SWCNT fabric to improve strain sensor performance. Within the manuscript, the authors provided an extensive characterization of the properties of the fabric, testing sensors with different shapes and structures. To demonstrate the potential of their sensors in practical applications, Vu & Kim proposed to attach the textile sensor to the skin of the neck, to monitoring pharynx motion, demonstrating that is possible to obtain consistent signals when speaking, coughing, and swallowing. Before them, Kim et al. [37] already explored the possibility of registering the movement of the pharynx with a textile sensor. They used a carbon nanotube ink drop-coated textile resistive sensor on a three-dimensional spacer structure, to monitor pharynx movement during speaking. In their experimental testing, authors demonstrated that the recorded signals exhibited distinct profiles when different words are pronounced, and the same word generated a similar wave profile in repeated tests. The same sensor was also tested attached to the cheek skin, demonstrating the ability to detect cheek bulging movements. Following these results, authors pointed out the potential applications of the sensor in human-machine interaction and as a face and speech recognition system.

Another important biomedical application, which is particularly suitable with wearable and textile-based electronics, is the measure of skin temperature. This is an important parameter for a variety of health monitoring applications, where changes in temperature can indicate changes in health. Embedding temperature sensors within textiles provides an easy method for directly measuring body temperature in defined areas. This is why many researchers, even though they do not have a focus in temperature-related health effects, integrated a temperature sensor into the devices they developed to add an additional information to the recorded health data. As first example, Lopez et al. [24,25] embedded a thermometer in the Wearable Data Acquisition Device to include the body temperature as a further parameter provided by the proposed healthcare monitoring system. Similarly, Tao et al. [30] exploited the temperature sensor integrated into the MEMS sensor chip they used for activity recognition purposes, to monitor user skin temperature. Ferreira et al. [15]

used an infrared thermopile sensor embedded in the wearable chest belt, to measure the body temperature of infants, adding this parameter to the other signals registered by the device and previously discussed in the subsections of this Review. Other examples are provided by the two works by Frydisiak & Tesiorowski [35,36]. They developed a system to remotely monitor elderly people by acquiring various physiological parameters including, in addition to those already mentioned in the previous sections, underclothing temperature. Moving to more specific textile-based sensors, Lugoda et al. [77] developed a temperature sensing yarn, using a micro thermistor covered with packing fibers and a warp knitted tube. The temperature sensing yarns were then used to create a series of temperature sensing garments: armbands, a glove, and a sock. The performances of the temperature sensing wearable devices were investigated and, from the outcomes of the analyses conducted, the authors found some limitations in measuring skin temperature due to the deformation of the yarn structure and also depending on the fit of the garment.

Jiang et al. [78] also proposed a wearable sensing device with embedded temperature and humidity sensors, the latter used as sweat sensor. However, the authors focused on the use of a textile based Near-Field Communication (NFC) antenna, which is able to power the system and transmit sensors data. The measurement results have shown that the textile NFC antennas can still perform properly under bending up to 150°, with a maximum range of 6 cm to access sensor data. This innovation figures to be a very attractive field of development towards self-powered wearable devices, to overcome the limitations of power supplies, very critical challenges for the e-textile field. Sweat volume monitoring on skin is also one of the topics of the work by Kiaghadi et al. [59]. Authors designed a triboelectric textile sensor to measure joint movement, but they noticed that the baseline signal varied due to sweat volume produced on the skin. The reason is that the sweat induces the wetting of the inner layers of the sensor, whereas the outer layers, that are close to air, remain drier. This results in a different impedance between the layers, causing a small DC offset that is amplified in the electronics circuits, creating an observable change at the output of the textile sensor. The baseline changes thus reflected the sweat volume production on the skin. The high performance of the proposed sensor were also demonstrated in real-world applications, by benchmarking its robustness in perspiration measurements during exercise, comparing the results with those of a GSR sensor for skin conductivity.

Many researchers also proposed sensor to analyze the chemical composition of sweat, to investigate its constituents, which could be related to the subject's physiological condition. Lactate and sodium are commonly analyzed markers in sweat, directly measured on body and, thus, very suitable for wearable textile application. On this research topic, Zhao et al. [80] presented a thread-based wearable biosensor to simultaneously measure concentration of lactate and sodium in sweat. To assess the performance of this wearable nanobiosensor, the authors developed an integrated smart headband to acquire data directly on the body. Tests were performed on a male volunteer subject during intense workout, and the sweat concentration was compared with the results obtained with standard methods, confirming the accuracy and stability of the biosensor in real use. Another electrochemical textile sensor was recently proposed by Liang et al. [32]. Fabricated via stencil printing Silk-Sericine Carbon Nanotube (SSCNT) ink and silver chloride paste on a PET film, the electrochemical sensor is capable to detect the concentration of hydrogen peroxide, which is an important intermediate in biological processes. The sensing mechanism is based on the electrocatalytic activity and conductivity of CNTs, very responsive to the change of concentration of hydrogen peroxide.

A very interesting application of textile electronics was presented by Mason et al. [79]. The authors investigated the response of a smart fabric, with integrated conductive pathways, strain gauges, and conductive pressure sensor points, at microwave frequencies region for data transmission of biomedical signals. The aim of this perspective research is to demonstrate the feasibility of the proposed smart sensing garments to detect dielectric changes directly on body. It is also shown how these sensing features can be exploited to monitor biomedical signals such as ECG and EMG, body temperature, sweat volume, etc. This novel sensor was even patented owing to the great potentialities shown in biomedical applications.

Finally, Rong Liu et al. [82] presented a peculiar application of e-textile, developing intelligent pants for monitoring incontinence status. The smart garment was developed incorporating conductive yarns in fabrics, using advanced circular seamless knitting technology. The presence of urine causes the variation of the measured electrical resistance of the conductive pathways, allowing to sense, monitor, and alert wearers and care providers on urinary incontinence status.

The overview proposed in this section demonstrates the wide range of biomedical applications that e-textile technologies can cover. The interest of researchers is not limited to the fields of medicine that are more easily explored by textile solutions, but also extends to apparently minor applications that, as demonstrated, can be developed and have great employment opportunities. In the works analyzed in this section, the focus is mainly on the development of new materials, which are sensitive to a certain physical quantity without losing the biocompatibility features. However, this prevailing focus on the development of the textile element means that less effort is invested in the clinical application of these products. For this reason, even in this case, the experimental procedures proposed are limited to proofs of concept on a limited cohort of healthy controls, while a structured clinical trial is never reported.

Table 6. Insights regarding e-textile literature in other fields: authors, aim, dataset, and data.

Authors	Aim	Dataset	Acquired Data
Lopez et al. (2010a) [24]	Describing a novel healthcare IT platform for localization and monitoring within hospital environments	5 PP	ECG; Heart rate; Angle of inclination; Activity index; Body temperature; Patient's location; Battery level; Alert code
Lopez et al. (2010b) [25]	Presenting a medical IT platform platform based on Wireless Sensor Networks and e-textile for patients' localization and monitoring	5 PP	ECG; Heart rate; Angle of inclination; Activity index; Body temperature; Patient's location; Battery level; Alert code
Healey et al. (2011) [76]	Presenting and validating performances of a novel e-textile sock for measuring GSR	1 HC	EDA
Liu et al. (2012) [82]	Manufacturing intelligent incontinence pants made of conductive yarns to monitor the incontinence status	HC [#]	Volume of leaked urine
Postolache et al. (2014) [14]	Presenting a wheelchair architecture equipped with e-textiles for ECG and SKC sensing	7 HC	ECG; EDA
Mason et al. (2014) [79]	Evaluating the performance of a flexible sensor with an embedded e-textile cloth for sensing applications	1 HC	Biomedical microwave sensing
Ferreira et al. (2016) [15]	Presenting the design and fabrication of SWSs to prevent infants' SIDS	HC [#]	Skin temperature; Respiratory rate; ECG
Frydisiak & Tesiorowski (2016a) [35]	Designing a smart textronic shirts for the health monitoring of elderly people	HC [#]	Blood Pulse; Breath Signal; Skin Temperature
Frydisiak & Tesiorowski (2016b) [36]	Designing a smart textronic shirts for the health monitoring of elderly people	HC [#]	Blood Pulse; Breath Signal; Skin Temperature
Golparvar & Yapici (2017) [72]	Acquiring EOG signals with graphene textile electrodes comparing the outcome with conventional Ag/AgCl electrodes	1 HC	EOG
Golparvar & Yapici (2018a) [73]	Detecting EOG signal using textile electrodes	HC [#]	EOG

Table 6. Cont.

Authors	Aim	Dataset	Acquired Data
Golparvar & Yapici (2018b) [74]	Characterization of graphene-coated electroconductive textile electrodes for EOG acquisition	4 HC 2 ME 2 HE	EOG
Lugoda et al. (2018) [77]	Fabricating temperature sensing yarns to manufacture temperature sensing garments	5 HC	Skin temperature
Chen et al. (2018) [81]	Fabricating a multifunctional e-textile for multi-detection of strain, pressure, and force maps	1 HC	Resistance signals
Haddad et al. (2018) [75]	Designing and integrating Ag/AgCl e-textile electrodes to monitor EDA comparing the outcome with standard electrodes	1 HC	EDA stimulus responses
Tao et al. (2018) [30]	Presenting a novel system—made up of a washable and wearable smart textile shirt, smartphone app and software desktop—for the acquisition of ECG signal, breathing rate, acceleration data for activity recognition and skin temperature	5 HC ^{ML} HC $^{\#}$	ECG; Skin temperature; Respiratory rate; Acceleration data
Kiaghadi et al. (2018) [59]	Developing of a wearable joint sensor	1 HC	Elbow Flexion Angles; Sweat Volume
Kim et al. (2019) [37]	Developing an all-textile based pressure/strain sensor for physiological signals using 3D spacer textile	HC $^{\#}$	Blood Pulse (wrist and neck); Finger flexion angles; Cheek motion; Pharynx motion
Sinha et al. (2019) [16]	Fabricating PEDOT:PSS coated electrodes to record EMG, ECG and EDA	4 HC ^{emg} 1 HC ^{eda} 1 HC ^{ecg}	EDA; ECG; EMG (biceps, triceps, tibialis, and quadriceps)
Vu & Kim (2020) [49]	Fabricating and optimizing the performance of e-textile strain sensors	1 HC	Finger flexion angles; Signal of pharynx motion
Jiang et al. (2020) [78]	Integrating textile NFC antennas with temperature and humidity sensors to enable battery-free wireless sensing for monitoring purposes	1 HC	Skin Temperature; Sweat Volume
Zhao et al. (2020) [80]	Presenting a thread-based wearable nanobiosensor to detect lactate and sodium concentrations during perspiration	1 HC	Sodium and lactate concentration in human sweat
Liang et al. (2020) [32]	Developing a stable and biocompatible silk sericine carbon nanotubes (CNT) ink and demonstrating its versatile applications in flexible electronics for monitoring human biosignals	HC $^{\#}$	ECG, Breath Signal; Hydrogen peroxide concentration

$^{\#}$ number of subjects not provided; ^{ecg}: Electrocardiographic acquisitions; ^{eda}: Electrodermal Activity acquisitions; ^{emg}: Electromyographic acquisitions; ^{ML}: Machine Learning training set. Abbreviations. ECG: Electrocardiogram; EDA: Electrodermal Activity; EMG: Electromyography; EOG: Electrooculography; HC: Healthy Controls; HE: Hypermetropic Eyes; IT: Information Technology; GSR: Galvanic Skin Response; ME: Myopic Eyes; NFC: Near Field Communication; PEDOT:PSS: Poly(3,4-Ethyelenedioxythiophne) Polystyrene Sulfonate); PP: Pathological Patients; SIDS: Sudden Infant Death Syndrome; SKC: Skin Conductivity; SWSs: Smart Wearable Systems.

4. Conclusions

This systematic review showed the development of e-textile applications in the medical field for a decade. Several specialties of medicine were analyzed in these years: cardiology, a particular emphasis on muscles, physiatry and orthopaedics, respiratory tract, and also sparse studies on other themes were found. The studies are variegated in purposes but there is one big common limitation that comes out from this review: most of the studies focused on the development and testing of new devices on a single healthy subject, and only few studies considered a dataset made of more than 10 s of HC. Therefore, researchers should consider validating their novel devices on a larger cohort of subjects (healthy and pathological) for further studies. Many of the analyzed studies did not even mention the number of subjects tested as a limitation for their research. Perhaps this is because the development of these technologies is still in an early phase and the aim of the researchers was to improve the technology itself, leading up to the potential future goal of an experimental campaign on larger datasets. Following this brief discussion, our review should help researchers understand that it is now the time for a second phase, in which the devices are tested on larger datasets.

Supplementary Materials: The following are available online at https://www.mdpi.com/article/10.3390/diagnostics11122263/s1, Table S1: Insights regarding the studies included in the Review: authors, aim, material and its configuration, dataset, acquired data and clinical application.

Author Contributions: Conceptualization, G.C., L.D., A.C., F.A. and C.R.; methodology, G.C., L.D. and C.R.; validation, G.C., L.D. and C.R.; formal analysis G.C., L.D., A.C., F.A. and C.R.; investigation, L.D., A.C. and F.A.; data curation, G.C., A.C. and F.A.; writing—original draft preparation, G.C., L.D., A.C. and F.A.; writing—review and editing, G.D. and C.R.; visualization, G.C., A.C. and F.A.; supervision, L.D., G.D. and C.R.; project administration, G.D. and C.R. All authors have read and agreed to the published version of the manuscript.

Funding: This research received no external funding.

Institutional Review Board Statement: Not applicable.

Informed Consent Statement: Not applicable.

Conflicts of Interest: The authors declare no conflict of interest.

Abbreviations

The following abbreviations are used in this manuscript:

ADL	Activities of Daily Living
Ag/AgCl	Silver/Silver Chloride
AgNW	Silver NanoWire
AI	Artificial Intelligence
CNTs	Carbon Nanotubes
ECG	Electrocardiogram
EDA	Electrodermal Activity
EMG	Electromyography
EOG	Electrooculography
FS	Forward Shift
GSR	Galvanic Skin Response
GO	Graphene Oxide
HE	Hypermetropic Eyes
IMUs	Inertial Measurement Units
IT	Information Technology
LEVOP	Lower Extremity Venous Occlusion Plethysmography
LL	Lateral Lean
ME	Myopic Eyes
MWCNTs	Multi-Walled Carbon Nano-Tubes
NFC	Near Field Communication
PDMS	PolyDiMethylSiloxane
PEDOT:PSS	Poly(3,4-Ethyelenedioxythiophne) Polystyrene Sulfonate)
PVDF	Polyvinylidene Fluoride
SBS	Styrene–Butadiene–Styrene
SCAs	Stretchable Conductive Adhesives
SEI	Skin-Electrode Impedance
sEMG	Surface Electromyography
SIDS	Sudden Infant Death Syndrome
SKC	Skin Conductivity

SNR	Signal-to-Noise Ratio
SSCNTs	Silk-Sericine Carbon Nano-Tubes
SWCNTs	Single-Walled Carbon Nano-Tubes
SWSs	Smart Wearable Systems
TATSA	Triboelectric All-Textile Sensor Array
TPU	Termoplastic PolyUrethane

References

1. Jung, Y.; Kim, S.; Choi, B. Consumer valuation of the wearables: The case of smartwatches. *Comput. Hum. Behav.* **2016**, *63*, 899–905. [CrossRef]
2. Stoppa, M.; Chiolerio, A. Wearable electronics and smart textiles: A critical review. *Sensors* **2014**, *14*, 11957–11992. [CrossRef] [PubMed]
3. Ghaffarzadeh, K.; Hayward, J. Stretchable and conformable electronics: Heading toward market reality. *Inf. Disp.* **2017**, *33*, 28–31. [CrossRef]
4. Majumder, S.; Mondal, T.; Deen, M.J. Wearable sensors for remote health monitoring. *Sensors* **2017**, *17*, 130. [CrossRef] [PubMed]
5. Amitrano, F.; Donisi, L.; Coccia, A.; Biancardi, A.; Pagano, G.; D'Addio, G. Experimental development and validation of an e-textile sock prototype. In Proceedings of the 2020 IEEE International Symposium on Medical Measurements and Applications (MeMeA), Bari, Italy, 1 June–1 July 2020; pp. 1–5. [CrossRef]
6. Amitrano, F.; Coccia, A.; Donisi, L.; Pagano, G.; Cesarelli, G.; D'Addio, G. Gait analysis using wearable e-textile sock: An experimental study of test-retest reliability. In Proceedings of the 2021 IEEE International Symposium on Medical Measurements and Applications (MeMeA), Lausanne, Switzerland, 23–25 June 2021; pp. 1–6. [CrossRef]
7. Lymberis, A.; Olsson, S. Intelligent biomedical clothing for personal health and disease management: State of the art and future vision. *Telemed. J. E-Health* **2003**, *9*, 379–386. [CrossRef] [PubMed]
8. Weng, W.; Chen, P.; He, S.; Sun, X.; Peng, H. Smart electronic textiles. *Angew. Chem. Int. Ed.* **2016**, *55*, 6140–6169. [CrossRef]
9. Coccia, A.; Amitrano, F.; Donisi, L.; Cesarelli, G.; Pagano, G.; Cesarelli, M.; D'Addio, G. Design and validation of an e-textile-based wearable system for remote health monitoring. *Acta Imeko* **2021**, *10*, 220–229. [CrossRef]
10. Erdmier, C.; Hatcher, J.; Lee, M. Wearable device implications in the healthcare industry. *J. Med. Eng. Technol.* **2016**, *40*, 141–148. [CrossRef]
11. Lewy, H. Wearable technologies—Future challenges for implementation in healthcare services. *Healthc. Technol. Lett.* **2015**, *2*, 2–5. [CrossRef] [PubMed]
12. Catarino, A.; Carvalho, H.; Dias, M.J.; Pereira, T.; Postolache, O.; Girão, P.S. Continuous health monitoring using E-textile integrated biosensors. In Proceedings of the 2012 International Conference and Exposition on Electrical and Power Engineering, Iasi, Romania, 25–27 October 2012; pp. 605–609. [CrossRef]
13. Kuroda, T.; Hirano, K.; Sugimura, K.; Adachi, S.; Igarashi, H.; Ueshima, K.; Nakamura, H.; Nambu, M.; Doi, T. Applying NISHIJIN historical textile technique for e-Textile. In Proceedings of the 2013 35th Annual International Conference of the IEEE Engineering in Medicine and Biology Society (EMBC), Osaka, Japan, 3–7 July 2013; pp. 1226–1229. [CrossRef]
14. Postolache, O.; Viegas, V.; Dias Pereira, J.M.; Vinhas, D.; Girão, P.S.; Postolache, G. Toward developing a smart wheelchair for user physiological stress and physical activity monitoring. In Proceedings of the 2014 IEEE International Symposium on Medical Measurements and Applications (MeMeA), Lisboa, Portugal, 11–12 June 2014; pp. 1–6. [CrossRef]
15. Ferreira, A.G.; Fernandes, D.; Branco, S.; Monteiro, J.L.; Cabral, J.; Catarino, A.P.; Rocha, A.M. A smart wearable system for sudden infant death syndrome monitoring. In Proceedings of the 2016 IEEE International Conference on Industrial Technology (ICIT), Taipei, Taiwan, 14–17 March 2016; pp. 1920–1925. [CrossRef]
16. Sinha, S.K.; Posada-Quintero, H.F.; Noh, Y.; Allen, C.; Daniels, R.; Chon, K.H.; Sloan, L.; Sotzing, G.A. Integrated dry poly(3,4-ethylenedioxythiophene):polystyrene sulfonate electrodes on finished textiles for continuous and simultaneous monitoring of electrocardiogram, electromyogram and electrodermal activity. *Flex. Print. Electron.* **2020**, *5*, 035009. [CrossRef]
17. Fouassier, D.; Roy, X.; Blanchard, A.; Hulot, J.S. Assessment of signal quality measured with a smart 12-lead ECG acquisition T-shirt. *Ann. Noninvasive Electrocardiol.* **2020**, *25*, e12682. [CrossRef] [PubMed]
18. Li, B.M.; Kim, I.; Zhou, Y.; Mills, A.C.; Flewwellin, T.J.; Jur, J.S. Kirigami-inspired textile electronics: K. I. T. E. *Adv. Mater. Technol.* **2019**, *4*, 1900511. [CrossRef]
19. Yao, S.; Yang, J.; Poblete, F.R.; Hu, X.; Zhu, Y. Multifunctional electronic textiles using silver nanowire composites. *ACS Appl. Mater. Interfaces* **2019**, *11*, 31028–31037. [CrossRef] [PubMed]
20. Le, K.; Servati, A.; Ko, F.; Servati, P. Signal quality analysis of electrocardiogram textile electrodes for smart apparel applications. In Proceedings of the 2019 IEEE International Flexible Electronics Technology Conference (IFETC), Vancouver, BC, Canada, 11–14 August 2019; pp. 1–3. [CrossRef]
21. Jin, H.; Nayeem, M.O.G.; Lee, S.; Matsuhisa, N.; Inoue, D.; Yokota, T.; Hashizume, D.; Someya, T. Highly durable nanofiber-reinforced elastic conductors for skin-tight electronic textiles. *ACS Nano* **2019**, *13*, 7905–7912. [CrossRef]
22. Acar, G.; Ozturk, O.; Yapici, M.K. Wearable graphene nanotextile embedded smart armband for cardiac monitoring. In Proceedings of the 2018 IEEE SENSORS, New Delhi, India, 28–31 October 2018; pp. 1–4. [CrossRef]

23. Wu, Y.Z.; Sun, J.X.; Li, L.F.; Ding, Y.S.; Xu, H.A. Performance evaluation of a novel cloth electrode. In Proceedings of the 2010 4th International Conference on Bioinformatics and Biomedical Engineering, Chengdu, China, 18–20 June 2010; pp. 1–5. [CrossRef]
24. Lopez, G.; Custodio, V.; Ignacio Moreno, J. Location-aware system for wearable physiological monitoring within hospital facilities. In Proceedings of the 21st Annual IEEE International Symposium on Personal, Indoor and Mobile Radio Communications, Istanbul, Turkey, 26–30 September 2010; pp. 2609–2614. [CrossRef]
25. López, G.; Custodio, V.; Moreno, J.I. Lobin: E-textile and wireless-sensor-network-based platform for healthcare monitoring in future hospital environments. *IEEE Trans. Inf. Technol. Biomed.* **2010**, *14*, 1446–1458. [CrossRef] [PubMed]
26. Akter Shathi, M.; Minzhi, C.; Khoso, N.A.; Deb, H.; Ahmed, A.; Sai Sai, W. All organic graphene oxide and Poly (3, 4-ethylene dioxythiophene) —Poly (Styrene sulfonate) coated knitted textile fabrics for wearable electrocardiography (Ecg) monitoring. *Synth. Met.* **2020**, *263*, 116329. [CrossRef]
27. Shathi, M.A.; Chen, M.; Khoso, N.A.; Rahman, M.T.; Bhattacharjee, B. Graphene coated textile based highly flexible and washable sports bra for human health monitoring. *Mater. Des.* **2020**, *193*, 108792. [CrossRef]
28. Arquilla, K.; Webb, A.K.; Anderson, A.P. Textile electrocardiogram (Ecg) electrodes for wearable health monitoring. *Sensors* **2020**, *20*, 1013. [CrossRef]
29. Zięba, J.; Frydrysiak, M.; Tesiorowski, L.; Tokarska, M. Textronic clothing to ECG measurement. In Proceedings of the 2011 IEEE International Symposium on Medical Measurements and Applications, Bari, Italy, 30–31 May 2011; pp. 559–563. [CrossRef]
30. Tao, X.; Huang, T.H.; Shen, C.L.; Ko, Y.C.; Jou, G.T.; Koncar, V. Bluetooth low energy-based washable wearable activity motion and electrocardiogram textronic monitoring and communicating system. *Adv. Mater. Technol.* **2018**, *3*, 1700309. [CrossRef]
31. Ko, Y.; Oh, J.; Park, K.T.; Kim, S.; Huh, W.; Sung, B.J.; Lim, J.A.; Lee, S.S.; Kim, H. Stretchable conductive adhesives with superior electrical stability as printable interconnects in washable textile electronics. *ACS Appl. Mater. Interfaces* **2019**, *11*, 37043–37050. [CrossRef]
32. Liang, X.; Li, H.; Dou, J.; Wang, Q.; He, W.; Wang, C.; Li, D.; Lin, J.; Zhang, Y. Stable and biocompatible carbon nanotube ink mediated by silk protein for printed electronics. *Adv. Mater.* **2020**, *32*, 2000165. [CrossRef] [PubMed]
33. Dabby, N.; Aleksov, A.; Lewallen, E.; Oster, S.; Fygenson, R.; Lathrop, B.; Bynum, M.; Samady, M.; Klein, S.; Girouard, S. A scalable process for manufacturing integrated, washable smart garments applied to heart rate monitoring. In *Proceedings of the 2017 ACM International Symposium on Wearable Computers*; ISWC '17; Association for Computing Machinery: Maui, HI, USA, 2017; pp. 38–41. [CrossRef]
34. Tang, Z.; Yao, D.; Du, D.; Ouyang, J. Highly machine-washable e-textiles with high strain sensitivity and high thermal conduction. *J. Mater. Chem. C* **2020**, *8*, 2741–2748. [CrossRef]
35. Frydrysiak, M.; Tesiorowski, L. Wearable textronic system for protecting elderly people. In Proceedings of the 2016 IEEE International Symposium on Medical Measurements and Applications (MeMeA), Benevento, Italy, 15–18 May 2016; pp. 1–6. [CrossRef]
36. Frydrysiak, M.; Tesiorowski, L. Health monitoring system for protecting elderly people. In Proceedings of the 2016 International Multidisciplinary Conference on Computer and Energy Science (SpliTech), Split, Croatia, 13–15 July 2016; pp. 1–6. [CrossRef]
37. Kim, K.; Jung, M.; Jeon, S.; Bae, J. Robust and scalable three-dimensional spacer textile pressure sensor for human motion detection. *Smart Mater. Struct.* **2019**, *28*, 065019. [CrossRef]
38. Jang, S.; Kim, J.; Kim, D.W.; Kim, J.W.; Chun, S.; Lee, H.J.; Yi, G.R.; Pang, C. Carbon-based, ultraelastic, hierarchically coated fiber strain sensors with crack-controllable beads. *ACS Appl. Mater. Interfaces* **2019**, *11*, 15079–15087. [CrossRef] [PubMed]
39. Fan, W.; He, Q.; Meng, K.; Tan, X.; Zhou, Z.; Zhang, G.; Yang, J.; Wang, Z.L. Machine-knitted washable sensor array textile for precise epidermal physiological signal monitoring. *Sci. Adv.* **2020**, *6*, eaay2840. [CrossRef]
40. Goy, C.B.; Dominguez, J.M.; Gómez López, M.A.; Madrid, R.E.; Herrera, M.C. Electrical characterization of conductive textile materials and its evaluation as electrodes for venous occlusion plethysmography. *J. Med. Eng. Technol.* **2013**, *37*, 359–367. [CrossRef] [PubMed]
41. Samy, L.; Huang, M.C.; Liu, J.J.; Xu, W.; Sarrafzadeh, M. Unobtrusive sleep stage identification using a pressure-sensitive bed sheet. *IEEE Sens. J.* **2014**, *14*, 2092–2101. [CrossRef]
42. Ozturk, O.; Yapici, M.K. Surface electromyography with wearable graphene textiles. *IEEE Sens. J.* **2021**, *21*, 14397–14406. [CrossRef]
43. Ozturk, O.; Yapici, M.K. Muscular activity monitoring and surface electromyography (Semg) with graphene textiles. In Proceedings of the 2019 IEEE SENSORS, Montreal, QC, Canada, 27–30 October 2019; pp. 1–4. [CrossRef]
44. Awan, F.; He, Y.; Le, L.; Tran, L.L.; Han, H.D.; Nguyen, L.P. Electromyography acquisition system using graphene-based e-textiles. In Proceedings of the 2019 International Symposium on Electrical and Electronics Engineering (ISEE), Ho Chi Minh City, Vietnam, 10–12 October 2019; pp. 59–62. [CrossRef]
45. Niijima, A.; Isezaki, T.; Aoki, R.; Watanabe, T.; Yamada, T. Biceps fatigue estimation with an E-textile headband. In *Proceedings of the 2018 ACM International Symposium on Wearable Computers*; ISWC '18; Association for Computing Machinery: Singapore, 2018; pp. 222–223. [CrossRef]
46. Niijima, A.; Isezaki, T.; Aoki, R.; Watanabe, T.; Yamada, T. Hitocap: Wearable emg sensor for monitoring masticatory muscles with pedot-pss textile electrodes. In *Proceedings of the 2017 ACM International Symposium on Wearable Computers*; ISWC '17; Association for Computing Machinery: Maui, HI, USA, 2017; pp. 215–220. [CrossRef]

47. Farina, D.; Lorrain, T.; Negro, F.; Jiang, N. High-density EMG E-Textile systems for the control of active prostheses. In Proceedings of the 2010 Annual International Conference of the IEEE Engineering in Medicine and Biology, Buenos Aires, Argentina, 31 August–4 September 2010; pp. 3591–3593. [CrossRef]
48. Choudhry, N.A.; Rasheed, A.; Ahmad, S.; Arnold, L.; Wang, L. Design, development and characterization of textile stitch-based piezoresistive sensors for wearable monitoring. *IEEE Sens. J.* **2020**, *20*, 10485–10494. [CrossRef]
49. Vu, C.C.; Kim, J. Highly sensitive e-textile strain sensors enhanced by geometrical treatment for human monitoring. *Sensors* **2020**, *20*, 2383. [CrossRef] [PubMed]
50. Heo, J.S.; Shishavan, H.H.; Soleymanpour, R.; Kim, J.; Kim, I. Textile-based stretchable and flexible glove sensor for monitoring upper extremity prosthesis functions. *IEEE Sens. J.* **2020**, *20*, 1754–1760. [CrossRef]
51. Ye, C.; Ren, J.; Wang, Y.; Zhang, W.; Qian, C.; Han, J.; Zhang, C.; Jin, K.; Buehler, M.J.; Kaplan, D.L.; et al. Design and fabrication of silk templated electronic yarns and applications in multifunctional textiles. *Matter* **2019**, *1*, 1411–1425. [CrossRef]
52. Fevgas, A.; Tsompanopoulou, P.; Lalis, S. Rapid prototype development for studying human activity. In *XII Mediterranean Conference on Medical and Biological Engineering and Computing 2010*; Bamidis, P.D., Pallikarakis, N., Eds.; Springer: Berlin/Heidelberg, Germany, 2010; pp. 643–646. [CrossRef]
53. Bartalesi, R.; Lorussi, F.; De Rossi, D.; Tesconi, M.; Tognetti, A. Wearable monitoring of lumbar spine curvature by inertial and e-textile sensory fusion. In Proceedings of the 2010 Annual International Conference of the IEEE Engineering in Medicine and Biology, Buenos Aires, Argentina, 31 August–4 September 2010; pp. 6373–6376. [CrossRef]
54. Toffola, L.D.; Patel, S.; Ozsecen, M.Y.; Ramachandran, R.; Bonato, P. A wearable system for long-term monitoring of knee kinematics. In Proceedings of the 2012 IEEE-EMBS International Conference on Biomedical and Health Informatics, Hong Kong, China, 5–7 January 2012; pp. 188–191. [CrossRef]
55. Raad, M.; Deriche, M.; Hafeedh, A.; Almasawa, H.; Jofan, K.; Alsakkaf, H.; Bahumran, A.; Salem, M. An iot based wearable smart glove for remote monitoring of rheumatoid arthritis patients. In Proceedings of the 12th International Joint Conference on Biomedical Engineering Systems and Technologies, Prague, Czech Republic, 22–24 February 2019; SCITEPRESS—Science and Technology Publications: Prague, Czech Republic, 2019; pp. 224–228. [CrossRef]
56. Vu, C.; Kim, J. Human motion recognition using e-textile sensor and adaptive neuro-fuzzy inference system. *Fibers Polym.* **2018**, *19*, 2657–2666. [CrossRef]
57. Zhang, X.; Wang, J.; Xing, Y.; Li, C. Woven wearable electronic textiles as self-powered intelligent tribo-sensors for activity monitoring. *Glob. Challenges* **2019**, *3*, 1900070. [CrossRef]
58. Li, M.; Torah, R.; Nunes-Matos, H.; Wei, Y.; Beeby, S.; Tudor, J.; Yang, K. Integration and testing of a three-axis accelerometer in a woven e-textile sleeve for wearable movement monitoring. *Sensors* **2020**, *20*, 5033. [CrossRef] [PubMed]
59. Kiaghadi, A.; Baima, M.; Gummeson, J.; Andrew, T.; Ganesan, D. Fabric as a sensor: Towards unobtrusive sensing of human behavior with triboelectric textiles. In Proceedings of the 16th ACM Conference on Embedded Networked Sensor Systems, Shenzhen, China, 4–7 November 2018; ACM: Shenzhen, China, 2018; pp. 199–210. [CrossRef]
60. Lorussi, F.; Lucchese, I.; Tognetti, A.; Carbonaro, N. A wearable system for remote monitoring of the treatments of musculoskeletal disorder. In Proceedings of the 2018 IEEE International Conference on Smart Computing (SMARTCOMP), Taormina, Italy, 18–20 June 2018; pp. 362–367. [CrossRef]
61. Amitrano, F.; Coccia, A.; Ricciardi, C.; Donisi, L.; Cesarelli, G.; Capodaglio, E.M.; D'Addio, G. Design and validation of an e-textile-based wearable sock for remote gait and postural assessment. *Sensors* **2020**, *20*, 6691. [CrossRef]
62. Hayashi, E.; Enokibori, Y.; Mase, K. Harmless line-oriented sensing point reduction for non-categorical sitting posture score. In Proceedings of the 2017 ACM International Joint Conference on Pervasive and Ubiquitous Computing and Proceedings of the 2017 ACM International Symposium on Wearable Computers, UbiComp '17. Maui, HI, USA, 11–15 September 2017; Association for Computing Machinery: Maui, HI, USA, 2017; pp. 61–64. [CrossRef]
63. García Patiño, A.; Khoshnam, M.; Menon, C. Wearable device to monitor back movements using an inductive textile sensor. *Sensors* **2020**, *20*, 905. [CrossRef] [PubMed]
64. Li, Y.; Li, Y.; Su, M.; Li, W.; Li, Y.; Li, H.; Qian, X.; Zhang, X.; Li, F.; Song, Y. Electronic textile by dyeing method for multiresolution physical kineses monitoring. *Adv. Electron. Mater.* **2017**, *3*, 1700253. [CrossRef]
65. Park, H.; Kim, J.W.; Hong, S.Y.; Lee, G.; Lee, H.; Song, C.; Keum, K.; Jeong, Y.R.; Jin, S.W.; Kim, D.S.; et al. Dynamically stretchable supercapacitor for powering an integrated biosensor in an all-in-one textile system. *ACS Nano* **2019**, *13*, 10469–10480. [CrossRef]
66. Huang, M.C.; Xu, W.; Liu, J.; Samy, L.; Vajid, A.; Alshurafa, N.; Sarrafzadeh, M. Inconspicuous on-bed respiratory rate monitoring. In *Proceedings of the 6th International Conference on PErvasive Technologies Related to Assistive Environments*; PETRA '13; Association for Computing Machinery: Rhodes, Greece, 2013; pp. 1–8. [CrossRef]
67. Liu, J.J.; Huang, M.C.; Xu, W.; Zhang, X.; Stevens, L.; Alshurafa, N.; Sarrafzadeh, M. Breathsens: A continuous on-bed respiratory monitoring system with torso localization using an unobtrusive pressure sensing array. *IEEE J. Biomed. Health Inform.* **2015**, *19*, 1682–1688. [CrossRef]
68. Zięba, J.; Frydrysiak, M.; Błaszczyk, J. Textronic clothing with resistance textile sensor to monitoring frequency of human breathing. In Proceedings of the 2012 IEEE International Symposium on Medical Measurements and Applications Proceedings, Budapest, Hungary, 18–19 May 2012; pp. 1–6. [CrossRef]
69. Frydrysiak, M.; Zięba, J. Textronic sensor for monitoring respiratory rhythm. *Fibres Text. East. Eur.* **2012**, *91*, 74–78.

70. Lian, Y.; Yu, H.; Wang, M.; Yang, X.; Li, Z.; Yang, F.; Wang, Y.; Tai, H.; Liao, Y.; Wu, J.; et al. A multifunctional wearable E-textile via integrated nanowire-coated fabrics. *J. Mater. Chem. C* **2020**, *8*, 8399–8409. [CrossRef]
71. Ramos-Garcia, R.I.; Da Silva, F.; Kondi, Y.; Sazonov, E.; Dunne, L.E. Analysis of a coverstitched stretch sensor for monitoring of breathing. In Proceedings of the 2016 10th International Conference on Sensing Technology (ICST), Nanjing, China, 11–13 November 2016; pp. 1–6. [CrossRef]
72. Golparvar, A.J.; Kaya Yapici, M. Wearable graphene textile-enabled EOG sensing. In Proceedings of the 2017 IEEE SENSORS, Glasgow, UK, 29 October–1 November 2017; pp. 1–3. [CrossRef]
73. Golparvar, A.J.; Yapici, M.K. Graphene-coated wearable textiles for EOG-based human-computer interaction. In Proceedings of the 2018 IEEE 15th International Conference on Wearable and Implantable Body Sensor Networks (BSN), Las Vegas, NV, USA, 4–7 March 2018; pp. 189–192. [CrossRef]
74. Golparvar, A.J.; Yapici, M.K. Electrooculography by wearable graphene textiles. *IEEE Sens. J.* **2018**, *18*, 8971–8978. [CrossRef]
75. Haddad, P.A.; Servati, A.; Soltanian, S.; Ko, F.; Servati, P. Breathable dry silver/silver chloride electronic textile electrodes for electrodermal activity monitoring. *Biosensors* **2018**, *8*, 79. [CrossRef]
76. Healey, J. Gsr sock: A new e-textile sensor prototype. In Proceedings of the 2011 15th Annual International Symposium on Wearable Computers, San Francisco, CA, USA, 12–15 June 2011; pp. 113–114. [CrossRef]
77. Lugoda, P.; Hughes-Riley, T.; Oliveira, C.; Morris, R.; Dias, T. Developing novel temperature sensing garments for health monitoring applications. *Fibers* **2018**, *6*, 46. [CrossRef]
78. Jiang, Y.; Pan, K.; Leng, T.; Hu, Z. Smart textile integrated wireless powered near field communication body temperature and sweat sensing system. *IEEE J. Electromagn. RF Microwaves Med. Biol.* **2020**, *4*, 164–170. [CrossRef]
79. Mason, A.; Wylie, S.; Korostynska, O.; Cordova-Lopez, L.E.; Al-Shamma'a, A.I. Flexible e-textile sensors for real-time health monitoring at microwave frequencies. *Int. J. Smart Sens. Intell. Syst.* **2017**, *7*. [CrossRef]
80. Zhao, C.; Li, X.; Wu, Q.; Liu, X. A thread-based wearable sweat nanobiosensor. *Biosens. Bioelectron.* **2021**, *188*, 113270. [CrossRef]
81. Chen, S.; Liu, S.; Wang, P.; Liu, H.; Liu, L. Highly stretchable fiber-shaped e-textiles for strain/pressure sensing, full-range human motions detection, health monitoring, and 2D force mapping. *J. Mater. Sci.* **2018**, *53*, 2995–3005. [CrossRef]
82. Liu, R.; Wang, S.; Lao, T.T. A novel solution of monitoring incontinence status by conductive yarn and advanced seamless knitting techniques. *J. Eng. Fibers Fabr.* **2012**, *7*, 155892501200700415. [CrossRef]
83. Serhani, M.A.; El Kassabi, H.T.; Ismail, H.; Nujum Navaz, A. Ecg monitoring systems: Review, architecture, processes, and key challenges. *Sensors* **2020**, *20*, 1796. [CrossRef]
84. Mohapatra, S.K.; Mohanty, M.N. Ecg analysis: A brief review. *Recent Adv. Comput. Sci. Commun. (Former. Recent Patents Comput. Sci.)* **2021**, *14*, 344–359. [CrossRef]
85. Hermens, H.J.; Freriks, B.; Disselhorst-Klug, C.; Rau, G. Development of recommendations for SEMG sensors and sensor placement procedures. *J. Electromyogr. Kinesiol.* **2000**, *10*, 361–374. [CrossRef]
86. Hogrel, J.Y. Clinical applications of surface electromyography in neuromuscular disorders. *Neurophysiol. Clin. Neurophysiol.* **2005**, *35*, 59–71. [CrossRef] [PubMed]
87. Stegeman, D.F.; Hermens, H. Standards for surface electromyography: The European project Surface EMG for non-invasive assessment of muscles (SENIAM). *Enschede Roessingh Res. Dev.* **2007**, 108–112.
88. Castano, L.M.; Flatau, A.B. Smart fabric sensors and e-textile technologies: A review. *Smart Mater. Struct.* **2014**, *23*, 053001. [CrossRef]
89. Donisi, L.; Pagano, G.; Cesarelli, G.; Coccia, A.; Amitrano, F.; D'Addio, G. Benchmarking between two wearable inertial systems for gait analysis based on a different sensor placement using several statistical approaches. *Measurement* **2021**, *173*, 108642. [CrossRef]
90. D'Addio, G.; Donisi, L.; Pagano, G.; Improta, G.; Biancardi, A.; Cesarelli, M. Agreement between opal and g-walk wearable inertial systems in gait analysis on normal and pathological subjects. In Proceedings of the 41st Annual International Conference of the IEEE Engineering in Medicine and Biology Society (EMBC), Berlin, Germany, 23–27 July 2019; pp. 3286–3289. [CrossRef]
91. Sama, A.J.; Hillstrom, H.; Daluiski, A.; Wolff, A. Reliability and agreement between two wearable inertial sensor devices for measurement of arm activity during walking and running gait. *J. Hand Ther.* **2020**. online ahead of print. [CrossRef] [PubMed]
92. Zheng, H.; Black, N.D.; Harris, N.D. Position-sensing technologies for movement analysis in stroke rehabilitation. *Med. Biol. Eng. Comput.* **2005**, *43*, 413–420. [CrossRef] [PubMed]
93. D'Addio, G.; Evangelista, S.; Donisi, L.; Biancardi, A.; Andreozzi, E.; Pagano, G.; Arpaia, P.; Cesarelli, M. Development of a prototype e-textile sock. In Proceedings of the 2019 41st Annual International Conference of the IEEE Engineering in Medicine and Biology Society (EMBC), Berlin, Germany, 23–27 July 2019; pp. 17498–1752. [CrossRef]
94. Rolfe, S. The importance of respiratory rate monitoring. *Br. J. Nurs.* **2019**, *28*, 504–508. [CrossRef]
95. Nicolò, A.; Massaroni, C.; Schena, E.; Sacchetti, M. The importance of respiratory rate monitoring: From healthcare to sport and exercise. *Sensors* **2020**, *20*, 6396. [CrossRef] [PubMed]
96. Liu, H.; Allen, J.; Zheng, D.; Chen, F. Recent development of respiratory rate measurement technologies. *Physiol. Meas.* **2019**, *40*, 07TR01. [CrossRef] [PubMed]
97. Vanegas Vásquez, E.; Igual Catalán, R.; Plaza García, I. Sensing systems for respiration monitoring: A technical systematic review. *Sensors* **2020**, *20*, 5446. [CrossRef] [PubMed]

MDPI AG
Grosspeteranlage 5
4052 Basel
Switzerland
Tel.: +41 61 683 77 34
www.mdpi.com

Diagnostics Editorial Office
E-mail: diagnostics@mdpi.com
www.mdpi.com/journal/diagnostics

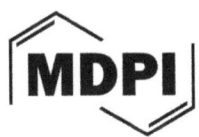

Disclaimer/Publisher's Note: The statements, opinions and data contained in all publications are solely those of the individual author(s) and contributor(s) and not of MDPI and/or the editor(s). MDPI and/or the editor(s) disclaim responsibility for any injury to people or property resulting from any ideas, methods, instructions or products referred to in the content.

www.ingramcontent.com/pod-product-compliance
Lightning Source LLC
LaVergne TN
LVHW070712100526
838202LV00013B/1078